Pocket Examiner in Medicine

Pocket Examiner in Medicine

Alexander Lawrence MB, ChB, MRCP(UK)
Zachary Johnson MRCPI, DTM & H, DCH, DPH, DObst

Churchill Livingstone

EDINBURGH LONDON MELBOURNE AND NEW YORK 1986

CHURCHILL LIVINGSTONE
Medical Division of Longman Group UK Limited

Distributed in the United States of America by Churchill Livingstone Inc., 1560 Broadway, New York, N.Y. 10036, and by associated companies, branches and representatives throughout the world.

First published 1983 (Pitman Publishing Ltd)
Reprinted 1984
Reprinted 1985
Reprinted 1986 (Churchill Livingstone)
Reprinted 1989

ISBN 0-443-03863-5

British Library Cataloging in Publication Data

Lawrence, C. A.
Pocket examiner in medicine.
1. Medicine—Problems, exercises, etc
I. Title II. Johnson, Z.
610'.76 R834.5

Library of Congress Cataloguing in Publication Data

Lawrence, C. A. (Charles Alexander)
Pocket examiner in medicine.

Bibliography: p.
Includes index
1. Internal medicine—Examinations, questions, etc.
I. Johnson, Z. (Zachary) II. Title [DNLM: 1. Medicine—Examination questions. WB 18 L419p]
RC58.L38 1983 616'.0076 83-2381
ISBN 0-272-79696-4

Text set in 8/9½ pt Century Schoolbook Roman,
Produced by Longman Singapore Publishers Pte Ltd
Printed in Singapore.

Contents

Preface

This book has been written for medical students preparing for examinations in clinical medicine, studying either alone or in groups. Its question and answer format lends itself to self-testing, but a special effort has been made to make the questions as well as the answers informative so that the questions themselves should be instructive.

The book can be used in two ways. Its material is set out in sections, like the chapters of a textbook, making it possible to revise system by system. Alternatively, specific topics can be checked by means of the very detailed index. This index has compiled for the reader with little time to spend browsing. Many subjects are listed under more than one heading and this should avoid too much searching.

The page references beneath each answer are a guide to further reading. As a general rule the larger textbooks (Price, Harrison, Cecil) devote more space to a subject but the smaller books tend to be concise and this may be more useful. However, all the smaller books suffer from having too short an index and looking things up can be a laborious task. We hope that by providing both a detailed index and page references we shall have helped readers to get the best possible use out of their textbooks.

We wish all our readers the very best of luck with their examiners!

CAL
ZJ

Acknowledgements

We would like to thank Dr Peter Abrahams for suggesting the book in the first place, Mrs Marietta Fenty of Border Secretarial Services who dealt with the whole business of producing the manuscript and Mr Willem van der Reijden of Borders Computing for sorting the index by word processor.

1 Key to references & further reading

A *A Short Textbook of Medicine*, Houston, J.C., Joiner, C.L. and Trounce, J.R., 7th edn (Unibooks, Hodder and Stoughton, Sevenoaks, 1982)

B *A Companion to Medical Studies*, ed. Passmore R. and Robson, J.S., Volume 3, parts 1 and 2 (Blackwell Scientific Publications, Oxford, 1974)

C *Davidson's Principles and Practice of Medicine*, ed. Macleod, J., 13th edn (Churchill Livingstone, Edinburgh, 1981)

D *Lecture Notes in Clinical Medicine*, Rubenstein, D. and Wayne, D., 2nd edn (Blackwell Scientific Publications, Oxford, 1980)

E *Modern Medicine, A Textbook for Students*, Read, A.E., Barritt, D.W. and Langton Hewer, R., 2nd edn (Pitman Medical Publishing Co. Ltd, Tunbridge Wells, 1979)

F *Price's Textbook of the Practice of Medicine*, ed. Bodley, Scott, 12th edn (Oxford University Press, Oxford, 1978)

G *Cecil Textbook of Medicine*, ed. Beeson, P.B., McDermott, W. and Wyngaarden, J.B., 15th edn (W.B. Saunders Company, Philadelphia, 1979)

H *Harrison's Principles of Internal Medicine*, ed. Isselbacher, K.J., Adams, R.D., Braunwald, E., Petersdorf, R.G. and Wilson, J.D., 9th edn. (McGraw Hill International Book Company, 1980).

2 Questions

Cardiovascular System

1 Cyanosis is a bluish discoloration of the lips and tongue, or of the extremities, which occurs when more than about 5 grams of haemoglobin per 100 ml of blood is deoxygenated.

What are the two major mechanisms by which inhaled oxygen fails to oxygenate the blood?

2 People can go blue from cold, or from very unusual causes such as methaemoglobinaemia, but in the vast majority of cases there is respiratory or cardiac disease, or both, as seen most commonly in the elderly chronic bronchitic who also has ischaemic heart disease.

What are the reasons why such an individual should become cyanosed?

3 The temperature of the hands and feet may be an important physical sign.

In a patient whose extremities become cold, what can you conclude?

4 Clubbing of the fingers is a physical sign in which thickening of the tissues at the base of the nail removes the angle between the nail and the adjacent skin. The normal longitudinal ridges disappear as the nail becomes curved not only from side to side but also from base to tip. In extreme cases, the finger tips look like drumsticks.

What are the three main groups of disease which cause clubbing?

5 Tachycardia is generally taken to be a heart rate faster than 100 beats per minute. In a sleeping patient with no heart disease, what causes of a tachycardia are there?

6 Bradycardia is a heart rate of less than 60 beats per minute. It is much less common than tachycardia but more often indicates disease. It is a normal finding in athletes, but may also occur in disorders such as hypothyroidism, obstructive jaundice and with raised intracranial pressure. It is most commonly caused by cardiac disorders.

What cardiac disorders are associated with bradycardia?

7 Extrasystoles are a very common arrhythmia in which the cardiac impulse arises in an abnormal site called an ectopic focus. They are commonly called 'ectopics'. They occur before the next expected beat, i.e. they are premature. The heart sounds may be softer or inaudible and the pulse wave may be reduced or impalpable at the wrist.

Why is this and what else might you or the patient notice?

8 Extrasystoles can originate in the atria, the AV node or most commonly in the ventricles. On the ECG, how can one distinguish atrial from ventricular extrasystoles?

9 Supraventricular tachycardia is due to a fast ectopic focus in the atria or AV node. On the ECG the QRS complexes are usually normal and there may be a P wave detectable.

What are the clinical features?

10 Unlike supraventricular tachycardia (SVT), ventricular tachycardia (VT) is nearly always associated with cardiac disease and it is important to institute the right treatment for VT without delay. The ECG may not positively identify a ventricular origin but there are physical signs of VT.

What are they?

11 You have a young adult patient with an attack of supraventricular tachycardia. There is a history of several previous attacks.

What underlying condition should you consider and what would you look for on the patient's ECG, especially when normal rhythm has returned?

12 Would you expect to encounter the sick sinus syndrome (a) in a patient who has suffered a myocardial infarction or (b) in an elderly person?

What would you do about it if you did?

13 What is the drug of choice for treatment of ventricular ectopics or ventricular tachycardia following myocardial infarction?

What doses are used and what is the main side-effect?

14 Procainamide is a drug used to control ventricular arrhythmias, especially after myocardial infarction. It can be given as a slow intravenous injection (100 mg per 5 minutes, maximum 1 g) but it is more often used orally to maintain antiarrhythmic therapy once the immediate problem has been treated with lignocaine.

What are its side-effects?

15 The anticonvulsant drug, phenytoin, has a place in the treatment of ventricular and also atrial arrhythmias.
For which cause of arrhythmia is it particularly appropriate?

16 Which of the following arrhythmias can be caused by digoxin: functional (AV nodal) rhythm; atrial tachycardia with block; bigeminal rhythm, i.e. a ventricular extrasystole following each normal impulse; multiform ventricular extrasystoles?

17 Apart from lignocaine and procainamide (the latter being less often used now) name two other drugs, valuable and increasingly used in the treatment of ventricular arrhythmias.

18 The treatment of cardiac arrhythmias, both atrial and ventricular, is one area in which propranolol and other beta-blockers are used. Can you name four other areas in which they are commonly used?
What are the side-effects of beta-blockers?

19 Practolol is a cardioselective beta-blocker that is very effective in controlling supraventricular tachycardia and, to a lesser extent, ventricular arrhythmias. It is no longer available in oral form.
Why is this?

20 Oxprenolol is a beta-blocker that is similar to propranolol in its action. In addition to slowing conduction through the AV node, these drugs have a depressant effect on the myocardium that helps to suppress ventricular arrhythmias.
Apart from this desirable action, what else might these drugs do to the heart that would make you think twice before giving them?

21 In which arrhythmias is digoxin the treatment of choice, and how would you give it?

22 Verapamil is a member of the recently discovered group of drugs which interfere with the passage of calcium ions across the cell membrane of cardiac tissue during the slow phase of depolarization. They are sometimes referred to as calcium blockers. The action of verapamil is mainly on the AV node.
For which arrhythmias is it particularly effective?

23 You find that a patient has a pulse and apex rate of 150. Next you prop the patient up at 45 degrees to

inspect the jugular venous pulse and find a rate of jugular pulsation of 300.

What is the likely arrhythmia?

24 The pulse in atrial fibrillation is completely irregular in volume and rhythm.

What two very important underlying conditions should it make you consider, what dangerous complication may occur two or three days after the onset of atrial fibrillation, and what drugs would you use in this situation?

25 What effect does atrial fibrillation have on cardiac function?

26 Atrial fibrillation can occur in normal hearts, either in attacks (paroxysmal) or in chronic form, so-called 'lone' atrial fibrillation. In this latter form, what sex is the patient likely to be and what underlying condition should be considered before instituting treatment?

27 What alternative to drug therapy is available for the treatment of atrial flutter, atrial fibrillation and other tachyarrhythmias?

28 If the ECG of a patient with a slightly irregular pulse showed that every fifth beat was simply missing, what would you conclude?

29 What are the clinical signs of first degree atrioventricular heart block?

30 Second degree atrioventricular block is the term used to describe the abnormality of conduction in which not all atrial impulses are conducted to the ventricles.

There are two varieties of this (sometimes referred to as Mobitz type 1 and type 2). The first is manifest by progressive lengthening of the PR interval until a P wave meets the AV node in its absolute refractory period and the impulse is blocked. The following P wave is conducted with a normal PR interval and the cycle starts again. This is the well known Wenkebach abnormality and it is relatively benign.

What are the features of the second type?

31 What is the cause of the Wenkebach conduction abnormality?

32 On examining an elderly patient you find that the pulse is slow (at a rate between 30 and 50), there is an occasional cannon wave in the jugular venous pulse and the first heart sound is very variable in intensity.

What conduction abnormality is likely to be present and what would you expect to find on the ECG?

33 Stokes–Adams attacks are episodes of cerebral ischaemia due to transient circulatory arrest. Ventricular asystole complicating complete heart block is one cause. Ventricular arrhythmias are another. The clinical features of S–A attacks were described long before electrocardiography was available.
What are they?

34 You are the second person to arrive on the scene of a cardiac arrest. You see a completely lifeless patient and a colleague trying to put up a drip.
What is he doing wrong and what should you do?

35 A defibrillator is a device for applying an electric shock across the heart.
What kind of shock is it, how big is it and does it matter how the shock is timed?

36 Calcium ions are needed for myocardial (and other muscle) contraction.
At what stages of the contractile process are they of clinical relevance?

37 Potassium is the main intracellular cation. The extracellular concentration of potassium is no guide to the body's total balance but is nevertheless of great importance since both hyperkalaemia and hypokalaemia can cause cardiac standstill. The toxic effects of a certain drug may be mitigated by giving potassium.
What drug is this?

38 Sodium bicarbonate is always used in cardiac arrest to correct the acidosis that results from circulatory arrest and anaerobic metabolism.
What strength would you use?

39 What alternative therapy is available for a patient with complete heart block that does not respond to atropine or isoprenaline?

40 The ECG of an asymptomatic patient shows an axis of +120°, QRS duration of 0.12 second, a wide S wave in standard lead I and in precordial leads V5 and V6 and a notched rSR pattern in V1.
Would you be worried about this patient's health?

41 Why do the ECG changes of left bundle branch block comprise a prolonged QRS, left axis deviation,

notching or slurring of the QRS complexes and a prolonged left ventricular activation time?

42 On the ECG, how would you distinguish between left anterior hemiblock and left axis deviation, and left posterior hemiblock and right axis deviation?

43 A man is admitted with crushing central chest pain, typical of myocardial infarction. His ECG shows ST elevation in leads I, aVL, V2–4 and also the changes of RBBB. His cardiac axis is +110°. On the ECG the next morning, the axis has changed to −45°.
What complication has occurred and what more serious development may follow this?

44 An elderly man with evidence of generalized arteriosclerosis gives a history of episodes of dizziness and occasional fainting. An ECG shows no evidence of heart block but 24 hour ambulatory monitoring shows that his dizziness coincides with sinus bradycardia, sometimes very marked.
What might be the diagnosis?

45 For which arrhythmias is atropine useful and what is its mode of action in this situation?

46 The pulse volume is a subjective assessment of the amount of blood flowing through the artery under one's palpating finger with each heart beat. It is influenced by the nature of the left ventricular contraction, the adequacy of the circulating volume and the resistance or compliance of the peripheral vasculature, and the conclusions one draws about the pulse volume depend on what one knows about these three factors. A patient with long-standing chronic bronchitis has an increased pulse volume.
What do you conclude?

47 You feel a collapsing (water-hammer) pulse in a patient with no symptoms, a blood pressure of 110/80 and no murmurs on cardiac auscultation.
What is the diagnosis?

48 A plateau pulse is a slowly rising pulse wave that increases little in amplitude and is prolonged. It is due to severe aortic stenosis.
What other physical signs would you expect to find?

49 What is pulsus bisferiens and when does it occur?

50 Failure of the left ventricle may be suspected from examination of the peripheral pulse.

What is the name of the abnormality of the pulse found under these circumstances, and what are its characteristic features?

51 You are feeling a patient's pulse and you notice that the pulse fades away when the patient breathes in and returns with each expiration. You then examine the JVP, find it raised and see it go even higher with inspiration.

What would you expect to see on this patient's chest X-ray?

52 The jugular venous pulse is often difficult to observe but it must always be examined. It consists of two positive waves and two negative troughs.

The dominant wave is the 'a' wave, which is due to atrial systole. The 'c' wave may be seen immediately afterwards, resulting from bulging of the tricuspid valve into the right atrium in the first part of ventricular systole. The 'x' trough follows with the 'v' wave occurring as the right atrium fills with blood before the tricuspid valve reopens, giving the 'y' descent.

What would you expect to see in atrial fibrillation?

53 When the atria contract against a closed tricuspid valve, a cannon wave (or accentuated 'a' wave) occurs.

What happens to the JVP in tricuspid regurgitation?

54 A patient known to be suffering from cor pulmonale, who has had several admissions for worsening oedema, is readmitted with a further episode of increasing dyspnoea and oedema. She also complains of abdominal pain and you find her liver tender and slightly enlarged. A colleague suggests she may have hepatitis.

What is your opinion?

55 What physical sign of congestive cardiac failure, indicating fluid retention, can be elicited even before the JVP becomes raised or oedema appears?

56 A common error in taking the blood pressure is to judge when the cuff pressure is above systolic by listening with the stethoscope as the cuff is inflated. In some patients this will give an erroneously low systolic reading, since there may be a 'quiet' zone of systolic pressure below the true and audible systolic level.

What factors may lead to a falsely elevated blood pressure reading being obtained?

57 In patients in whom it is visible and/or palpable, the apex beat may be a very informative physical sign. Normally it is located at the fourth or fifth intercostal spaces, and medial to the midclavicular line. Not only the position is important, however.

What would you expect to see in a patient with an anterior wall infarct?

58 A thrill in medicine is a palpable murmur. This is best palpated with the open palm and the proximal surface of the fingers is often the best part with which to feel the vibrations. Over the cardiac apex the murmurs of mitral stenosis and mitral regurgitation may be felt.

What murmurs would you be feeling for with your hand over the front of the chest in the midline?

59 When listening to the heart sounds it is important to assess their intensity and also to check for splitting of either sound. You are listening to the heart sounds of a 53-year-old man who has been admitted for control of severe hypertension. As the patient breathes in the second heart sound becomes single and as he breathes out you hear splitting of the second sound.

Is this normal?

60 A 20-year-old clerk is referred to you for a pre-employment physical check-up. On listening to the heart sounds, you hear a low-pitched sound in diastole, loudest over the apex and best heard with the bell of the stethoscope.

What is it?

61 A normotensive man with an acute myocardial infarction has an extra, low-pitched heart sound occurring immediately before the normal first heart sound. He is in sinus rhythm.

What is this extra sound, what does it indicate and in what other conditions might you hear it?

62 A pericardial friction rub may be heard in both diastole and systole but when present only in systole it may be confused with a murmur.

What features would help you to recognize a rub?

63 As a patient recovers from congestive cardiac failure you notice on daily auscultation of the heart that a faint systolic murmur is gradually becoming louder. The murmur is loudest in midsystole and radiates to the base of the neck.

What may the murmer be due to, and why is it getting louder?

64 Pansystolic murmurs occur when there is a large systolic pressure difference between two chambers, such as between the left ventricle and the left atrium or the right ventricle.

What lesions can give rise to pansystolic murmurs?

65 Hypertrophic obstructive cardiomyopathy is a condition, sometimes familial and a cause of sudden death, in which hypertrophy of the left ventricular outflow tract causes obstruction and a murmur. The intensity of the murmur is greater the closer the walls of the outflow tract approximate.

What would you expect to happen to the murmur when the patient stands up?

66 Not all heart murmurs indicate cardiac pathology. The diagnosis of so-called innocent murmurs is very often based on circumstantial evidence and the absence of other signs of cardiac abnormality. For instance, a soft midsystolic or ejection murmur heard in the pulmonary area of a young thin man is likely to be innocent.

Name two conditions in which mere increase in flow over normal valves may cause murmurs.

67 A 32-year-old man is admitted with a stroke. In view of his age, cerebral embolus seems likely and you are therefore anxious to examine very carefully for any mitral stenosis.

In what position would you place the patient and what would you listen for?

68 In severe aortic regurgitation there may be another diastolic murmur in addition to the early diastolic decrescendo aortic murmur. It can be mid-diastolic or presystolic and is caused by blood rushing back from the aorta mixing with the blood flow from the left atrium, setting up vibration of the anterior mitral valve leaflet.

What is this murmur called and with which more common murmur is it likely to be confused?

69 A patient gives a history of dyspnoea and angina on exertion and also nocturnal angina. Her pulse is collapsing in nature and BP estimation reveals a wide pulse pressure. The apex beat is displaced laterally and inferiorly. As you put your stethoscope to the chest you are thinking of aortic regurgitation.

What should you expect to hear?

70 In interpreting the electrocardiogram, it is essential to know the position and polarity of the electrodes, so that a full interpretation of the tracing can be made

without resorting to set patterns learnt parrot-fashion. The position of the limb leads and augmented limb leads is always the same and described according to the angle they make with the horizontal, which is assigned the value of 0°. Lead I is at 0°.

What are the angles of leads II, aVF and aVL?

71 It can be disheartening to watch more senior colleagues make rapid diagnoses from only a cursory glance at the ECG. The temptation to emulate this, however, must be resisted. There is no substitute for using a set routine for going through the major points of the tracing so that nothing important is missed.

What should this routine consist of?

72 In the following conditions, what non-invasive technique can help you diagnose or assess cardiac impairment: mitral stenosis, hypertrophic obstructive cardiomyopathy, left atrial myxoma, mitral rugurgitation due to a prolapsing mitral leaflet, left ventricular hypertrophy, pericardial effusion?

73 Much information about the heart can be obtained from a chest X-ray, including an indication of the size of the four chambers. It is important to know which chamber is responsible for each part of the cardiac silhouette.

On a normal PA view where are the left atrium and right ventricle?

74 Compression or posterior displacement of the barium-filled oesophagus on a right anterior oblique chest X-ray indicates enlargement of which chamber of the heart?

75 You find a patient with cold hands and feet, a fast low volume pulse, low blood pressure, a falling urine output over the last few hours and a slight temperature. The patient is a little confused. There is no sign of haemorrhage. Blood gases show a metabolic acidosis.

What is this patient's immediate problem?

76 A 45-year-old man is admitted to hospital with chest pain, and acute myocardial infarction is diagnosed. His pain subsides but in the following days his blood pressure remains low at 85/60. He slowly develops a positive hepatojugular reflux followed by a raised JVP, ankle oedema and bilateral pulmonary oedema.

What is his condition due to, in haemodynamic terms?

77 Congestive cardiac failure is the term used for heart failure that has become complicated by fluid retention. This develops because of the failure of the heart to deliver adequate quantities of oxygenated blood to the tissues.

What are the main symptoms and signs of this fluid retention?

78 What explanation can you give for the occurrence of paroxysmal nocturnal dyspnoea, in which condition the patient typically describes having not only to sit up, but get out of bed, walk to an open window and breathe deeply to get relief?

79 Left ventricular failure of acute or recent origin is typically marked by pulmonary oedema resulting from elevation of end diastolic pressure causing raised left atrial pressure and back pressure on the pulmonary capillaries.

When faced with a patient with left ventricular failure, what underlying conditions should you consider?

80 In heart conditions in which the abnormality causing failure is on the right side, pulmonary oedema and fluid retention occur comparatively late in the course of the condition.

What is the main symptom earlier on?

81 In heart failure, what is the effect of digoxin on the heart rate (chronotropic effect), the force of contraction (inotropic effect), conduction through the SA and AV nodes and on peripheral vasculature?

82 Which of the following statements about digoxin are correct? It is a cause of arrhythmias. It is a cause of nausea and vomiting. It is a cause of visual disturbance—blurring, flashing or xanthopsia.

83 In the majority of subjects digoxin produces changes in the ECG which indicate the presence of the drug but not the degree of its therapeutic effect or its toxicity.

What are these changes?

84 The thiazides, like other diuretics, cause a diuresis by interfering with cation handling in the renal tubules. Water is lost as a result of sodium excretion but the thiazides also promote potassium excretion, as do frusemide and ethacrynic acid.

In what situation may this be harmful?

85 Frusemide, bumetanide and ethacrynic acid are all powerful diuretics with a rapid onset of action and

shorter-lasting effect than the thiazides. Frusemide is the most commonly used although ethacrynic acid is occasionally effective where frusemide fails and has the distinction of promoting a diuresis when mannitol has failed to stave off acute renal failure.

Apart from causing a diuresis, what other effects does frusemide have that enhance its usefulness?

86 Frusemide is very widely used and the incidence of undesirable effects is relatively low. There are, however, some drug interactions of importance.

What are they?

87 It has been shown that potassium supplements are not necessarily required in all the situations where thiazide diuretics are used.

What is the reason for this and in what condition may omission of potassium supplements be safely tried?

88 Vasodilators are becoming increasingly used in the treatment of heart failure. Those that dilate the vessels on the venous side of the heart, principally the nitrates, reduce venous return, thereby reducing left ventricular end diastolic pressure. Other drugs, such as hydralazine and prazosin, reduce peripheral resistance.

What is sublingual glyceryl trinitrate commonly used for?

89 Cheyne–Stokes respiration is a form of cyclical respiration in which periods of apnoea alternate with hyperventilation. It can occur in heart failure, particularly in elderly patients who have associated cerebrovascular disease.

What is the underlying abnormality?

90 In congestive cardiac failure, pleural effusion is common, more often occurring on the right side.

What is the mechanism of its formation and what is the explanation for its right-sided frequency?

91 Ascites does not only occur in liver disease. A 55-year-old woman gives a history of a few months' dyspnoea on exertion, general weakness and epigastric discomfort. Examination shows distended neck veins, smooth hepatomegaly and a pansystolic murmur loudest at the lower sternal border.

The two cardiac conditions which particularly give rise to ascites are tricuspid incompetence and constructive pericarditis.

What features would help you to distinguish between these two conditions?

92 The majority of cases of hypertension do not have an identifiable cause, and are called essential hypertension. In those 10 per cent of patients in whom the hypertension is secondary, what are the possible underlying causes?

93 Most cases of hypertension are asymptomatic. Even severe hypertension may not cause the patient any trouble in the earlier stages. Signs of the condition may be present on examination, however. The left ventricle may be enlarged as demonstrated by finding a displaced apex beat, or cardiomegaly on chest X-ray if a displaced apex beat is not detected clinically. A fourth heart sound may be present, indicating the decreased compliance of the left ventricle. Further confirmation of the effect on the left ventricle may be found on the ECG.

What would you look for?

94 Hypertension accelerates arteriosclerosis and the damage to the vasculature can be detected clinically.

What signs would you routinely look for in a hypertensive patient?

95 The value of inspecting the fundi cannot be overstated. In the case of hypertension the appearance of the retinal vessels and the presence of exudates, haemorrhages or papilloedema gives an indication of the duration and a precise demonstration of the severity of the condition.

What are the four grades of hypertensive retinopathy?

96 The effects of hypertension on the brain are common and often catastrophic. Cerebral thrombosis and cerebral haemorrhage tend to strike without warning, but sometimes there are antecedent neurological symptoms which might point to hypertension.

What are they?

97 The damage that hypertension may cause to the kidneys is of particular importance since renal damage may itself further elevate the blood pressure.

What are the renal effects of hypertension?

98 For the asymptomatic patient with mild to moderate hypertension, what is the usual treatment, bearing in mind that it may need to be life-long?

99 In moderate to severe hypertension, one drug is usually not sufficient to give adequate control. Many drug combinations are possible but the most effective appears to be that of a beta-blocker with a vasodilator.

An example would be propranolol combined with hydralazine.
What is it that makes this combination effective and attractive?

100 Thiazide diuretics, propranolol and other beta-blockers, alpha-methyldopa and hydralazine, are all commonly used antihypertensives. Their side effects are also quite common.
What are they?

101 Acute rheumatic fever is the name given to some of the inflammatory processes that occur following infection with group A streptococci. The exact link with the streptococcus is disputed, but the tissue damage appears to be via an autoimmune mechanism.
What sort of streptococcal infection is implicated and how long after may features of acute rheumatic fever occur?

102 The manifestations of acute rheumatic fever have been classified 'major' or 'minor' according to the degree to which they support the diagnosis. These Duckett Jones criteria are necessary because there are no absolutely confirmatory tests by which to be sure of the diagnosis. The minor manifestations comprise a history of previous rheumatic fever or pre-existing rheumatic heart disease, arthralgia, fever, elevated ESR or C-reactive protein and ECG changes.
What are the major manifestations and how many of each are required for diagnostic confidence?

103 Acute rheumatic fever may be difficult to diagnose because of the various presentations. For instance, arthritis or chorea may occur, apparently alone, or the carditis may present as congestive heart failure. The characteristically serpiginous skin rash, erythema marginatum, occurs in only 5 per cent of cases, as do the subcutaneous nodules.
What are the features of the arthritis?

104 Carditis is the commonest and the most serious manifestation of acute rheumatic fever because of the damage it can cause to the heart muscle and valves. One attack of carditis also predisposes to recurrences of rheumatic fever, and patients with carditis should go on long-term antibiotic prophylaxis.
What are the diagnostic findings of rheumatic carditis?

105 What is the treatment for acute rheumatic fever and what antibiotic should be used to prevent recurrences?

106 Post-streptococcal or Sydenham's chorea carries a good prognosis and gets better, causing no residual intellectual impairment. Nevertheless, it may be disturbing to the patient and her family (it is commoner in girls than in boys).

What are the distinctive features of choreiform movements and how does Sydenham's chorea differ from Huntington's chorea?

107 In rheumatic heart disease, the mitral valve is most commonly affected, followed by aortic, tricuspid and pulmonary valves in decreasing order of frequency. Rheumatic lesions of the pulmonary valve are rare. There is a logical explanation for this pattern of involvement.

What is it?

108 The physical signs of mitral stenosis depend on the severity of the lesion. Cyanosis and the well-known malar flush indicate a severe lesion as do the congestive signs of fluid retention—ankle oedema, pleural effusion, hepatomegaly, ascites.

On auscultation, a loud pulmonary heart sound indicates pulmonary hypertension. In what way would you interpret the sounds arising from the mitral valve itself?

109 In mitral stenosis, the clinical picture is largely determined by the degree of pulmonary hypertension. If pulmonary artery pressure is normal, all the auscultatory signs of the stenosis may be audible but the patient is likely to have normal or near-normal exercise tolerance. As the pulmonary artery pressure rises, exercise tolerance diminishes.

What is the cause of the pulmonary hypertension?

110 A 55-year-old woman presents with haemoptysis. On examination you feel a thrill over the apex and auscultation reveals an accentuated pulmonary sound, a snap immediately following the second heart sound and a low-pitched diastolic murmur most easily heard over the apex with the patient on her left elbow.

Are these findings relevant to the haemoptysis?

111 One of the greatest hazards of mitral stenosis is systemic embolization due to the formation of thrombi in an enlarged left atrium and atrial appendage. This is more likely when atrial fibrillation is present (atrial arrhythmias are a common complication of long-standing stenosis).

Is this the only thromboembolic hazard of this lesion?

112 Which non-invasive investigation can provide considerable information on the state of the mitral valve and indicate the degree of stenosis?

113 The typically low-pitched rumbling diastolic murmur of mitral stenosis may be accompanied by other murmurs.
What are they?

114 The ECG of a patient with mitral stenosis shows sinus rhythm with a wide, diphasic mainly negative P wave in V1 and notched P wave in standard leads I and II. The sum of the S wave in V1 and the R wave in V5 is 45 mm and there is sagging ST depression in V4, 5 and 6. Is this what you would expect or is some other problem also present?

115 You are shown a patient's chest X-rays, including some films with barium in the oesophagus (so a cardiac problem is likely). You notice on the PA view that the left upper border of the cardiac silhouette is straight, and the pulmonary vessels at the hila are prominent as are the vessels in the upper lobes. On the right anterior oblique view, the barium-filled oesophagus is pushed backwards as it passes the left atrium.
What do these X-ray findings indicate, what lesion could account for them all and what would you look for in the lower lung zones near the periphery?

116 Under what circumstances would you treat a patient with rheumatic valve disease with antibiotics?

117 When would you advise your patients with mitral stenosis to undergo cardiac surgery, and what surgical procedures are available?

118 Whereas the predominant symptom of mitral stenosis is dyspnoea, mitral regurgitation is marked by fatigue, weakness and weight loss due to the fall in cardiac output.
What are the most common physical signs of mitral regurgitation?

119 Rheumatic heart disease is not the only cause of mitral regurgitation, in fact it now accounts for only about half of the cases. Ischaemic heart disease can also cause mitral regurgitation.
How?

120 Calcification of the mitral valve leaflets quite often occurs in patients with combined mitral stenosis and regurgitation, but not with pure mitral regurgitation.

What are the X-ray findings of mitral regurgitation?

121 Mitral valve prolapse, in which the posterior leaflet prolapses into the left atrium, is a relatively common abnormality, occurring in up to 15 per cent of the general population. The physical signs include a click in midsystole and a mid- or late systolic murmur. In some cases, there are associated ECG changes.

What are they?

122 Tricuspid regurgitation seldom occurs as an isolated lesion but usually develops secondary to mitral valve disease or chronic lung disease, the common factor being pulmonary hypertension.

What are the signs of tricuspid regurgitation?

123 Tricuspid stenosis is usually rheumatic in aetiology and therefore often accompanied by mitral stenosis. The neck veins will be distended, 'A' waves in the jugular venous pulse will be prominent and hepatomegaly, ascites and oedema may be present. These physical signs are shared by mitral valve lesions and cor pulmonale.

What findings would distinguish tricuspid stenosis?

124 Aortic stenosis is usually present for many years before symptoms develop. Conversely, once symptoms do develop, life expectancy in the majority of cases is less than 4 years. The lesion is commoner in men.

There are three main causes of aortic valve stenosis and three main symptoms.

What are they?

125 The plateau pulse is a well-known feature of aortic stenosis but it develops only in the later stages of the condition. While the blood pressure and pulse pressure are still normal, what changes would you expect to find on examination?

126 In aortic stenosis, the obstruction to outflow usually develops gradually, giving the left ventricle time to adapt. The response to an increasing pressure load is muscle hypertrophy and usually resting stroke volume remains normal until a late stage of the disease. There are some penalties for myocardial hypertrophy, however, including reduced compliance, increased oxygen needs and increased coronary artery compression. Atrial arrhythmias are poorly tolerated.

Why is this?

127 When the main symptoms of aortic stenosis develop, namely angina, syncope and dyspnoea, the outlook is

not very good. What can be offered to these patients that carries a lower mortality than conservative management?

128 Aortic regurgitation is mainly due to rheumatic heart disease, and this is even more true of lesions where there is significant haemodynamic disturbance. Some cases are due to congenital valve abnormalities. But there are also other conditions which may cause or be accompanied by aortic regurgitation.
Can you name four?

129 Increased force of left ventricular contraction is one of the features of aortic regurgitation felt by the patient as an uncomfortable awareness of the heart beat.
The murmur of aortic regurgitation is typically high-pitched and decrescendo and best heard with the patient leaning forward in forced expiration.
What other murmurs may be heard?

130 In a patient with suspected aortic regurgitation, the ECG shows depressed ST segments and inverted T waves in leads I, aVL, V5 and V6. There is also a deep S wave in V1 and a tall R wave in V5, the sum of which exceeds 35 mm.
Do these findings support your clinical diagnosis?

131 The angina that occurs in aortic regurgitation is unusual in that it can occur at rest or at night and is not very effectively relieved by nitroglycerin.
What is the explanation for this?

132 Aortic aneurysms may occur anywhere along the aorta. They are commonest in the abdomen but the associated symptoms and signs are more dramatic in intrathoracic cases.
The causative agent of syphilis, *Treponema pallidum*, has a predilection for the ascending aorta and following a latent period of 10 years or more from the primary infection and provided antibiotics have not been given, the inflammatory process of syphilitic aortitis may lead to aneurysm formation.
Cardiovascular syphilis is now rare, however. What is the common aetiology of fusiform or saccular aortic aneurysms?

133 A 60-year-old patient presents with a few months' history of gradually increasing cough, difficulty swallowing, hoarseness and a vague sensation of chest discomfort. While talking to him you observe a left-sided Horner's syndrome and you correctly suspect that all these symptoms and the Horner's syndrome could be caused by one lesion, namely an upper

mediastinal mass. He is a non-smoker and there is no clubbing. Neither of these facts excludes carcinoma, but what vascular lesion could he have?

134 The treatment of aortic aneurysm is surgical and often it is possible to remove or bypass the diseased section of aorta and replace it with a dacron graft. The dacron has holes in it which are large enough to let blood through.
How therefore does it work?

135 Dissecting aneurysm is the name for the usually catastrophic event of aortic blood splitting the intima and forcing a false passage through the layers of the media, which have been weakened by necrosis. The false passage may be blind or it may reopen into the aortic lumen further along the aorta. Dissections are classified according to the site and length of aorta involved.
What is the cause of the underlying medial necrosis?

136 The clinical features of aortic dissection include the pain of the initial event and the symptoms and signs resulting from the occlusion of vascular branches that can follow. The pain is often indistinguishable from that of acute myocardial infarction, but a sudden onset between the shoulder blades and maximum intensity at the beginning may be helpful clues.
What other features would you look for?

137 What are the radiological and electrocardiographic features of a dissecting aortic aneurysm and how do they affect management?

138 A cardiomyopathy is a subacute or chronic disorder of heart muscle, of unknown or unusual cause, often with associated endocardial and sometimes pericardial involvement. By convention, damage due to coronary artery disease, hypertension or valvular disease is not included. Primary cardiomyopathies are those in which the main disorder is of the heart itself.
There are four main kinds. Can you name them?

139 Secondary cardiomyopathies are those in which the heart is involved in a generalized disorder. There are many of these and worldwide the commonest is that associated with malnutrition. More than 10 years' heavy drinking is a qualification for alcoholic cardiomyopathy. Haemochromatosis, amyloidosis and sarcoidosis are important examples of infiltrations in which arrhythmias are common. Myocardial damage may accompany the muscular dystrophies.

Can the heart be involved in the collagen vascular diseases?

140 In hypertrophic obstructive cardiomyopathy, in which there is thickening of the left ventricular outflow tract, digoxin makes things worse.
Is propranolol helpful?

141 A patient is admitted with several weeks' history of general malaise, fever and weight loss. Three weeks earlier the patient had a mild stroke of sudden onset from which he appears to have made a full recovery. The reason for this admission is severe, sharp upper abdominal pain, also of sudden onset. He also describes some fainting episodes and occasional breathlessness. Examination is unremarkable except for a low-pitched diastolic murmur best heard with the patient on his left elbow and stethoscope over the apex. Investigations reveal a raised ESR and raised gammaglobulins. Clearly this man has a cardiac problem.
What is it?

142 For reasons that are not clear, some, but not all, heavy drinkers are susceptible to myocardial cell damage.
What is the clinical picture of alcoholic cardiomyopathy?

143 The thyroid has a powerful influence on the heart as on other parts of the body. Even when the diagnosis of hyperthyroidism is not apparent from eye signs or gland enlargement, the following cardiac features must arouse suspicion: persistent tachycardia, high-output cardiac failure in the absence of an obvious cause, refractory cardiac failure, atrial fibrillation (paroxysmal or chronic) with an apparent resistance to the ventricular slowing effect of digoxin.
What are the cardiac manifestations of hypothyroidism?

144 What advice would you give regarding the safety of pregnancy to (a) a woman with a heart lesion but no symptoms and no signs of cardiac enlargement, (b) a woman who has had heart failure and who has severe exercise intolerance, and (c) a woman who has mild symptoms and some exercise intolerance?

145 Coarctation of the aorta is an uncommon but important cause of hypertension. In one-third of cases there is an associated heart lesion, such as bicuspid aortic valve, patent ductus arteriosus or ventricular septal defect. It is commonly present in Turner's

syndrome. The coarctation is usually just distal to a normally closed ductus arteriosus.

What are the clinical features, ECG and X-ray findings in this condition?

146 The division of congenital heart disease into cyanotic and acyanotic is more than just a textbook description. There are distinctive clinical consequences of having cyanotic heart disease, apart from the cyanosis.

What are they?

147 The ECG finding of all negative deflections in lead I, all positive in aVR and increasing negativity across the precordial leads should alert you to the presence of dextrocardia.

Usually situs inversus is present and the heart is normal. If the dextrocardia is an isolated malposition, then an abnormality is likely to be present. If the heart is in the normal position but there is situs inversus of the abdominal organs, then serious cardiac abnormality can be expected.

What is the name of the syndrome of bronchiectasis, sinusitis and dextrocardia?

148 Bicuspid aortic valve is a congenital abnormality.

What tends to happen to the valve with this condition?

149 Pulmonary stenosis is nearly always congenital in origin and it is the commonest congenital cause of right ventricular outflow tract obstruction. Surgery is indicated if there is evidence of right ventricular hypertrophy or of a gradient across the valve of approximately 100 mmHg.

What are the physical signs?

150 Patent ductus arteriosus is an anomaly that is usually compatible with survival to adult life. It is commoner in girls. The physical signs depend on the pressure gradients across the ductus between the aorta and the pulmonary artery.

What are the signs?

151 Atrial septal defect is the commonest congenital cardiac anomaly in adults. Women are more often affected.

What are the typical physical findings and ECG features of ASD in the asymptomatic stage?

152 Ventricular septal defect is the commonest congenital heart lesion. In uncomplicated cases, there is a left-to-right shunt which produces a pansystolic murmur loudest in the third and fourth left intercostal

spaces. The maladie de Roger is a defect causing no symptoms and no ECG or X-ray changes.

What are the ECG changes of larger defects with significant shunts?

153 What is the place of surgery in the treatment of ventricular septal defect?

154 Fallot's tetralogy is a relatively common form of cyanotic heart disease that has, as its name suggests, four components: a VSD, obstruction to right ventricular outflow, over-riding of the aorta over both ventricular outflow tracts, and right ventricular hypertrophy. The haemodynamic and clinical picture is determined by the degree of right ventricular outflow tract obstruction.

What are the main clinical features?

155 What is the outlook for children with Fallot's tetralogy and what is the treatment?

156 In congenital heart lesions, antibiotic prophylaxis to prevent infective endocarditis is only necessary if the lesion is causing significant haemodynamic disturbance.

Would you agree with this statement?

157 Angina pectoris is pain resulting from myocardial hypoxia. It commonly occurs on exertion or with emotion and is usually felt in the central chest area. It may radiate to the neck, jaw, left or right arm. Occasionally it is felt initially in the left hand or elbow alone. In western societies, the commonest cause is coronary artery narrowing or obstruction due to atheroma. But there are other important causes.

What are they?

158 The epidemiology of coronary artery disease shows that although certain populations or ethnic groups may be particularly spared or prone to disease, the general picture is of a very low prevalence in so-called developing countries, a high prevalence in westernized societies and a rising prevalence where the cultural and dietary habits of western societies are being acquired.

Which countries have the highest incidence of coronary artery disease?

159 The exact aetiology of human atheromatous plaques is not known for certain. Theories abound, the best-known being that incriminating dietary fat, especially an excess of saturated fats. Despite considerable investigation, proof is still not

forthcoming although a high serum cholesterol is accepted as being a marker or risk factor for coronary artery disease.
Give three other theories for atheroma.

160 While the aetiology of atherosclerosis remains uncertain, the clinician can make some assessment of the likelihood of coronary atherosclerosis (and also other cardiovascular diseases) developing from the presence of what are called risk factors.
What are they and how important are they relative to each other?

161 Where is Framingham and what is its medical significance?

162 In the field of coronary artery disease, much effort has gone into primary prevention, that is, preventing myocardial infarction in a healthy but at risk population, and secondary prevention, namely seeking to prevent further infarctions in people who have already suffered (and survived) one.
Can you give examples of trials that have been conducted in these areas?

163 The myocardial hypoxia or ischaemia that causes angina may give rise to ECG changes. These may be present only when angina occurs, or only during exercise or they may be seen on a resting tracing.
What ECG changes would you look for in angina?

164 A common diagnostic problem is deciding whether or not coronary artery disease is present in patients who have normal resting ECGs and cardiac enzymes in the presence of typical or atypical chest pain.
What two tests, one functional and one radiological, should enable one to decide?

165 Many patients with angina have stable and predictable pain, but some give a history of recent increase in symptoms; either the angina comes on at lesser degrees of activity or it comes on at rest. There are many terms for this, including unstable angina, crescendo angina, pre-infarction angina, impending myocardial infarction etc. Studies of these patients have revealed no way of reliably predicting which patients will go on to infarction.
How should such a patient be managed?

166 The rationale of existing treatment for angina is to reduce the work done by the myocardium so that it conforms to the limited oxygen supplies. One group of drugs does this by reducing venous return, thereby

decreasing end diastolic pressure in the left ventricle. A second group achieves it by a negative inotropic action, reducing the force of muscle contraction. A third group has a similar effect but by a more direct mechanism.

What are the three groups of drugs?

167 The only corrective treatment for coronary artery disease is surgical, in the form of vessel grafting—usually of saphenous vein—to bypass the sites of severest narrowing or obstruction. The operation goes by the letters CABG.

What does the operation involve for the patient and what results can he expect?

168 In some patients, definite angina occurs at rest and without any association with exertion. During an attack, the ECG shows elevation of the ST segments.

What is the name for this kind of angina and what would you look for on a coronary angiogram?

169 In myocardial infarction, acute deprivation of oxygen, either due to coronary artery narrowing or to abnormalities of the blood or both, causes irreversible damage to an area of cardiac muscle. The integrity of the cell membrane is lost and the muscle cells become 'stuffed with blood'.

What are the usual clinical features of myocardial infarction?

170 Confirmation of the clinical suspicion of a myocardial infarction rests on ECG and biochemical evidence. The common three ECG changes that indicate infarction are Q waves, ST segment elevation especially with an upward convexity, and inverted T waves. Subendocardial infarcts may only cause symmetrical T wave inversion. It is a curious fact that the ECG changes may take several hours to develop. The importance of serial ECGs is therefore very great.

What is the biochemical evidence for infarction?

171 The ECG is very useful not only to confirm the diagnosis of a myocardial infarction but also to localize it. Anterior wall infarction will show in I, aVL and the precordial leads corresponding to the affected area. Inferior (diaphragmatic) infarction shows in II, III and aVF and also in V5 and V6 if there is apical extension, while true posterior infarction may be revealed by tall R waves in leads V1 and 2.

For each of these three examples, which coronary artery is likely to be involved?

172 While an initial ECG in a patient with pain suggestive of myocardial infarction may show equivocal changes, such as minor T wave inversion or borderline ST changes, repeating the ECG at 12 or 24 hourly intervals for the first few days may reveal progressive changes that indicate definite infarction. Another reason for serial ECGs is to observe the healing of an infarct.

What changes characteristically occur as an infarct heals?

173 The two most common complications of myocardial infarction are those of a weakened pump, i.e. heart failure, and electrical disturbance, i.e. arrhythmias. Whereas pump failure is associated with a relatively large area of muscle damage, this is usually not the case with arrhythmias, for which the myocardial damage matters more by its site than by its size. The arrhythmia most commonly causing death is ventricular fibrillation.

What can be done to prevent it?

174 What are the clinical features of ventricular aneurysm following myocardial infarction?

175 'All patients with acute myocardial infarction should be admitted to hospital.'

Is this statement true?

176 Interference with electrical conduction leading to arrhythmias is probably the commonest complication of myocardial infarction. In the acute stages, the hospital patient is likely to be attached to a continuous monitor with some form of arrhythmia detector and alarm system.

What are the technical possibilities for monitoring arrhythmias subsequently?

177 When hypotension occurs due to a weakened myocardium (pump failure) what treatments may be tried to maintain the circulation?

178 Secondary prevention is the term given to the attempt to protect survivors of heart attacks from subsequent infarction. Much attention has focused on the correction of risk factors, especially hypercholesterolaemia, although in this case there is not much evidence that lowering serum cholesterol confers secondary protection. Another aspect is the use of long-term therapy. Antiplatelet agents and beta-blockers have been the subjects of a large number of conflicting studies.

Of at least equal importance is what is actually said to the patient when he or she goes home.

What should this include as a minimum?

179 Four weeks after suffering a myocardial infarction, a man presents with fever, pain on inspiration and on swallowing, a dry cough and mild dyspnoea. Examination reveals some dullness to percussion and reduced breath sounds over the left lower zone of the chest, some crepitations over both lower zones and the heart sounds are not well heard. His white cell count and ESR are both elevated.

What is the likely diagnosis?

180 Four weeks after a D and C for intermenstrual bleeding, a 32-year-old woman with mitral valve disease is referred to hospital in heart failure. She has been having night sweats and a fluctuating fever and her husband has noticed she has become mentally dull.

What is the likely diagnosis, why the mental dullness and what would you expect to find in a fresh specimen of urine?

181 In what condition do microscopic haematuria, subconjunctival and splinter haemorrhages, Osler's nodes, Roth's spots and Janeway lesions occur?

How would you confirm the diagnosis and what is the treatment?

182 A 35-year-old woman complains of precordial chest pain that alters with movement, and is found to have pericarditis. Echocardiography demonstrates the presence of a loculated effusion.

What associated symptoms and signs would help pinpoint the aetiology?

183 A 55-year-old lorry driver who is a heavy smoker presents with retrosternal chest pain that varies with position and is felt more when he takes a deep breath or swallows food. A few days before, while in the cab, he had felt a heavy sensation in his chest and had had to open the window to get more air, but he thought nothing of it. His ECG shows a Q wave in leads I, aVL, V2 and V3 and marked ST elevation in the chest leads with an upward concavity to the ST segments.

What is wrong with him and name two other primarily cardiac conditions in which this development can occur.

184 A 50-year-old man with chronic renal failure, who has failed to keep his last two outpatient appointments, is admitted with some chest discomfort and dyspnoea. He

has tachycardia with cold peripheries and looks unwell and slightly restless. When he breathes in, the radial pulse gets weaker and his jugular venous pulse rises. Heart sounds are quiet.

What would you expect to find on the chest X-ray and ECG?

185 Chronic constrictive pericarditis is a condition that causes dyspnoea on exertion and orthopnoea with congestion of neck veins but little or no cardiac enlargement. Like tricuspid valve disease, it commonly causes hepatomegaly with ascites but little peripheral oedema. The usual cause used to be tuberculosis but it has now been observed following other forms of pericarditis.

What is the treatment?

186 The occurrence of venous thrombosis and pulmonary embolism in patients immobilized by fractures, operations or severe illness is predictable enough, but pulmonary embolism is met in some other conditions.

What are they?

187 Post-mortem studies show that less than a third of pulmonary emboli are diagnosed before death. Thinking of the diagnosis is half the battle. The only consistent symptom is dyspnoea and the only consistent physical sign is tachycardia. The patient may complain of an oppressive feeling in the chest or of pleuritic pain subsequently.

What physical signs should you look for that would support the diagnosis?

188 In the diagnosis of pulmonary embolism, the definitive investigation is pulmonary angiography. This is seldom available outside specialist centres. The next most direct method is a lung perfusion scan using a radioisotope but interpretation of any defects is unreliable unless a simultaneous ventilation scan is done. This too may not be available. On most occasions, doctors have to make the diagnosis with the aid of chest X-ray and ECG and arterial blood gases.

What findings would support the diagnosis of PE?

189 The majority of cases of pulmonary embolism are treated with intravenous heparin followed by an oral anticoagulant such as warfarin. Heparin blocks several of the factors in the coagulation pathway but its most potent action is on factor X. Its undoubted effectiveness in reducing the mortality from PE is not fully understood, although one of its properties is to block the reflex bronchospasm that occurs in acute embolism.

What is the mode of action of warfarin?

190 The list of commonly used drugs which do not interact with warfarin is short and easy to remember, namely diazepam and paracetamol. The list of commonly used drugs that do interact is very long. Nevertheless, it must be learned in some form, since too much or too little warfarin effect may be catastrophic.

What are the main kinds of interaction and the main culprits?

191 Most pulmonary emboli are treated with anticoagulants. In acute, massive embolism in which the circulation is severely compromised, doctors with access to appropriate facilities can assess the patient for urgent embolectomy.

What alternative treatment is there?

192 There are some patients, often women in middle age, who describe dyspnoea on exertion for which routine tests of heart and lungs reveal no cause. Many of them, unfortunately, are labelled as neurotic.

What condition must be considered and excluded before organic pathology can be ruled out?

193 Peripheral vascular disease is common in western communities, and is a consequence of heavy cigarette smoking and a complication of diabetes. The commonest symptom is intermittent claudication, which is pain occurring in calf muscle on exercise but subsiding within a minute or two of resting. More severe disease is marked by rest pain, usually in the toes or foot, which is typically relieved by hanging the leg out of bed or getting up and walking. Both these manoeuvres enlist gravity to aid flow, but walking may deprive the foot of blood flow altogether, rendering it anaesthetic.

What signs would you look for?

194 What are the main points of management in peripheral vascular disease?

195 A 35-year-old man complains of pain in the insteps of both feet that comes on with walking and subsides with rest. He admits to smoking 50 cigarettes daily and also reports that his fingers sometimes become white and numb especially in winter. Examination reveals, apart from nicotine-stained fingers, absent pulses in both feet and an absent radial pulse at the right wrist.

What disease has he got and what must he do to save his feet and hands?

196 A 65-year-old man presents with sudden onset of pain in his left arm, followed by an increasing sensation of cold and numbness from the elbow down. What is the most likely diagnosis and cause?
What treatment is indicated and how soon?

197 Raynaud's disease is the isolated entity that most commonly effects young adult women, with symmetrical involvement of both hands and usually without tissue necrosis. When Raynaud's phenomenon starts later in life, affects men, progresses rapidly to tissue necrosis or affects just one or two digits, then there is considerable likelihood of an underlying disorder.
What may this be?

198 A 23-year-old primary school teacher reports increasing weakness and easy tiring of her arms. On a few occasions after exercise she has found herself close to fainting. Examination reveals absent pulses in her arms, although femorals and foot pulses are normal, and there is a systolic murmur heard best at the base of the neck.
What is the likely diagnosis?

199 What procedures exist to help confirm the presence of deep venous thrombosis?

200 Superficial thrombophlebitis and deep venous thrombosis are both very common in the western world. The former gives rise to pain, redness and local swelling but seldom causes embolization, whereas the latter is often silent. DVTs that produce oedema, increased girth and increased temperature of the calf and a positive Homan's sign may not cause pulmonary embolism, whereas silent DVT may be associated with massive pulmonary embolism.
What would you expect to find when examining the leg of someone who had had a DVT some years previously?

Respiratory System

201 The fissures between the lobes of the lungs are of clinical interest because they are often visible on posteroanterior and lateral chest X-rays and their displacement may provide valuable diagnostic clues.
What are the normal positions of the fissures of the right lung?

202 Knowledge of the bronchopulmonary segments is important for localizing disease correctly and for

getting the best results from bronchography or physiotherapy and postural drainage.

On the right side, the upper lobe consists of anterior, apical and posterior segments. The middle lobe has lateral and medial segments while the lower lobe has an apical, anterior, lateral, posterior and a small medial segment.

What are the segments of the left lung?

203 A chest X-ray can be a goldmine of information, but in order not to miss anything it is important to have a sytematic way of checking the main points of the film. This seems slow and laborious at first, but with practice, it takes little time.

What is the first thing to check?

204 On a chest X-ray, 40 per cent of the lung is hidden by overlying shadows, of which the largest area is the heart. In order to see all of the lungs it is essential to do a lateral view, normally a left lateral unless there is particular interest in the right lung field.

What are the lung markings due to?

205 A chest X-ray is good for anatomy but gives no information at all about lung function.

There are a large number of tests of lung function, some of which are widely available but others require much equipment. In the first category is included the vitalograph.

What does this measure?

206 Tidal volume is the volume of air expired during a normal breath which in the normal adult is approximately 450 ml.

What is the vital capacity?

207 Abnormalities of lung function can be usefully divided into two kinds. In obstructive disease there is a ventilatory defect due to narrowing of the airways (which is variable in asthma but usually fixed in chronic bronchitis and emphysema). In restrictive disease, the defect lies in reduced lung compliance causing 'stiff' lungs. Airways resistance is normal or may even be low.

Measurement of forced vital capacity (FVC) and of forced expiratory volume in one second (FEV_1) usually distinguishes these two abnormalities.

What values would you expect?

208 At the bedside, two valuable measurements of pulmonary function are the peak flow rate and the minute volume.

What instruments are used to measure these and when are they of particular interest?

209 Changes in breathing and ventilation can have rapid and profound effects on acid–base balance. Measurement of arterial blood gases gives one the pH, Po_2, Pco_2, plasma bicarbonate, corrected values for the bicarbonate (for a theoretical Pco_2 of 40 mmHg or 5.3 kPa) and oxygen saturation of haemoglobin.

A 23-year-old medical student presents with attacks of emotional lability accompanied by spasms of her limbs. She does not lose consciousness but immediately after an attack, Chvostek's sign is positive. Between attacks, her blood gases are as follows: pH 7.42, Po_2 14.7 kPa (110 mmHg), Pco_2 3.8 kPa (28.5 mmHg) and plasma bicarbonate 18 mmol/l.

What is the probable diagnosis?

210 Transfer factor is the name of the test of lung function which gives an approximate indication of the surface available for gas exchange in the lung. Its symbol is T_L and because its value is routinely measured using carbon monoxide, it is often written T_LCO. The term 'diffusing capacity' is, for practical purposes, synonymous.

During childhood the transfer factor increases with the growth of the lung and in adult life is related to body size.

What causes a reduction in transfer factor?

211 What is the effect of smoking on lung function?

212 What is meant by purulent sputum and what does it usually indicate?

213 Haemoptysis has both pulmonary and cardiac causes. It occurs in pulmonary infarction and is quite commonly seen in bronchiectasis. Fully treated and healed TB can give rise to haemoptysis, sometimes massive (this is one of the ways in which TB still causes death). In between a third and a half of cases of a small haemoptysis, no cause is found despite careful follow-up.

What are the main cardiac causes of haemoptysis?

214 Pleuritic pain is usually sharp and stabbing in character and aggravated by deep inspiration or coughing. Often it is well localized, although it may be referred to the abdomen or to the shoulder tip.

Many of these features are shared, however, by other conditions.

What are they and how would you distinguish between them?

215 A 32-year-old unmarried woman, taking the oral contraceptive pill, was seen by a locum GP because of

an uncomfortable chest pain that was exacerbated by breathing. Within a few hours she had been admitted to hospital, started on a heparin drip and told that she must never take the pill again. The following day she had a ventilation/perfusion lung scan and was told that there was nothing wrong with her, the drip was discontinued and she was discharged. She still had her pain.

In a state of considerable confusion and anxiety she again went to the surgery. Her GP listened to the story, examined her thoroughly and reached the right diagnosis—with his hands.

How?

216 What happens to the expiratory phase of respiration in airways obstruction?

217 What pulmonary conditions cause clubbing?

218 Changes in chest shape may not only result from lung disease, as in the barrel chest of the chronic bronchitic, they may be the cause of lung disease.

While examining a 16-year-old student you note a marked thoracic kyphoscoliosis.

What may be the effect of this in later life?

219 While examining a 30-year-old asthmatic with an attack of breathlessness of sudden onset, you note the movement of his accessory muscles of respiration and also the hunched-up position of his shoulders, making a right angle between his neck and his shoulders.

What does this fixed position of his shoulders indicate and what observation about the right and left chest wall movements would tell you that this is not primarily an asthmatic attack?

220 Disease of the upper lobes can effect the position of the trachea at the thoracic inlet. A 45-year-old Chinese seaman with fully treated pulmonary TB is seen for a check-up. His trachea is noted to be displaced to the right.

On which side was his disease?

221 In percussion of the chest, the note obtained depends on the amount of air in the chest under one's percussing fingers. In addition, an effusion has a particularly 'stony' dullness.

What three common conditions cause increased resonance?

222 What does bronchial breathing sound like and what does it indicate?

223 What are the physical signs of a pleural effusion?

224 Rhonchi originate in the trachea and bronchial tree at sites of narrowing. The pitch gives an indication of the size of bronchus involved, from the low-pitched noise of a partially obstructed main bronchus to the high-pitched squeaks of small bronchioles. Another separation of rhonchi is into inspiratory and expiratory.

What is the significance of this?

225 How are râles produced and what does their presence indicate?

226 Hay fever is one variety of allergic rhinitis but some allergic rhinitis sufferers get their persistently runny nose, sneezing and nasal obstruction in the winter, when the windows are shut and extra blankets are on the beds.

Why is this?

227 The common cold is medically termed acute coryza. Some sufferers go on to develop secondary infections of the upper respiratory tract, such as sinusitis, otitis media and laryngitis.

What viruses cause coryza?

228 Although hoarseness is most commonly a short-term consequence of acute laryngeal infection, it can also result from serious disease and any hoarseness lasting longer than 3 weeks must be investigated.

What might you suspect in the presence of a chronic cough and hoarseness? How can doctors cause hoarseness?

229 The prescribing of antibiotics for 'flu', and relatively trivial viral infections of the lower respiratory tract is frowned upon, yet it is widespread and expected by large numbers of patients.

In which groups of patients is the practice entirely justified?

230 Chronic bronchitis is defined as the presence of a cough with expectoration for at least 3 months of a year for more than 2 consecutive years.

What are the anatomical changes in the bronchi that signify the condition?

231 What are the main symptoms of chronic bronchitis and what would you expect to find on clinical examination and on the chest X-ray?

232 The main principles in the treatment of chronic bronchitis are to prevent further deterioration, and to treat any reversible elements of the condition (such as accompanying bronchospasm) and to maximize exercise tolerance by fitness training.

The first includes giving up smoking, avoiding polluted atmospheres (e.g. fog), and having a course of antibiotics ready in the home to take at the first sign of an acute respiratory tract infection.

What other drugs might be useful?

233 In emphysema, there is dilatation or destruction of the walls of alveoli and respiratory bronchioles. When the alveolar damage predominates panacinar emphysema results. When the respiratory bronchioles bear the brunt of the damage, a centrilobular pattern results.

What are the main causes of emphysema and what effects does emphysema have on lung function?

234 Patients with emphysema suffer primarily from dyspnoea.

What would you expect to find on physical examination?

235 In what condition may all of the following chest X-ray features occur: flattened diaphragms with loss of the normal costophrenic angles; thin, vertical heart; prominence of the right and left pulmonary arteries but reduced vessel markings and hypertranslucency in the lung fields; bullae?

What abnormalities would you expect on lung function studies?

236 What can be done for a patient with emphysema?

237 You see a chest X-ray with unilateral translucency of a lung field.

What are the possible causes?

238 When a patient is on a ventilator, or, more precisely, on intermittent positive pressure ventilation, why is it advisable to give a sigh or deeper breath every so often, e.g. four per hour?

What are the things that threaten a patient on a ventilator?

239 A 56-year-old man is involved in a road traffic accident in which he suffers bilateral rib fractures and fractures of the left forearm and femoral shaft. It is some hours before he is brought to hospital and when he arrives you note him to be obese, exhausted, in pain and very dyspnoeic. His chest shows some paradoxical

movement. Blood gases show hypoxaemia with 60 per cent oxygen saturation and a carbon dioxide level at the upper limit of normal.

How should his respiratory problem be managed?

240 A 55-year-old man, known to be a heavy smoker and to have had chronic bronchitis for many years, comes into hospital with an acute exacerbation of his bronchitis. He is dyspnoeic and cyanosed with warm extremities. The veins on his hands are prominent and his pulse has an increased volume. The JVP is raised, oedema reaches up his calves and there is a heave felt to the left of the sternum. Auscultation reveals a triple rhythm.

What complication of his chronic lung disease has occurred?

241 What is the main haemodynamic factor that leads to cor pulmonale in chronic lung disease and what brings it about?

242 Comparison of ECG records with post-mortem studies show that by no means all cases of cor pulmonale manifest diagnostic ECG changes.

But what would you look for on the ECG and what are the chest X-ray features of the heart in this condition?

243 A patient with cor pulmonale secondary to chronic bronchitis and emphysema is treated with diuretics (and appropriate potassium supplements), digoxin, bronchodilators, 28 per cent oxygen given by Ventimask and, as recovery begins, with physiotherapy. Ampicillin is also given in view of the presence of an acute infection.

Is this the right treatment?

244 Which patients will retain carbon dioxide if given too much oxygen and how may a doctor inadvertently assist such a patient to his demise?

245 Bronchiectasis is a condition in which sections of the bronchi in one or more parts of the lungs are dilated, chronically inflamed and may be a continuing source of infected secretions.

What are the causes?

246 A 30-year-old man is admitted with haemoptysis. He gives a history of cough for several years, productive of large quantities of purulent sputum. He has had haemoptysis in the past and also attacks of pneumonia and bronchitis. On examination, he is underweight and has clubbing.

What is the likely cause of his haemoptysis?

247 What investigations would you routinely do on a new case of bronchiectasis and how would you assess suitability for surgery (to remove the affected parts of the lung)?

248 In bronchiectasis, what features would make you consider surgery and what would you do to the patient before performing bronchography?

249 While the medical treatment for bronchiectasis resembles that for chronic bronchitis, the most important aspect is postural drainage. To drain the lower lobes, which are the most commonly affected, the foot of the bed is elevated 18 inches and the patient lies face down or on his side depending on the segments involved.

How long should the patient spend in postural drainage each day and how is the right middle lobe drained?

250 Asthma is a condition characterized by airways obstruction. Asthmatics behave as if the beta-adrenergic receptors in their bronchi (which mediate dilation) are partly blocked all the time, rendering them vulnerable to any factors which can cause bronchospasm.

What are the important factors?

251 In an acute asthmatic attack, the patient is breathless, the lung compliance is reduced and the residual lung volume is increased.

What else invariably happens?

252 When an acute attack of asthma has continued for several hours, in addition to the initial bronchospasm there will be oedema of the bronchial mucosa (plus the inflammation resulting from any infection), and the patient may be tired, anxious, dehydrated and hypoxaemic.

What are the main lines of treatment?

253 The development of disodium cromoglycate has made a big difference to the management of asthma. The drug works by inhibiting mast cell degranulation and is effective in extrinsic (allergic), exercise-induced and occasionally other cases of asthma.

It is important that the patient appreciates that it does not relieve an attack. After starting with one inhaled capsule four times daily its beneficial effect may eventually be maintained with two or even one capsule daily.

What other drugs and techniques are employed in preventing attacks?

254 What is the time interval between exposure to an allergen and the onset of an asthmatic attack, and how long does the allergic reaction last?

255 What is the main reason for patients with bronchospasm failing to get benefit from nebulized aerosols of salbutamol and other bronchodilators?

256 In detecting an allergen, what is the relative value of skin testing, RIST (radioimmunosorbent test) and RAST (radioallergosorbent test)?

257 What are the main factors implicated in the causation of bronchogenic carcinoma?

258 The main histological types of bronchogenic carcinoma are: squamous cell, anaplastic, adenocarcinoma, alveolar cell carcinoma. State one important fact about each type.

259 A 55-year-old man, a non-smoker, presents with a cough with green, mucopurulent and occasionally blood-streaked sputum and a fever. Chest X-ray shows an irregular and streaky area of shadowing in the right midzone and a diagnosis of pneumonia is made. Four weeks later, the patient is well but a little shadowing on the chest X-ray remains. Tomography reveals no distinct shadow and sputum cytology is three times negative.

Could this man nevertheless have a carcinoma?

260 It is not uncommon for bronchogenic carcinoma to have occluded a main bronchus and caused a whole lung to collapse by the time the patient seeks medical help. The chest X-ray may show a homogeneous ground-glass appearance over the collapsed lung field and the mediastinum may have shifted towards the collapsed lung. If the mediastinum is central, a malignant pleural effusion may also be present.

Before attempting aspiration, how could you demonstrate the presence of fluid?

261 A centrally situated bronchial carcinoma can involve one or more of the many components of the mediastinum. A patient has oedema of the face and arms with engorged neck veins and prominent veins over the upper thorax. He complains of an unpleasant feeling of fullness in the head.

What is being obstructed?

262 What are the five most common sites of metastasis for bronchogenic carcinoma?

263 Bronchogenic carcinoma is responsible for several neurological lesions and syndromes, both by direct spread and by non-metastatic effects.

In the thorax, encroachment on the brachial plexus from the apex of the lung causes painful weakness and wasting in the hand and arm. This is a Pancoast's tumour. The recurrent laryngeal and phrenic nerves are vulnerable to direct involvement.

What are the extrathoracic neurological effects?

264 Carcinoma of the bronchus is well known for its non-metastatic endocrine effects, due to the production of peptides and amines that closely resemble native hormones.

What are the main syndromes?

265 What does hypertrophic pulmonary osteoarthropathy look like and what other non-neurological, non-endocrine signs and syndromes can be due to non-metastatic effects of a bronchogenic carcinoma?

266 If a pulmonary lesion is suspected to be malignant but cytology is negative, the next step is likely to be bronchoscopy. Another reason for bronchoscopy is to assess the extent of a growth to see if surgery is possible.

What should be done before bronchoscopy and surgery are considered?

267 The results of treatment for bronchogenic carcinoma are extremely disappointing. Of those that are eligible for surgical removal, only 20 per cent survive 5 years. Much longer survival is common for single alveolar cell carcinomas, but these account for a minority of cases.

What is the place of radiotherapy?

268 Can cytotoxic drugs be useful in the treatment of bronchogenic carcinoma?

269 Is it possible to have false positives when looking for malignant cells in the sputum?

270 A 30-year-old woman presents with haemoptysis. Chest X-ray shows a small well-defined coin shadow in the centre of her right lung field.

The patient does not smoke and is in any case young for bronchogenic carcinoma.

Assuming this is a growth, what endocrine syndrome might she be suffering from?

271 What are the radiological features of a pulmonary hamartoma? Would you be able to diagnose one before the pathologist examines the surgical specimen?

272 As a general rule, lobar pneumonia occurs in fit people encountering a virulent organism, whereas bronchopneumonia affects the very young, the old and others with impaired resistance and involves common pathogens which may even be normally carried in the upper respiratory tract.

What are the main organisms in these two types of pneumonia?

273 What is Mendelson's syndrome?

274 In bacterial pneumonias, the severity of the illness is usually commensurate with the clinical and radiological extent of the lesions.

In the group of pneumonias known as 'atypical' this is not so. Malaise, fever and other symptoms may far exceed the detectable evidence of the pulmonary lesions and large, radiologically abnormal areas of pneumonitis may be relatively silent.

What are the main organisms in the atypical group?

275 The classical features of pneumococcal pneumonia—abrupt onset with a rigor, dyspnoea, pleuritic pain, high fever, rusty sputum, herpes labialis—are familiar.

But what are the possible complications of pneumococcal pneumonia and which three groups of patients have an increased susceptibility to pneumococcal infection?

276 Staphylococcal pneumonia, which tends to lead to a cavitating abscess (multiple abscesses if a septicaemia is present) usually responds well to antibiotic therapy. Sometimes, however, it can be a fulminating illness with a significant mortality.

When would you be particularly on the look-out for staphylococcal pneumonia?

277 *Klebsiella* pneumonia is not very common but is usually serious. In presentation it resembles the acute febrile illness of pneumococcal pneumonia, although it shows some tendency to affect the upper lobes. Sometimes an acute attack is followed by a chronic infection leading to thin-walled cavities in the upper lobes (mimicking tuberculosis).

What conditions predispose to *Klebsiella* infection and what antibiotics would you use?

278 A 20-year-old Indian woman from East Africa presents with a febrile illness of recent onset in which the main symptom is a cough, producing purulent, occasionally blood-tinged sputum. Chest X-ray shows consolidation of the right middle lobe and a diagnosis of lobar pneumonia is made.

After five days there is no response to penicillin. What would you do?

279 *Mycoplasma pneumoniae* is an uncommon cause of pneumonia but an important pathogen of the respiratory tract. School children meet it more often than adults. It may cause pharyngitis, tracheobronchitis and bullous myringitis as well as pneumonia. Cough is a common symptom as is fever.

In pneumonia, what features on a chest X-ray would make you think of *Mycoplasma* and what laboratory test is particularly useful with this organism?

280 The main features of psittacosis are a history of even brief contact with budgerigars (or any other birds), fever, unproductive cough and headache. The physical signs in the chest are usually slight but the malaise may be great. The spleen may enlarge. The radiological appearances can mimic all other forms of pneumonia and the best diagnostic test is a complement fixation test carried out on paired sera. Treatment is with tetracycline.

What are the main features of Q fever?

281 The lungs, like the skin, can manifest acute or chronic adverse reactions to drugs. The list of culprits is long and includes some commonly used antibiotics, diuretics, antihypertensives and cytotoxic drugs. Temporal relationship to drug administration, withdrawal and re-exposure may be the only diagnostic test, although in the acute reactions, there may be eosinophilia.

What would you expect the symptoms to be in the acute and chronic forms of this disease?

282 A patient with fever and an unproductive cough abruptly begins to cough up quantities of foul-smelling pus.

What is the likely source and what should you do with the pus?

283 A patient with a lung abscess shows some initial improvement both clinically and radiologically when treated with penicillin but within a few days improvement ceases and expectoration of foul-smelling sputum continues.

What may be happening and how would you change the antibiotic treatment?

284 A 60-year-old woman is admitted as a surgical emergency with a perforated diverticular abscess and undergoes laparotomy and drainage.

Postoperatively she develops an ileus. On the third day you are asked to see her regarding some chest discomfort and dyspnoea. She tells you that she had a bad cold on the day of admission.

What should this alert you to?

285 Infected congenital cyst of the lung is an uncommon cause of lung abscess and usually requires surgical treatment. Acquired cysts are a fairly common part of emphysema or healed pulmonary tuberculosis.

What organism produces a characteristically cystic disease that can involve the lung (as well as the liver), and how would you diagnose it?

286 The causative organism of pulmonary tuberculosis is *Mycobacterium tuberculosis* also known as AFB, which stands for acid-fast bacillus (an abbreviation of acid–alcohol-fast bacillus), referring to its staining properties.

Are there any other mycobacteria that may cause lung infection?

287 There are ethnic differences in the incidence of chronic and fulminating pulmonary TB, that appear to be partly related to the period of time for which the ethnic group has been exposed to the bacillus.

Caucasians and Mongolians have a higher resistance, on the whole, and tend to run a more chronic course.

In which ethnic groups is acute disease more common?

288 Haemoptysis used to be a death sentence and there are many literary accounts of the dying consumptive. It is a popular misconception that deaths from TB no longer occur now that chemotherapy is available. But the late effects of extensive pulmonary TB may be severely incapacitating or fatal, and are of equally great literary value.

What are they?

289 What is a Ghon focus and what is the primary complex?

Does the Mantoux test become positive after primary tuberculosis infection?

290 Miliary tuberculosis is the name for infection that has been disseminated via the blood stream, usually as a result of erosion of a blood vessel by a caseating focus. It results in multiple tiny lesions resembling grains of wheat. It is incorrect to use the term for pea-sized nodules and other larger multiple shadows, which originate by transbronchial spread or other means.

What are the clinical and diagnostic features of miliary disease?

291 In what ways may abdominal tuberculosis come to light?

292 Although lymph nodes are part of host defences, they may themselves be overwhelmed by infection and this can occur with TB, commonly affecting the cervical lymph nodes.

What are the clinical features?

293 Can one tell whether pulmonary tuberculosis is active or healed from its radiological appearance?

294 The tubercle bacillus is a strict aerobe and it appears to be this taste for oxygen that leads it to the upper zones of the lungs where alveolar oxygen tension is highest.

Tuberculosis should be the first illness to come to mind when confronted with apical disease, but what other conditions can affect the upper lobes?

295 Pleural effusions are common in post-primary tuberculosis. The fluid is straw-coloured, not blood-stained, and isolation of tubercle bacilli from it is unusual.

Why is this?

296 How are tubercle bacilli demonstrated on a direct smear and how long does it take to culture the bacilli?

297 How is a Mantoux test performed and what is the difference btween old tuberculin and PPD (purified protein derivative)?

298 The initial phase of treatment for pulmonary tuberculosis in the UK consists of isoniazid, rifampicin and ethambutol for 2 months.

What does the continuation phase consist of?

299 How do the different antituberculosis drugs compare for bactericidal or bacteriostatic activity and what are the main factors influencing the success of treatment?

300 What is BCG and how important has it been relative to other factors in reducing the incidence of tuberculosis?

301 All the antituberculous drugs have side-effects. Most patients complete their treatment safely but side-effects may require adjustments in dose or complete alteration of regimen.

In which situation is treatment very difficult?

302 *Cryptococcus neoformans* is a yeast-like organism that principally causes a meningoencephalitis. It can also cause pulmonary disease.

What are the features of this and where does the organism usually come from?

303 What are the five ways in which species of the *Aspergillus* fungus can cause lung disease?

304 What is a mycetoma and what is the usual treatment?

305 What is bronchopulmonary aspergillosis, who is at risk from it and what are the late consequences?

306 Immunosuppression, which is commonly the result of chemotherapy for malignancy, autoimmune disease, or following organ transplantation, can have unusual or dire consequences in the form of opportunistic infections.

Notorious examples of opportunistic lung infection are *Pneumocystis carinii*, *Nocardia asteroides* and *Candida albicans*.

How would you diagnose each of these and what is the appropriate chemotherapy?

307 Coal-miners, quarry workers, sand-blasting workers and those in similar occupations are exposed to dusts of fine silica particles which lodge in the distal airways and set up a chronic, progressively fibrotic reaction. The earliest radiological change is a fine mottling, but each small focus may enlarge into a nodule and gross impairment of lung function results.

What may bring a patient with silicosis into hospital?

308 What clinical entities can result from exposure to asbestos, of which blue asbestos or crocidolite is the most dangerous form?

309 Pneumoconiosis results from coal dust inhalation in miners. Sufferers are eligible for compensation and the assessment of severity is based on radiological appearance, not on clinical features.

What are the radiological types?

310 The pathological process in simple pneumoconiosis centres around deposits of carbon dust in the respiratory bronchioles. The initial inflammatory process causes bronchiolar dilatation and centrilobular emphysema. A reticular pattern is seen on the chest X-ray. The formation of nodules up to 5 mm in size marks the subsequent stage. If dust exposure ceases, so does the inflammatory process.
This is in contrast to progressive massive fibrosis. What are the features of this?

311 Some patients with pneumoconiosis develop seropositive rheumatoid arthritis and multiple pulmonary nodules. The nodules are histologically rheumatoid.
What is the name for this combination of symptoms and signs?

312 'Monday dyspnoea' is a feature of byssinosis, the disease of workers exposed to cotton dust.
What is the cause of it and what X-ray changes would you expect to see in acute and chronic byssinosis?

313 What are the main causes of a combination of pulmonary infiltration and a significantly raised blood eosinophil count (>1000 per mm^3), that is, pulmonary eosinophilia?

314 In sarcoidosis, the Mantoux test is usually negative, due to depressed cellular immunity.
What is the Kveim–Siltzbach test?

315 Acute sarcoidosis can present in many different ways but the commonest is the combination of erythema nodosum, bilateral hilar adenopathy and fever. Polyarthralgia or polyarthritis may also be present.
In this and other forms of active disease, which blood test will help confirm the diagnosis?

316 Sarcoidosis can be a chronic condition of many years' duration.
Apart from chronic lung disease what are the other clinical features of long-standing sarcoidosis?

317 Uveoparotid fever (Heerfordt's syndrome) is one of the acute presentations of sarcoidosis. Uveitis, bilateral parotid (and other salivary gland) enlargement, fever, facial palsy and keratoconjunctivitis sicca (dryness of the eyes, also of the mouth) can all occur together.

The sicca syndrome occurs in another disease process with which sarcoidosis may initially be confused but which histological examination readily distinguishes.

What is this?

318 Pulmonary involvement is the commonest feature of sarcoidosis. Approximately one-third of patients with hilar lymphadenopathy develop pulmonary infiltration. Many of these cases remit spontaneously and most are asymptomatic, but steroid therapy is considered if remission is not evident after a year. About one per cent of cases progress inexorably to severe pulmonary fibrosis and death from cor pulmonale.

Would you expect to have pleural effusions in sarcoidosis?

319 Increased gut sensitivity to vitamin D is a feature of sarcoidosis which can cause hypercalciuria with or without hypercalcaemia. Sarcoidosis comes into the differential diagnosis of hypercalcaemia and is one of the group of conditions in which serum calcium levels are lowered by steroids.

As far as treatment of this abnormality in sarcoidosis is concerned, steroids are effective but expose the patient to side-effects.

What safer alternative is there?

320 Fibrosing alveolitis can occur as part of a generalized connective tissue disorder, e.g. rheumatoid arthritis, SLE, or—in isolation—cryptogenic fibrosing alveolitis.

What are the clinical and radiological features and what is the Hamman–Rich syndrome?

321 What is the name of the allergic lung disease in which dyspnoea begins 3–6 hours after exposure or re-exposure to the causative agent but rhonchi are absent, a restrictive lung defect is present and the diagnosis can be confirmed by blood test?

322 What condition causes recurrent episodes of fever and haemoptysis in company with iron-deficiency anaemia and with what other condition is it sometimes combined in whose syndrome?

323 The two cardinal signs of pleurisy are pleuritic chest pain and a friction rub.

What are the main causes?

324 In diagnosing the cause of a pleural effusion, the age of the patient and the presence of disease in any other

system are two important considerations. In a 30-year-old woman the two main diagnostic possibilities are TB and SLE. In a 65-year-old man, malignancy is likely although TB is also an occasional cause.

What tests would you routinely request when sending a specimen of pleural fluid to the laboratory?

325 What is the definition of empyema and what are the causes?

326 The successful treatment of an empyema is based partly on giving the appropriate chemotherapy but also on draining the pus and collapsing the empyema cavity before the walls become so fibrotic and stiff as to be permanent. Drainage is by means of a tube and rib resection may be necessary to get adequate drainage.

What possibilities should you consider if an empyema cavity won't close?

327 The commonest cause of spontaneous pneumothorax is rupture of a cyst or bleb on the surface of the lung. These may be multiple and the pneumothorax may recur.

What underlying lung diseases predispose to pneumothorax and how may doctors be responsible for this condition?

328 The effects of a pneumothorax depend not only on its size but also on the state of the lungs. A young healthy adult may tolerate complete collapse of a lung without undue distress, while an elderly man with pulmonary fibrosis may be rendered acutely dyspnoeic by a pneumothorax barely visible on the X-ray.

What are the physical signs?

329 Small, asymptomatic pneumothoraces are usually kept under observation and reabsorb spontaneously.

Larger ones require insertion of a chest catheter which is connected by rubber tubing to an underwater seal usually on the floor under the bed.

How is the patient subsequently managed?

330 The nature of a mediastinal mass can usually be correctly predicted by its position in the mediastinum.

What are the common pathologies of mid-mediastinal, anterior and posterior mediastinal shadows?

Alimentary Tract, Liver & Pancreas

331 Certain metabolic and neurological disorders may present with abdominal pain and should be considered

in the differential diagnosis of the acute abdomen. These include diabetic ketoacidosis, acute intermittent porphyria, tabes dorsalis, herpes zoster and thoracic disc prolapse.

An important feature of episodic abdominal pain is its relationship to meals.

Which condition would you consider in a man aged 65 years who experienced paraumbilical pain about 2 hours after meals?

332 It is important to distinguish between pain due to peritoneal irritation and colic i.e. pain arising from the muscular contractions of a hollow viscus. A patient with peritoneal irritation lies still whereas colic usually causes a patient to change position in search of comfort.

Which sources of abdominal pain produce radiation to the groin and genitalia?

333 Early morning sickness is a symptom of both pregnancy and alcoholism.

What is the name of the condition in which vomiting leads to fresh haematemesis from a tear of the mucosa at the gastro-oesophageal junction?

334 Heartburn, a burning discomfort or pain felt between the epigastrium and the back of the throat is a common symptom of hyperacidity and gastro-oesophageal reflux.

An overweight 50-year-old woman describes heartburn when bending or lying down.

What condition does she have and what would you advise her to do? What other gastrointestinal conditions may she have?

335 In a case of chronic non-blood-stained diarrhoea in which bacteriological studies have excluded an infectious cause, radiology of the gastrointestinal tract is normal, faecal fat content is normal and both diabetes and thyrotoxicosis have been excluded, which other diagnostic possibilities remain?

336 A change in bowel habit is a symptom of great importance, and, in an older patient, should always arouse suspicion of malignancy.

Some commonly used, long-term medications can alter bowel habit.

Which drugs can cause diarrhoea and which can cause constipation?

337 Small intestinal biopsy is useful in the differential diagnosis of steatorrhoea.

Which special tests can demonstrate the presence of (a) bacterial overgrowth of the small intestine and (b) lactase deficiency?

338 Inspection of the tongue, gums, teeth and oropharyngeal mucosa can provide diagnostic information for many systemic conditions.
What signs of anaemia, leukaemia, Addison's disease, pemphigus, ulcerative colitis and infectious mononucleosis may be seen in the oropharyngeal area?

339 The Plummer–Vinson syndrome is the same as the Patterson–Kelly syndrome. Both eponyms refer to atrophy of the oral mucosa with the formation of a membrane or web at the upper end of the oesophagus which causes dysphagia.
What is the aetiology of this condition and what changes would you expect in the nails?

340 Achalasia of the cardia is due to defective cholinergic innervation of the lower two-thirds of the oesophagus. The gastro-oesophageal sphincter fails to relax and peristalsis in the oesophagus disappears. In contrast to benign oesophageal stricture (due to reflux oesophagitis) pain is not a prominent symptom.
In alchalasia of the cardia what is the natural history of the dysphagia?

341 A 50-year-old man describes increasing retrosternal discomfort and regurgitation after swallowing solids over the last 3 months. He has lost weight but still drinks and smokes heavily.
This history suggests carcinoma of the oesophagus, but physical examination reveals no lymph node or liver enlargement.
Does this make the diagnosis of oesophageal carcinoma any less likely?

342 Oesophageal varices at the lower end of the oesophagus occur in portal hypertension. Their appearance on barium swallow is mimicked by oesophageal moniliasis (as occurs in the immunosuppressed) and by heavy *Ascaris* infestation (as occurs in some tropical areas).
What radiological feature distinguishes varices from these other two conditions?

343 Critically ill or injured patients often develop acute gastric erosions and gastric haemorrhage. The cause seems to be microinfarction of the mucosa due to ischaemia, combined with the action of acid.

Prophylactic treatment with antacids and cimetidine is consequently often given in such cases.

What are the causes of acute gastritis in the population at large?

344 Alcohol irritates the gastric mucosa. Acute gastritis is common in drinkers, as is peptic ulceration. Alcoholics are also susceptible to retching and vomiting and they show an increased incidence of the Mallory–Weiss syndrome.

What is the drinker's remedy for early morning nausea and vomiting and what does this symptom signify?

345 In the pathogenesis of duodenal and gastric ulceration, increased acid production tends to be associated with duodenal ulcer while gastric ulceration is linked with impaired mucosal resistance.

What other factors are related to peptic ulceration?

346 Epigastric pain is common to both duodenal and gastric ulceration but whereas food tends to relieve duodenal ulcer pain, it may have the opposite effect in gastric ulcer patients. Weight loss is consequently unusual in the former but common in the latter.

How do duodenal and gastric ulcers differ with regard to (a) pain at night and (b) vomiting?

Is there considerable overlap between duodenal and gastric ulcers in their symptomatology?

347 Ninety per cent of peptic ulcers are visualized on barium meal X-ray. Of those that are not shown by X-ray, endoscopy will detect the majority. Ulcers missed on endoscopy may show on X-ray.

In what situations is measurement of gastric acid production of diagnostic help?

348 The three major complications of peptic ulceration are haemorrhage, perforation and pyloric stenosis. Most cases of haemorrhage are managed medically but it is customary to have a surgeon following the case. Rebleeding increases the mortality.

What are the signs and acid–base changes of pyloric stenosis?

349 In the treatment of peptic ulcer symptoms (which are commoner than proven peptic ulcers), antacids are the first line of treatment. In the opinion of many they are still the first line of treatment for proven peptic ulcer.

What is an effective dose of antacid and what is the milk–alkali syndrome?

350 Histamine receptors on the gastric parietal cells, designated H_2 receptors, are blocked by cimetidine with a marked reduction in gastric acid production. A typical regimen is 200 mg three times a day with meals and 400 mg at bedtime for 6 weeks.

What happens to gastric acid production when the drug is stopped?

351 There are treatments for dyspepsia and peptic ulceration other than antacids and H_2 receptor antagonists. The antiemetic, metoclopramide, increases gastric emptying and improves some patients' symptoms. Carbenoxolone has been shown to increase the healing of ulcers, but sodium and water retention limit its usefulness.

What general and dietary advice should ulcer patients receive? For which kind of ulcer is colloidal bismuthate effective?

352 Elective surgery for benign gastric ulcer usually consists of partial gastrectomy with direct gastroduodenal anastomosis (Billroth I operation).

For duodenal ulcer, the most commonly performed operation is vagotomy and pyloroplasty.

What is the effect of vagotomy on gastrin release?

353 A mild degree of malabsorption results from surgical procedures for peptic ulcer. In the years following surgery anaemia and osteomalacia can develop, due to defective absorption of iron, B_{12} or folate, and calcium and vitamin D respectively.

What are the early and late dumping syndromes?

354 For practical purposes, duodenal ulcers are never malignant. Malignancy should be suspected when a gastric ulcer occurs on the greater curvature, or when a gastric ulcer fails to show clear evidence of healing after 4 weeks' medical treatment. Healing with cimetidine should be followed up especially closely since a malignant ulcer may appear to heal.

Which factors predispose to carcinoma of the stomach?

355 Anaemia is common in carcinoma of the stomach, partly because of occult blood loss and partly because pernicious anaemia is a predisposing factor. It is also common for metastasis to predate the onset of symptoms.

How is the diagnosis of gastric malignancy made?

356 Carcinoma arising in the cardia of the stomach may spread to the lower end of the oesophagus, resulting in dysphagia.

Haematogenous spread is most commonly to the liver, while lymphatic spread involves the nodes in the supraclavicular fossa on the left side. These nodes are named after Virchow who first made this sinister observation.

In what other way may carcinoma of the stomach metastasize?

357 Loss of normal peristalsis in the small intestine allows bacterial overgrowth to occur. In tropical sprue, however, the reason for bacterial overgrowth of the small intestine is not clear.

What is the treatment for tropical sprue?

358 In coeliac disease, the jejunal villi become blunted or flattened, crypts decrease in depth and the epithelial cells become irregular with a reduction or loss of the brush border. Inflammatory cells infiltrate the lamina propria. These changes are due to gluten intolerance and cause malabsorption.

(a) Which skin condition is associated with gluten-sensitive enteropathy and (b) which malignancy has an increased incidence in patients with coeliac disease?

359 Malabsorption is a cause of weight loss, general malaise and diarrhoea.

What symptoms result from interference with absorption of specific factors?

360 The Zollinger–Ellison syndrome is the eponym for the symptoms caused by a gastrinoma. In the majority of cases the tumour is in the pancreas. Failure of hyperacidity and peptic ulceration to respond to both medical and surgical treatment is the most prominent feature. Diarrhoea occurs in about half the cases.

What is the definitive diagnostic test?

361 Whipple's disease and intestinal lymphoma are two rare causes of malabsorption. In Whipple's disease arthralgia and lymphadenopathy are often present and biopsy of the intestinal mucosa shows replacement of the lamina propria by PAS-positive macrophages. Microorganisms are also present and many cases respond to long-term antibiotic therapy.

What features should arouse suspicion of intestinal lymphoma?

362 Faecal fat measurement, xylose absorption and the Schilling test for B_{12} absorption are helpful tests in confirming the presence of malabsorption.

Barium follow-through studies of the small bowel may show a malabsorption pattern.

What are the features of this malabsorption pattern?

363 The inflammatory process in Crohn's disease extends through all layers of the bowel wall. Histology in many cases shows non-caseating granulomas and depressed cell-mediated immunity is found in patients with Crohn's disease.

What is the aetiology of Crohn's disease?

364 Crohn's disease can affect any part of the intestinal tract but the two commonest sites are the terminal ileum and the colon. An important feature of the disease is the occurrence of normal bowel between diseased segments, so-called skip lesions.

In which age group does Crohn's disease most commonly occur, and what are the radiological features of the disease?

365 Crohn's disease commonly causes abdominal pain and diarrhoea, but fever, weight loss and malabsorption also occur. Another problem is intestinal obstruction but this settles in many cases without surgical intervention.

What is the treatment of Crohn's disease?

366 Fistula formation and intestinal obstruction are the main abdominal complications of Crohn's disease. The perianal area is the most common site for fistulae.

What other features may occur in Crohn's disease?

367 In contrast to Crohn's disease, rectal bleeding is a common symptom of ulcerative colitis. Diarrhoea is usual in ulcerative colitis and the stools contain pus and mucus. The presentation may be similar to bacillary dysentry.

In which age group is the incidence of ulcerative colitis highest and what other conditions can cause bloody diarrhoea?

368 Ulcerative colitis commonly involves the rectum and sigmoid colon and is sometimes confined to this part of the large bowel. When the disease is limited in this way, corticosteroids by enema is an effective method of treatment.

What are the radiological features of long-standing ulcerative colitis?

369 In the acute attack of ulcerative colitis, bed rest, correction of fluid and electrolyte abnormalities, correction of anaemia, parenteral nutrition and corticosteroids comprise the main lines of medical management. Toxic megacolon and failure of serious

disease to respond to medical management are indications for surgery. Sulphasalazine helps maintain remissions.

What is pyoderma gangrenosum and what is the risk of malignant change in ulcerative colitis?

370 Irritable bowel syndrome is a very common disorder of large bowel motility. Motility may be increased as in patients suffering with constipation and lower abdominal pain, or decreased as in patients with painless diarrhoea. In many patients there is alternating constipation and diarrhoea.

Which investigations must be normal for the diagnosis of irritable bowel syndrome to be made with certainty?

371 Diverticular disease of the colon is a very common acquired disorder, believed to be connected with the low fibre content of the average Western diet. Most cases are asymptomatic but patients who at the same time have the irritable bowel syndrome can be relieved of their symptoms by bran or other inert bulk agents.

What serious complications can result from diverticular disease?

372 Sigmoidoscopy should be performed before barium enema because the last 25 cm of the bowel are difficult to visualize clearly radiologically. Sigmoidoscopy also provides the chance to biopsy abnormal areas. In ulcerative colitis the friability of the mucosa may be readily apparent on sigmoidoscopy while the barium enema may be normal.

In which inflammatory bowel condition are ulcers visible with the naked eye? What proportion of large bowel malignancy occurs within reach of the sigmoidoscope?

373 In normal people, the lower border of the liver may be just palpable below the right costal margin on inspiration. In emphysema, a normal-sized liver may appear to be enlarged unless the position of the upper border of the liver is checked by percussion.

In what conditions causing hepatomegaly can treatment cause a rapid reduction in liver size?

374 Biochemical tests to assess the severity of liver damage comprise the serum total bilirubin, serum albumin, prothrombin time and serum transaminases. When cholestasis is present alkaline phosphatase levels rise, and this also occurs when the liver is infiltrated by malignancy or lymphoma.

Which enzyme provides a sensitive indicator of alcoholic damage?

375 A liver scan is performed by giving an intravenous dose of radioisotope (usually technetium-99) and then scanning the liver with a gamma camera. The spleen and bone marrow also take up the isotope.

A generalized disorder of the liver, such as cirrhosis, gives a diffuse decrease in uptake whereas cysts, abscesses, or tumours will appear as filling defects.

What other non-invasive techniques are available for investigating the structure of the liver?

376 If a gall bladder is normally visualized on an oral cholecystogram and no stones are present then it is extremely likely that the gall bladder is normal. Oral cholecystography cannot be expected to show the gall bladder, however, if hepatocellular disease is present or if the total serum bilirubin level is greater than 35μmol/l. A similar proviso applies to intravenous cholangiography.

What other techniques are there for demonstrating or visualizing the biliary tree?

377 In chronic liver cell failure it is common to find general weakness, loss of flesh and anorexia. There may be cyanosis due to pulmonary arteriovenous shunting. Jaundice and ascites are variable but vascular spiders, palmar erythema and white nails are all common. Men may show testicular atrophy and gynaecomastia.

What are the main points in the management of patients with chronic liver failure?

378 Features of hepatic encephalopathy range from slight alterations in mood or behaviour to deep coma. The most characteristic neurological sign is asterixis, i.e. the flapping tremor of the outstretched, dorsiflexed hands.

In a patient with fulminant hepatic failure who has some degree of hepatic encephalopathy what are the main lines of management?

379 Portal (vein) hypertension by itself does not cause ascites. Hypoproteinaemia must also be present for ascites to develop.

What is the treatment for ascites in portal hypertension?

380 In portal hypertension, a collateral circulation develops. This is responsible for portal–systemic shunting of which the two main consequences are

encephalopathy and septicaemias due to intestinal organisms.

What are the physical signs of portal hypertension?

381 Liver cells are easily damaged by hypoxia and ischaemia and a period of hypotension may cause massive elevation of hepatic enzymes in the blood.

In congestive cardiac failure and cor pulmonale, what are the causes of a raised bilirubin level?

382 Jaundice is simply classified into prehepatic, hepatic and cholestatic types. Examples of each type are haemolysis, viral hepatitis and carcinoma of the head of pancreas respectively.

How may the three types of jaundice be distinguished before resorting to investigation?

383 Type A viral hepatitis is usually a mild illness and often anicteric. There is no tendency to chronicity.

In Type B viral hepatitis, however, there is a greater chance of serious illness including fulminant hepatic failure and 10 per cent of cases become carriers of the surface antigen, HB_sAg (Australia antigen).

What are the different antigens and particles belonging to the type B hepatitis virus, and what is their significance?

384 Chronic hepatitis, which is defined as persistence of biochemical liver abnormality longer than 6 months, tends to occur in immunosuppressed patients and in patients whose attack of hepatitis was mild or anicteric.

What are the main types of chronic hepatitis and how are they distinguished from each other?

385 Cirrhosis of the liver is histologically defined by the presence of both fibrosis and nodules. When making a clinical assessment it is important to note the degree of liver cell failure, the degree of portal hypertension and whether the condition is improving, deteriorating or static.

Which forms of cirrhosis are commonly associated with high titres of smooth muscle and mitochondrial antibodies?

386 Women are considerably more susceptible than men to the liver toxicity of alcohol. Steady drinking is more closely associated with cirrhosis than is spree drinking. Spree drinking, however, is often implicated in acute alcoholic hepatitis.

What is Zieve's syndrome?

Which clinical features would suggest an alcoholic aetiology to a patient's cirrhosis?

387 Haemochromatosis is marked by cirrhosis and diabetes mellitus, due to iron deposits in the liver and pancreas respectively. However, impaired glucose tolerance is a common feature of cirrhosis in general.

Which clinical features would support the diagnosis of haemochromatosis?

388 The commonest cause of jaundice in pregnancy is viral hepatitis. The next commonest is cholestatic jaundice of pregnancy. What are the features and treatment of cholestatic jaundice of pregnancy?

Why must tetracyclines never be given to a pregnant woman?

389 A 45-year-old woman with a history of ulcerative colitis for 20 years presents with steadily deepening jaundice of a few weeks' duration.

Which two diagnoses would be relevant to her history of ulcerative colitis?

390 Primary hepatocellular carcinoma shows marked geographical variation in incidence. It is particularly common in the East African Bantu and in the Chinese. The symptoms include pain in the epigastrium or right upper quadrant, weight loss and low-grade fever.

Non-metastatic features are common.

What are they?

391 Lithogenic bile, containing an excess of cholesterol relative to the quantity of bile salts, is one prerequisite for the formation of gall stones. It is a factor which cholecystectomy does not alter.

Advancing age, multiparity and obesity confer an increased risk of cholelithiasis.

What drugs increase the formation of gall stones?

392 The main symptom of acute pancreatitis is severe pain. This is felt in the epigastrium and typically radiates through to the back.

The main differential diagnosis of acute pancreatitis is a perforated ulcer.

What conditions predispose to acute pancreatitis?

393 A history of biliary tract disease or alcoholism and the presence of diabetes mellitus, steatorrhoea and pancreatic calcification are all features of chronic pancreatitis.

How can further diagnostic evidence of exocrine pancreatic failure be obtained?

394 Carcinoma of the head of the pancreas is commoner in men than in women and has its peak incidence in the

sixth and seventh decades. There is a statistical association with coffee consumption.

Common symptoms are pain, weight loss and general malaise, but the tumour is usually advanced before it attracts attention.

Which investigations should be performed to make the diagnosis?

395 In which condition is pancreatic exocrine failure associated with bronchiectasis, recurrent pulmonary infections, a sweat chloride content greater than 60 mmol/l and male infertility?

Which aspect of the condition mainly determines morbidity and mortality?

Nervous System

396 The commonest causes of loss of smell, or anosmia, are colds and heavy smoking. Anosmia comprises loss of ability to detect flavours as well, since most flavours have an aromatic component. The only ones that do not are salt, sweet, bitter and acid. Infrequently, anosmia is due to damage to the olfactory bulb or tract.

What are the likely causes of this?

397 Defects in visual acuity are commonly due to refractive errors or to lens opacities, but optic nerve damage is also an important cause. Patients usually report loss of acuity but may not be aware of the other aspect of visual defect, namely loss of visual fields. Examination of visual fields can be of enormous diagnostic value.

Tunnel vision is the term used when the peripheral visual fields are lost.

Where is the damage likely to be?

398 A defect of vision comprising one half of the visual field is called a hemianopia. If both eyes are affected in the corresponding side of the visual field, the hemianopia is described as homonymous. Loss of a quarter of a visual field is called a quadrantanopia and less than this a scotoma.

A patient develops blindness in one eye and is found to have a temporal hemianopia in the other eye.

Where is the lesion?

399 A patient with a bitemporal hemianopia must have a lesion causing damage to the fibres from the nasal half of each retina at the same time.

What is the condition that typically causes this?

400 Lesions behind the optic chiasma will cause some form of homonymous hemianopia or quadrantanopia. A patient has a non-congruous quadrantic hemianopia.

Where is the lesion and what may be causing it?

401 After visual fibres have reached the lateral geniculate body of the thalamus, they fan out in the optic radiations on their route to the occipital cortex.

What is it about the arrangement of the fibres in the optic radiation that may make it possible to distinguish a lesion there from one in the optic tract?

402 In the optic tracts, fibres from the lower part of the retinae run in proximity to the temporal lobe and those from the upper part of the retina in proximity to the parietal lobes.

What visual field defect would you expect to result from a right parietal lesion, and from a left temporal lesion?

403 The optic nerve is subject to inflammation from a number of causes, principally disseminated (multiple) sclerosis, tabes dorsalis, deficiency of vitamin B_{12} or other B vitamins and toxic causes including methanol, lead and quinine. Optic neuritis may consist of papillitis, when the inflammation affects the disc and is visible on fundoscopy, and retrobulbar neuritis, when the nerve is affected behind the eyeball. The result to the patient is the same, however.

What would you expect to find in optic neuritis?

404 Papilloedema is oedema of the optic disc. In the earliest stages, the swelling begins in the optic cup, the depression in the optic nerve head that runs down to the cribriform plate and which should be visible in the normal eye. As the oedema progresses, the margins of the disc become blurred and in advanced papilloedema, the disc is swollen and the blood vessels become heaped up at the edges.

What is the outcome of long-standing papilloedema?

405 Optic atrophy represents scarring of the optic nerve head. It is the final result of a variety of insults including optic neuritis, long-standing papilloedema, glaucoma and optic nerve compression. The Foster–Kennedy syndrome consists of the combination of optic atrophy in one eye with papilloedema in the other. It is due to compression of one optic nerve by a frontal brain tumour, which also causes a rise in intracranial pressure leading to papilloedema in the other eye.

The normal optic disc varies in its degree of pinkness or pallor. How would you distinguish between a pale normal disc and a mild degree of optic atrophy?

406 A 35-year-old woman is admitted with a severe headache of sudden onset and examination reveals abnormal signs in the left eye. She has ptosis, a dilated unreactive pupil and the eye deviates inferolaterally.

What lesion does she have and what is the probable cause?

407 The trochlear (IV) nerve emerges from the midbrain, and in company with the oculomotor and abducent nerves and the ophthalmic division of the trigeminal nerve, it traverses the cavernous sinus and lies in the superior orbital fissure. It is susceptible to damage from meningitis or meningioma, cavernous sinus thrombosis or internal carotid artery aneurysm and lesions within the orbit. In all these conditions, the adjacent nerves are usually also damaged.

There is a lesion, however, in which the trochlear nerve alone may be damaged. What is it and what is its effect?

408 The abducent sixth nerve arises from the pons and has a long intracranial course before passing through the superior orbital fissure to the eye. This makes it vulnerable to a large number of lesions, including raised intracranial pressure alone, but usually a clue to the site and therefore the nature of the lesion is provided by involvement of other cranial nerves.

What is the result of a sixth nerve palsy and what is the cause likely to be if the patient also has involvement of the trigeminal, facial and acoustic–vestibular nerves?

409 What are the distinctive features of a concomitant squint?

410 When examining a patient to decide which muscle weakness is responsible for double vision, it is important to know the actions of the extraocular muscles and to remember that diplopia is maximal when the eye is looking in the direction of pull of the paralysed muscle and that the more peripheral image of the two is from the eye with the weak muscle. Covering one eye at a time will distinguish which eye has the weak muscle.

What palsy is present if the patient has maximal double vision on looking up and to the right and the more peripheal image is in the left eye?

411 The constrictor pupillary muscle is supplied by parasympathetic fibres which travel in the oculomotor nerve. The dilator pupillary muscle is innervated by sympathetic fibres originating in the cervical sympathetic chain. In the light reflex, the afferent fibres travel in the optic nerve to the midbrain nuclei responsible for pupillary constriction. These are situated close to the oculomotor nuclei. In the more complex accommodation reflex the afferent side of the reflex probably arises in the cortex.

What happens to the pupil reflexes in cortical blindness?

412 A 25-year-old woman is referred to you because her symptom of headaches has been found to be accompanied by an abnormal pupil. The pupil is slightly larger than its normally reacting companion, and it does react to light and accommodation but only very slowly. No other cranial nerve signs are present.

What else would you look for on examination?

413 Horner's syndrome consists of ptosis, a constricted pupil which does not dilate to shade, slight sinking-in of the eye in the orbit or enophthalmos, and decreased sweating over the same side of the face. The syndrome indicates damage to the sympathetic fibres.

Where is the lesion and what is it likely to be?

414 A 63-year-old man has abnormal pupils. They are irregular, small and somewhat depigmented. The response to accommodation is preserved but there is no light reflex.

What is the name of these pupils and what conditions may this patient be suffering from?

415 A patient has mild, bilateral ptosis. There are no other neurological signs and, in particular, no evidence of Horner's syndrome, tabes dorsalis or hysteria. In any case these are usually causes of unilateral ptosis. The problem is clarified when the patient is visited by his family.

How?

416 An interesting fact about the different sensory modalities on the face is that while the trigeminal fibres carrying touch and proprioception cross the midline as soon as they enter the brain stem to join the medial lemniscus, those fibres carrying pain and temperature first descend to the upper cervical cord (to C3) before crossing the midline to join the lateral spinothalamic tract. The fibres that reach the lowest level in this descending tract are those derived from the upper part of the face.

What is the clinical significance of this anatomical fact?

417 The facial nerve emerges from the lateral aspect of the lower border of the pons and crosses the cerebellopontine angle in the particular company of the nervus intermedius (carrying taste and secretomotor fibres) and the eighth nerve, to reach the internal auditory meatus from where it travels in its own bony canal to the stylomastoid foramen.

Between entering and leaving the canal it gives off two nerves and is joined by another. What are they?

418 Facial nerve palsy is a common occurrence and it is very useful to be able to localize the site of the lesion. This is done partly from the distribution of the facial weakness and partly from the presence of damage to other nerves.

How would you tell an upper motor neurone lesion from a Bell's palsy, and a cerebellopontine angle lesion from Bell's palsy?

419 Bell's palsy is a facial nerve palsy of unknown aetiology. Usually the facial weakness is the only sign but occasionally loss of taste and hyperacusis indicate that the lesion is high up in the facial canal.

If there is some sign of recovery a week after the event, what can you tell the patient?

420 The facial nerve may be affected by herpes zoster when this virus attacks the geniculate ganglion. The combination of facial palsy and herpetic vesicles on the anterior wall of the external auditory canal and sometimes on the soft palate is called the Ramsay Hunt syndrome.

Bilateral facial palsy can occur in uveoparotid fever in which there is accompanying parotid gland enlargement and uveitis as well as fever. This combination of features is also called Heerfordt's syndrome.

Of what systemic disease is it a feature?

421 Conductive (middle ear) deafness is commonly caused by secretory otitis media (glue ear) in children, otosclerosis in later life and infection at any age.

What are the two tuning-fork tests of hearing that enable one to distinguish conductive from perceptive deafness?

422 In nerve deafness, although acuity is reduced, air conduction is still better than bone conduction. As in the examination of other cranial nerves, localizing the

site of an eighth nerve lesion depends on the presence of other signs and palsies.

What would you look for and how would you interpret your findings? How can cochlear deafness be distinguished from nerve deafness?

423 Vertigo is a subjective sensation of movement of oneself or one's surroundings accompanied by a disturbance of balance. The causes are numerous and the diagnosis is usually to be made on a careful investigation. The frequency, duration, time of occurrence and associated features are all important.

Many of the less common causes are neurological or labyrinthine but before considering these areas, what five simple steps would exclude common causes of this symptom?

424 There are three forms of nystagmus. In one form (a), not often seen, the two phases of movement are equal in speed.

In another form (b), there is a slow phase and a rapid phase but no matter in which direction the patient looks, the direction of the slow and rapid phases remains the same.

In the third form (c), the slow phase is directed towards the rest position of the eyes so that the direction of the slow and rapid phases alters with full excursion of the eyes.

Where are the lesions in these three cases?

425 One of the less common but more serious causes of vertigo is a condition in which there is also tinnitus and deafness. The tinnitus may be more or less continuous but the vertigo comes in attacks that last from a few minutes to a few hours. Women are more often affected and it occurs more commonly in later life. There may be long intervals between attacks.

Some patients notice a change in their tinnitus and a sensation of pressure in the ear about half an hour before an attack begins, and can stop driving or lie down or take other appropriate steps to prepare for the attack.

What condition is this?

426 Vestibular neuronitis, as its name indicates, is an inflammation of the vestibular part of the eighth nerve. It is marked by a sudden onset of vertigo that lasts usually for a few days. Sometimes there is an associated upper respiratory tract infection, suggesting a viral aetiology. Tinnitus and deafness are not part of the clinical picture.

The main test of vestibular function is abnormal in this condition. What is this test?

427 The glossopharyngeal, vagus and accessory (ninth, tenth, eleventh) nerves all arise from the medulla, lie close together and all pass through the internal jugular foramen. Consequently it is common for them to be damaged together, e.g. by meningioma or nasopharyngeal tumour.

What does the glossopharyngeal nerve supply?

428 The vagus nerve carries nerve fibres of great variety. Motor fibres supply the levator palati, the vocal cords and other muscles of the pharynx and larynx. Sensory fibres supply parts of the meninges and the ears as well as the larynx. The parasympathetic fibres supply the organs in the chest—bronchi, heart—and abdomen—intestines, pancreas, biliary tract.

What is the course of the vagus after entering the internal jugular foramen?

429 What is the origin of the motor nerve fibres that supply the sternomastoid and trapezius muscles (the accessory nerve)?

430 The tongue is supplied by the hypoglossal (twelfth) nerve. This nerve arises in the medulla and may be involved together with the ninth, tenth and eleventh nerves in posterior fossa disease.

The tongue is easy to examine and the effects of damage to its innervation are striking. How do you distinguish between upper and lower motor neurone lesions of the hypoglossal nerves?

431 Dysarthria means difficulty with the articulation of speech. Although articulation is a complex process, the classification of its abnormality as with that of any muscle activity is simple, namely upper motor neurone lesions, lower motor neurone lesions, cerebellar disturbance of coordination, and muscle lesions (e.g. myopathies). Give one example from each of these four groups for dysarthria.

432 Aphasia is the name for loss of speech while dysphasia means difficulty with speech. The parts of the brain concerned with speech, collectively called the speech centre, are usually in the dominant cerebral hemisphere. For right-handed and many left-handed people this means the left hemisphere. What is the difference between expressive and receptive dysphasia (sometimes called motor and sensory respectively)?

433 A 31-year-old labourer is noted by his colleagues on returning from a holiday to have become very

quiet and to be behaving in an odd and quite uncharacteristic way. He is referred to a psychiatrist, who diagnoses severe depression and treats him with ECT. After two treatments there is no response, the patient remaining completely mute. A physician is called in to exclude organic disease. Physical examination is normal, but lumbar puncture shows 25 white cells per mm^3 of CSF.

What is the probable diagnosis?

434 What is the pathway of the upper motor neurones?

435 Enormous importance attaches to correctly identifying the kind of neurological lesion present as well as its localization.

What are the salient features of an upper motor neurone (UMN) lesion of gradual onset and what differences would you expect if the onset is sudden?

436 The fact that the different sensory modalities are carried in different tracts in the spinal cord and brain stem is of great anatomical interest and clinical value, since disease processes tend to affect particular sites, e.g. subacute combined degeneration of the cord affects the posterior columns, syringomyelia affects the spinothalamic tracts.

What is the pathway for each sensory modality?

437 Most of the common causes of peripheral neuritis, either polyneuropathy or mononeuritis multiplex are disorders with manifestations in other parts of the body.

What are the distinguishing features of a peripheral neuritis (neuropathy)?

438 The dorsal (posterior) roots, more commonly damaged by disease than the ventral roots, are the site of degeneration in tabes dorsalis and of inflammation in herpes zoster. Meningitis or disease of the spine may also damage them. The commonest cause of posterior root damage is compression by a prolapsed intervertebral disc, especially in the lumbar region.

What are the characteristic features of a dorsal root lesion?

439 A very important situation, constituting a neurological emergency, is spinal cord compression. The source may be extradural and disease of the vertebrae is a common cause which can be diagnosed initially with simple X-rays.

A 60-year-old heavy smoker presents with a girdle of hyperalgesia (increased pain) at the sensory level of T12, and sensory loss below this. AP and lateral X-rays of his spine show collapse of the eighth and ninth thoracic vertebrae. What is the probable diagnosis?

440 In what ways can pressure on the spinal cord give rise to symptoms and signs?

441 In spinal cord compression, unless there is evidence of vertebral disease, it can be very difficult to distinguish between extradural, extramedullary and intramedullary lesions.

Factors in favour of an extradural lesion, such as an abscess or lymphoma, include bilateral and symmetrical symptoms with motor changes occurring early and only a slight rise in CSF protein.

What features might help distinguish intramedullary from extramedullary lesions?

442 A 45-year-old woman presents with a 6-month history of increasing weakness and burning pains of the left leg. Examination reveals wasting of the left quadriceps with loss of the left knee jerk but an increased ankle jerk and extensor plantar response on the left side. Vibration and position sense are impaired in the left leg while there is a patchy loss of touch, pain and temperature sensation of the right leg.

Where is the lesion and what is the name of the syndrome?

443 The brain stem contains so many tracts and nuclei that lesions here often produce florid neurological deficits. Generally, lateral lesions will damage the spinothalamic tracts and the medial lemniscus. Other signs and symptoms will depend on the level of the lesion.

In the medial medullary syndrome, there is ipsilateral wasting of the tongue, contralateral UMN damage to arm and leg (but not face) and contralateral impairment of touch and proprioception.

What features occur in the lateral medullary syndrome?

444 The thalamic syndrome is usually the result of cerebrovascular disease.

What are the features of this syndrome?

445 The sensory cortex is concerned with the discrimination of different sensations and with appreciation of position and spatial orientation.

How are all of these tested at the bedside?

446 The cerebellum is mainly concerned with coordination of muscle activity. This applies to the maintenance of posture and limb position as much as to active movements. The cerebellum provides a damping influence without which the alternate contractions of opposing muscle groups result in oscillating movements. Nystagmus, an obvious example of this, is an important sign of cerebellar disease.

What are the other signs?

447 The basal ganglia are a group of nuclei situated close to the junction of midbrain and cerebrum. Together, they comprise the extrapyramidal system.

Lesions in different parts of the system can result in what clinical pictures?

448 Normal cerebrospinal fluid (CSF) is at a pressure of 60–150 mm of CSF when the patient is lying down.

The protein content is not more than 0.4 g/l, glucose is approximately 60 per cent of the accompanying blood level and should be more than 2.8 mmol/l, and the chloride concentration is 120–130 mmol/l. There should not be more than 5 lymphocytes per mm^3.

What does an abnormal Queckenstedt's test indicate?

449 Certain factors are associated with a predisposition to epilepsy. A family history is one. Others include perinatal injury or illness, head injury, inflammatory and vascular damage, all of which can result in a scar which acts as a centre of epileptic activity. Neurosurgery can also cause this. Some brain tumours present with epilepsy.

What factors can actually precipitate an attack?

450 A common diagnostic problem is to distinguish between fits and faints.

What features would suggest epilepsy?

451 Before a grand mal fit, there may be an aura, but loss of consciousness coincides with the tonic stage which lasts for about a minute. The patient stops breathing and the face becomes engorged with blood (in contrast to a Stokes–Adams attack). This is followed by the clonic stage, and then by postictal coma which usually lasts less than an hour.

What is the sequence of events in status epilepticus?

452 Petit mal epilepsy consists of transient absences or blank spells, almost invariably beginning in childhood, and associated with a characteristic EEG pattern.

Focal, or Jacksonian epilepsy, refers to attacks that involve only one part of the brain and body. It may be motor or sensory and is commonly a sign of organic disease.

What are the features of psychomotor (temporal lobe) epilepsy?

453 In the treatment of epilepsy it is important to avoid multiple therapy and to limit the frequency of medication to the minimum necessary. For example, phenytoin need only be given once or twice a day and phenobarbitone once, ideally at night.

It is also important not to stop or change anticonvulsants abruptly.

What would be an average adult treatment regimen for phenytoin and for carbamazepine?

454 The anticonvulsants all have undesirable side-effects.

Phenytoin in overdosage causes symptoms of cerebellar impairment—ataxia, nystagmus and slurred speech. In chronic use it can cause a variety of syndromes including acne and coarse facies, lymphadenopathy, gingival hypertrophy, drug fever, folate deficiency with megaloblastic anaemia and osteomalacia due to altered vitamin D metabolism.

What are the side-effects of carbamazepine?

455 The initial symptom of shingles (herpes zoster) is pain, and this may precede the appearance of erythema and the vesicular eruption. It may lead to a suspicion of myocardial ischaemia or intra-abdominal disease.

What other features of shingles are clinically important?

456 In gasserian herpes, the zoster virus involves the ophthalmic division of the trigeminal nerve. The eye is usually involved and keratitis or panophthalmitis may cause blindness.

A 60-year-old man presents with a lower motor neurone facial palsy and pain in the ear. Examination reveals a vesicular eruption in the ear canal and on the earlobe and deafness in the affected ear.

Would you be right to diagnose herpes zoster? What is the name of the syndrome?

457 There is reluctance to prescribe opiates or similarly potent analgesics for post-herpetic neuralgia because the chronic, severe nature of the pain makes addiction a possibility.

What alternative methods of pain relief are enjoying current popularity?

458 Migraine is one form of recurring headache. Its name is derived from the word 'hemicranium', illustrating the property of this condition to affect one side of the head or face at a time. An important diagnostic point is that the pain can affect either side. Persistently one-sided pain raises the possibility of a tumour or other pathology.

What are the main stages in an attack of migraine?

459 The actual cause of a migraine is difficult to pin down. Migraine sufferers are often said to be obsessional, and attacks may occur at times of relaxation after a period of stress, e.g. weekends. Hunger may provoke an attack. Some women have migraine in the premenstrual phase of their cycle. Pregnancy, on the other hand, confers protection from migraine. Dietary factors are being increasingly implicated, particularly foods rich in amines.

What are these?

460 Treatment for a migraine attack is more effective the sooner it is given. A well established attack may be resistant to treatment. In the early stages, a rapidly absorbed form of simple analgesic such as paracetamol may be sufficient. Otherwise, some form of ergotamine which has a vasoconstrictor effect on the vessels of the head, is usually necessary. It is important not to take excess ergotamine for this can itself cause a headache.

What drugs are available for the prophylaxis of migraine?

461 Some patients, often elderly men, describe a form of headache which wakes them at about 2 o'clock in the morning with severe pain on one side of the face, with marked reddening and watering of the eye. This headache recurs for several nights or days in succession but then remits for a few weeks or longer until a fresh bout occurs.

What is this condition called and what is the treatment?

462 Head injuries can have immediate and delayed effects. Immediate effects are usually due to some degree of brain contusion for which there is no surgical treatment, only supportive management.

Intracranial bleeding is a very important delayed effect in which surgery should be life-saving.

What is the clinical picture of extradural haemorrhage?

463 Chronic subdural haematomas are more common in older people and a history of head injury may be vague

or even absent. Sometimes the injury may have occurred weeks or months earlier.

What is the sequence of events and the clinical picture?

464 Haemorrhage into the subarachnoid space, which tends to present with a sudden, severe headache and/or neurological deficit and coma, can be detected by lumbar puncture, usually not less than 6 hours after the event. It takes 24 hours for xanthochromia to develop.

Many cases of subarachnoid haemorrhage are due to ruptured berry aneurysm. When would you seek neurosurgical help with a case of subarachnoid haemorrhage?

465 The commonest cause of a stroke is a cerebral artery thrombosis. Other causes include cerebral embolus, cerebral haemorrhage and a space-occupying lesion.

How would you distinguish between these on clinical grounds?

466 A 25-year-old secretary with a history of mainly unilateral headaches for a few years, and focal epilepsy involving the left arm for 2 years, presents with a more severe and generalized headache of sudden onset. Neck stiffness is present and lumbar puncture the following day reveals blood-stained, xanthochromic CSF.

What is the likely cause of all her symptoms and what specific physical sign would you look for?

467 Transient ischaemic attacks, which by definition do not last longer than 24 hours, may occur in the territory of either the internal carotid or vertebrobasilar arteries.

Monocular blindness and contralateral hemiparesis or sensory disturbance occur in internal carotid disease.

What are the features of vertebrobasilar attacks?

468 An 80-year-old woman presents with dementia and incontinence. The relatives describe a step-like deterioration over the previous few years with transient episodes of confusion, loss of speech and unilateral weakness.

What is the likely cause of her condition?

469 Following a large boil on the right side of her nose, a 15-year-old girl presents with severe pain in her right eye and over the forehead, oedema of the eyelids and periorbital tissues and a non-reactive pupil. There is a slight squint and movements of the right eye are

virtually absent. She has a marked pyrexia and a neutrophil leucocytosis.

What has happened and where else could a similar sequence of events occur?

470 Acute pyogenic meningitis is usually a serious illness of rapid onset but occasionally its presentation is altered by antibiotic therapy given for some other infection.

What are the main symptoms and signs and what are the common pathogens involved?

471 Tuberculous meningitis is usually more gradual in onset than pyogenic meningitis. Headache is a prominent symptom. Fever is variable. Encephalitic symptoms—confusion, drowsiness—may be more common than signs of meningeal irritation, i.e. neck stiffness. There may be cranial nerve and other neurological deficits. Occasional patients lapse into coma with rapidity.

It is uncommon to see tubercle bacilli in the cerebrospinal fluid, and confirmation by culturing the organism may take 6 weeks.

What are the usual CSF findings and what else about the patient could give a clue to the diagnosis?

472 Most infections with the polio virus never reach the preparalytic or paralytic stages. In the paralytic stage, however, what are the cardinal physical signs and what would your management be?

473 Tabes dorsalis is characterized by inflammation in the posterior roots of the cord and wasting and demyelination of the posterior columns.

What are the physical signs of tabes?

474 What are the symptoms of tabes dorsalis?

475 General paralysis of the insane (GPI) is the condition caused by syphilitic meningoencephalitis. The early changes include dementia and personality change. It is rarely seen nowadays but it used to be suspected when a patient never stopped praising his doctors!

What forms of neurological disease can syphilis cause, other than tabes dorsalis and GPI?

476 A minority of brain tumours and other space-occupying lesions cause headache and vomiting.

What other symptoms may occur?

477 Apart from the specific neurological deficits related to the site of the lesion, brain tumours can also cause an elevation of intracranial pressure which leads to

papilloedema. This may be due to the mere size of the tumour, or to obstruction of the cerebrospinal fluid pathways, as is particularly the case with posterior fossa tumours.

What evidence of a space-occupying lesion can one obtain from skull X-rays?

478 A 17-year-old girl, who is taking an oral contraceptive, develops recurrent headaches which persist despite frequent analgesics. Examination of her fundi reveals marked papilloedema. She is investigated extensively but no intracranial space-occupying lesion is found.

What is the probable diagnosis?

479 Where computerized axial tomography (CAT scan) is available, this test may clearly demonstrate the site and size of an intracranial space-occupying lesion, especially if enhancement techniques are used.

In the absence of CAT scanning, what other investigations may provide useful information?

480 Neurosurgery, radiotherapy and chemotherapy are the three forms of treatment for brain tumours.

What chance do they offer of cure or of correcting the neurological defect?

481 Spinal cord compression is a neurological emergency. The main symptoms are pain, spastic weakness of the legs and sphincter disturbance. The most important physical sign is the finding of a motor, sensory or reflex 'level'.

What are the main causes of cord compression?

482 In a patient with suspected spinal cord compression what plain X-rays would you request?

483 In the absence of CAT scanning, the definitive radiological investigation for spinal cord compression is myelography. This can demonstrate whether the lesion is extradural, extramedullary or intramedullary.

It may also aggravate the symptoms since the procedure involves tapping the cerebrospinal fluid. It should only be done where there is rapid access to appropriate neurosurgical facilities.

What is Froin's syndrome?

484 In motor neurone disease, there is degeneration of the anterior horn cells, the motor nuclei of the medulla, and the upper motor neurones of the cord and brain stem. There is no sensory impairment, the disease does not occur under the age of 40, the sphincters are not affected, and the condition invariably progresses.

What are the main clinical presentations?

485 What condition causes progressive muscle wasting of the hands and feet, extending up to the distal third of the forearms and thighs without much loss in power?

What other neurological signs are present in this condition?

486 Neurofibromatosis (von Recklinghausen's disease) is inherited as an autosomal dominant condition although expression of the gene is very variable. There is an association with phaeochromocytoma.

What are the two cardinal signs of the condition?

487 The commonest early symptoms of syringomyelia are wasting and weakness of the hands, and the onset is usually insidious.

What neurological findings would be in keeping with this diagnosis?

488 One of the abnormalities in Parkinsonism is a deficiency of dopamine in the pathways connecting the basal ganglia. The predominant clinical features are rigidity, slowness of movement and a tremor which is present at rest and relieved by movement and sleep.

What other clinical features may be present?

489 Parkinsonism may be due to spontaneous degeneration affecting the basal ganglia (Parkinson's disease), some cases of which are familial. Many cases of Parkinsonism resulted from epidemics of encephalitis lethargica between 1915 and 1925 but this is now a rare cause. Carbon monoxide poisoning, manganese poisoning and repeated or severe head injury may all cause Parkinsonism.

How may doctors cause it?

490 L-Dopa (dihydroxyphenylalanine), the precursor of dopamine, improves the slowness and paucity of movement in approximately 60 per cent of patients with Parkinsonism. The anticholinergic drugs, benzhexol, benztropine and orphenadrine have more effect on the tremor and rigidity.

What is the rationale for combining L-dopa with a decarboxylase inhibitor?

491 Huntington's chorea is inherited as an autosomal dominant condition, but the choreiform movements do not appear until the 30s. The face is usually particularly involved.

What is the other main feature of the condition?

492 Friedreich's ataxia usually first manifests itself between the ages of 5 and 15. The principal symptom is ataxia, due to degeneration of both spinocerebellar and posterior column fibres, and with this goes loss of vibration sense and loss of reflexes. There is also spasticity due to involvement of the pyramidal tracts. Pes cavus and scoliosis are commonly present and a cardiomyopathy may be the eventual cause of death.

What eminently treatable condition can also cause damage to the posterior columns and pyramidal tracts in an older age group?

493 Myasthenia gravis, the hallmark of which is fatiguability of voluntary muscle, usually appears between the ages of 15 and 50, and most commonly affects the eyelids and external eye muscles first. Any muscles may be involved. The course of the disease is usually one of remissions and relapses.

What is the underlying pathological process?

494 The weakness of myasthenia gravis responds to administration of anticholinesterase drugs. The short-acting edrophonium is used intravenously as a diagnostic test, while longer-acting neostigmine and pyridostigmine are used as oral medication.

What else may improve the condition?

495 Multiple sclerosis, also called disseminated sclerosis, is characterized by lesions of the central nervous system which are disseminated both in site and in time. The most common picture is for the initial episode to remit completely only to be followed by further episodes which gradually produce a cumulative neurological deficit.

At what age does it occur and what are the common lesions?

496 The cerebrospinal fluid is abnormal in the majority of cases of multiple sclerosis. The abnormalities comprise a raised cell count and an elevated gammaglobulin fraction of the total CSF protein which is usually normal. Over 90 per cent of MS cases demonstrate oligoclonal bands on CSF electrophoresis. These findings are common but are not specific for this disease.

What other test can support the diagnosis of multiple sclerosis? How would you distinguish between MS and hysteria in a patient presenting with giddiness, weakness and paraesthesiae?

497 Supportive management is very important in multiple sclerosis, but there is no specific treatment. Prognosis is very variable. If retrobulbar neuritis is the first

lesion there can be a long interval before the next lesion occurs and this in turn is often a feature of a more benign course. Complete recovery from the presenting lesion is a good sign, whereas incomplete recovery is a sinister one.

What geographical fact affects the incidence of the disease?

498 Like multiple sclerosis, neuromyelitis optica, or Devic's disease, is a demyelinating disease but the pattern of the lesions and the clinical course are different.

What are they?

499 The degenerative and osteoarthritic changes of cervical spondylosis consist mainly of disc prolapse and osteophyte formation. Cervical spine X-rays may be normal in a younger person with an acute disc prolapse. Osteophyte formation indicates chronic disease, is common in the elderly and often symptomless.

What types of symptoms would make you include cervical spondylosis in your differential diagnosis?

500 In root compression, pain can be felt in the motor, sensory or visceral distribution of the root. Sensory loss is much less common. When the first sacral root is compressed by a prolapsed disc, the patient complains of pains passing down the back of the thigh into the calf and into the outer border of the foot. The pain is exacerbated by coughing and sneezing.

What signs would you expect to find? What is Lasègue's sign?

501 A 55-year-old man complains of pains in the front of his right thigh which spread down the inner aspect of his right leg and are aggravated by coughing or straining. Examination reveals loss of the knee jerk and weakness of knee extension (quadriceps) and ankle inversion (tibialis posterior).

These symptoms and signs could be due to compression of the nerve root of L4. If the cause of this is prolapse of the intervertebral disc, which disc is involved?

502 A cervical rib (arising from C7) may cause vascular, sensory or motor symptoms, all of which are typically improved by raising the arm above the head.

Pressure on the subclavian artery may be indicated by a bruit behind the clavicle and reduction or disappearance of the radial pulse on lowering the arm or retracting the shoulder.

Which nerves are involved in this syndrome?

503 The radial nerve may be compressed in the axilla through use of a crutch, or by the edge of a chair or railing when drunk, or by the edge of the operating table if the arm of an anaesthetized patient is allowed to hang down. Midshaft fractures of the humerus may also damage this nerve.

The ulnar nerve is commonly damaged at the elbow where it may be felt to be thickened.

What signs result from lesions of these two nerves?

504 In the carpal tunnel the median nerve may be compressed by changes in the wrist joint (rheumatoid arthritis, acromegaly), soft tissue swelling (myxoedema), or fluid retention (pregnancy). The symptoms are usually worse after a night's rest and improve as activity mobilizes extracellular fluid.

One of the hand muscles supplied by the median nerve, and consequently weakened, is abductor pollicis brevis. How is this muscle tested?

505 Nerve entrapment syndromes in the leg include meralgia paraesthetica (lateral cutaneous nerve of the thigh), and lateral popliteal palsy due to pressure on the nerve where it winds around the upper end of the fibula. In this latter condition, a flaccid foot drop occurs with loss of eversion and dorsiflexion of foot and toes. Sensation over the lateral aspect of the leg and dorsum of the foot may also be affected.

What are the symptoms of meralgia paraesthetica?

506 The difference between mononeuritis multiplex and polyneuritis is largely one of distribution. Many conditions can cause both but the important aspect of a polyneuritis is that it is symmetrical.

What are the features of acute infective polyneuritis?

507 Polyneuritis can be caused by a large number of metabolic, toxic, vasculitic and infective conditions. Diabetes is the most common.

What other disease process, more common in older people, can cause a neuropathy as well as other neurological disturbance?

508 Thiamine (vitamin B_1) is required for carbohydrate metabolism. Alcoholics, whose diet may consist almost exclusively of carbohydrate and contains no thiamine, are particularly prone to thiamine deficiency. This causes polyneuritis with marked muscle tenderness, Wernicke's encephalopathy and Korsakoff's psychosis.

How can adults encounter pyridoxine deficiency?

509 Riboflavin and nicotinic acid are both water-soluble B vitamins but riboflavin deficiency does not affect the nervous system. Nicotinic acid deficiency causes pellagra, in which dementia is accompanied by chronic diarrhoea and dermatitis.

What does cyanocobalamin (B_{12}) deficiency cause?

510 Trigeminal neuralgia, also called tic douloureux, does not occur before the age of about 50. Either the maxillary or mandibular division of the fifth cranial nerve is usually affected first.

What physical signs are found?

Kidney Function & Disorders; Water, Electrolyte & Acid–Base Balance

511 What is the size of normal kidneys and what can you deduce if the renal margin overlies the psoas shadow rather than lying next to it?

512 In each glomerulus, the endothelial cells are the lining cells of the capillaries. They lie on the glomerular basement membrane, on the other side of which the epithelial cells of Bowman's capsule rest their podocytes.

What and where are the mesangial cells?

513 What is the juxtaglomerulus apparatus of the kidney, where is it and what does it produce?

514 Creatinine clearance is a measurement of the amount of plasma being filtered by the glomeruli each minute. A patient has a urine output of 1008 ml in 24 hours. The plasma creatinine level during that 24 hours is 368 μmol/l and the 24 hour urinary creatinine excretion is 10.6 mmol (10 600 μmol).

What is the creatinine clearance and how does creatinine clearance compare with inulin clearance?

515 In a glucose tolerance test, urine glucose is measured at the same time as blood glucose in order to determine at what level glucose 'spills' into the urine. This level is often called the renal threshold.

What is its proper name in terms of the actual process involved?

516 Renal plasma flow (ERPF—the E standing for estimated) is another aspect of renal function, based on the behaviour of substances like para-aminohippuric acid (PAH) which are secreted by the tubular cells, as well as being filtered by the

glomeruli. The calculation of this is based on the Fick principle.

What is the formula for this, and what is the meaning of the term 'filtration fraction'?

517 70–80 per cent of the water present in the glomerular filtrate is reabsorbed in the proximal tubule, accompanying the active uptake of sodium ions.

Where else in the renal tubule does reabsorption of water occur and what controls this reabsorption?

518 The loop of Henle operates as a counter-current multiplier system. This technological title hides the simple facts of the system which are:

(a) there is sodium transfer from the ascending limb across the tubular wall to the descending limb;

(b) urine arriving in the distal convoluted tubule is always hypotonic as a result; and

(c) the blood supply to the tips of the loops of Henle, lying in the hypertonic medulla, is sluggish, thus preserving the hypertonicity generated by the system.

Why is loss of urine concentrating ability one of the first signs of renal impairment?

519 Approximately 75–80 per cent of the sodium in the glomerular filtrate is reabsorbed in the proximal tubule, most of this as sodium bicarbonate by an active, energy-requiring process, while some sodium passively follows chloride.

A further 10 per cent is absorbed in the ascending limb of the loop of Henle by means of a sodium pump in the tubular cells.

Further sodium absorption occurs in the distal convoluted tubule and the collecting ducts, partly by active transport and partly by ion exchange involving hydrogen or potassium ions.

How is potassium handled by the tubule?

520 What is the action of antidiuretic hormone (ADH, vasopressin) on the collecting ducts?

521 Normal urine may contain up to 150 mg of protein per 24 hours and this consists of albumin, IgG, Tamm–Horsfall protein from the tubules, microglobulin and lower urinary tract proteins.

What are Bence Jones proteins and how can they be detected?

522 Proteinuria is an indication of renal disease—with a few exceptions. What are they?

523 In glomerular disease, urine protein always contains albumin with the quantities of other proteins depending on the degree of damage and the pore sizes in the diseased basement membrane.

In tubular disorders the protein composition is different.

How?

524 On a normal protein intake, plasma urea begins to rise when creatinine clearance is down to 25 ml/min. However, on a low protein diet, plasma urea may remain normal until the creatinine clearance is as low as 5 ml/min.

Plasma creatinine, on the other hand, is independent of dietary protein, and generally begins to rise when its clearance falls below 25 ml/min.

In what circumstances, other than renal disease, may the plasma urea be elevated?

525 In renal impairment, the level of protein intake affects the plasma urea level.

What effect does a low protein diet have on the function of normal kidneys?

526 Insensitivity to ADH (nephrogenic diabetes insipidus) may be inherited as an X-linked recessive condition or it may occur as a result of acquired factors including hypokalaemia, hypercalcaemia, pyelonephritis or hydronephrosis.

The convenient test for this is the vasopressin test.

How is this done and what are its shortcomings?

527 A patient's urine pH never drops below 6. Is this normal or could there be a failure of acidification?

How would you test for it?

528 What is a renogram and what can it tell you about renal function?

529 You want to examine a specimen of urine by microscopy.

How would you prepare it?

530 The main object of urine microscopy is to identify and count the types of cells and casts.

There are four types of cell found: red blood cells, polymorphs, tubular epithelial cells and squamous epithelial cells. There should not be any confusion between polymorphs and tubular epithelial cells, the latter being larger but with a more compact nucleus.

What are the different casts and what do they signify?

531 You want a patient to have an intravenous pyelogram (IVP).

How should the patient be prepared and for which patients could it be hazardous?

532 Both chronic pyelonephritis and urinary tract obstruction may cause blunting of calyces on IVP.

What other features on IVP may help distinguish between these two conditions?

533 On an IVP you see distortion and elongation of the calyces with loss of the normal cupping of the pyramids throughout both kidneys. The kidneys are $4\frac{1}{2}$ vertebrae in length.

What is the diagnosis and what might it be if the kidneys were $3\frac{1}{2}$ vertebrae in length and the calyceal distortion was confined to half of one kidney?

534 What are the indications for doing retrograde pyelography?

535 In what conditions is renal arteriography helpful, and, in view of its invasive nature, what alternatives are there?

536 Renal biopsy is more likely to cause bleeding than liver biopsy. Uraemia will increase this likelihood as will hypertension, and biopsy should not be undertaken unless the blood pressure is controlled. Other contraindications to biopsy include suspicion of tumour, abscess or TB or the presence of a single kidney.

In what circumstances may biopsy be helpful?

537 The incidence of acute glomerulonephritis following group A streptococcal type 12 infection is between 2 and 30 per cent. Although type 12 is most commonly implicated, other types can also cause this, and viruses have also been incriminated, including hepatitis B.

How soon after streptococcal infection does the nephritis begin and which patients are at greatest risk of developing nephritis?

538 The main clinical features of acute glomerulonephritis are oliguria, haematuria, hypertension and oedema, particularly of the face, since patients with this condition can tolerate lying flat.

Adults can be affected but the disease is more common in infants and primary school children.

What is the immunological process involved?

539 Acute glomerulonephritis has some features in common with malignant hypertension, pyelonephritis,

Henoch–Schönlein purpura, focal nephritis and some milder cases of the nephrotic syndrome.

How would you distinguish it from each of these other conditions?

540 The uncomplicated case of acute glomerulonephritis usually undergoes complete recovery within 2 weeks.

What should the treatment consist of?

541 Approximately 5 per cent of cases of acute glomerulonephritis go on to develop subacute glomerulonephritis and a further 5 per cent develop chronic glomerulonephritis.

The subacute form consists of a continuation of oedema, hypertension, haematuria and the development of anaemia. Terminal renal failure usually ensues within 18 months. Treatment is symptomatic and immunosuppressive.

What is the typical pattern of events with chronic glomerulonephritis?

542 With chronic glomerulonephritis, the patient can present in a number of ways. There may be asymptomatic proteinuria. Hypertension may occur alone. Approximately half the patients go through a nephrotic phase at some stage of their illness, with heavy proteinuria, hypoalbuminaemia and oedema. In others, renal failure steals on unannounced, except perhaps by nocturia.

For some histological types, steroids and immunosuppressive drugs may be effective. Which types?

543 The nephrotic syndrome, as its name suggests, is not a disease in its own right but a constellation of clinical and biochemical changes with many causes.

Proteinuria (more than 5 g daily), oedema, hypoalbuminaemia (less than 3 g/dl) and hypercholesterolaemia are the main diagnostic features, although a raised cholesterol level is not invariable.

What are the causes?

544 Disturbance of lipid metabolism is very common in the nephrotic syndrome. Plasma lipids tend to show increased levels of total cholesterol, free cholesterol and beta lipoproteins and the elevation is universally related to the severity of the hypoalbuminaemia. The urine may contain free fat globules or tubular epithelial cells laden with fat.

What are the clinical complications that occur with this chronic hyperlipaemia?

545 The metabolic derangements of the nephrotic syndrome are not limited to albumin and cholesterol.

What happens to aldosterone, serum thyroxine and glucose?

546 When chronic glomerulonephritis causes the nephrotic syndrome the pathological lesion can be inferred from the age of the patient. Most children have a 'minimal change' lesion. Some adults have this too but most adults have either a membranous or a proliferative lesion.

What is the relevance of this to treatment?

547 Proliferative glomerulonephritis is known to result from streptococcal infection. What are the known causes of membranous glomerulonephritis?

548 To detect the involvement of complement in a disease process, it is generally convenient to measure the levels of C3 and C4, since assays of the other factors are difficult to perform. There are two patterns of abnormal results. Both C3 and C4 may be low, or C3 alone may be low while C4 remains normal. How do you interpret these?

549 The kidneys are commonly involved in amyloidosis. Amyloid is laid down in the walls of the capillaries, gradually encroaching on the lumen until it is obliterated.

Proteinuria without symptoms is usual, but some cases deteriorate into the nephrotic syndrome with heavy proteinuria or renal failure. Renal vein thrombosis is a common complication.

There is no treatment for amyloidosis other than that of the underlying cause. What are the underlying causes?

550 Renal vein thrombosis is a common complication of the nephrotic syndrome because of elevated levels of fibrinogen, platelets and other clotting factors that accompany the syndrome.

Conversely, renal vein thrombosis can cause the nephrotic syndrome. What is the usual clinical picture in renal vein thrombosis?

551 What is the treatment for the nephrotic syndrome?

552 The life expectancy of a patient with the nephrotic syndrome ranges from a few months to normal, depending on the underlying cause and on the renal lesion.

What is the life expectancy for 'minimal change', membranous glomerulonephritis and proliferative glomerulonephritis when there is no spontaneous remission or response to treatment?

553 While acute pyelonephritis is usually not difficult to diagnose, underlying conditions predisposing to this infection may not be so obvious and should be kept in mind. What are they?

554 With careful cleansing of the external urinary meatus it is not difficult to collect a satisfactory urine specimen for culture. What number of organisms is regarded as significant for bacterial infection and for yeast infection of the urine?

555 Chronic pyelonephritis is characterized histologically by the presence of lymphocytes and plasma cells in the renal tissue, and bacterial antigens can also be detected although positive cultures are not so common.

Its relationship to acute pyelonephritis is poorly defined. Sometimes there is a clear history of recurrent acute pyelonephritis and this emphasizes the importance of detecting and treating any underlying predisposing condition. In other cases there is hypertension, in others renal failure of insidious onset.

How would you support a diagnosis of chronic pyelonephritis?

556 Acute renal failure can occur with almost any major insult including trauma, major surgery, haemorrhage or myocardial infarction. In most of these cases, the renal failure is totally reversible if the patient can be kept alive until renal function is re-established.

What are the first biochemical changes of acute renal failure?

557 A patient with acute renal failure may be oliguric because little urine is being produced. What other explanation is there for oliguria and what should alert you to it?

558 In acute renal failure, fluid overload and hyperkalaemia are two of the factors that may kill the patient. How would you prevent them and what are the other important aspects of management?

559 Peritoneal dialysis is a very useful measure, but it cannot be used after abdominal surgery (when the peritoneum would leak) nor in hypercatabolic states when the plasma urea rises by 10–20 mmol/l daily thus exceeding the capacity of PD for urea removal.

What are the complications of peritoneal dialysis?

560 In chronic renal failure, the intact nephron hypothesis has been put forward to explain why the kidneys lose their ability to retain sodium.

What does the hypothesis say and what does one do about the patient's sodium?

561 Chronic normochromic, normocytic anaemia is a prominent feature of chronic renal failure although patients with polycystic disease tend to have slightly higher blood counts than those with other forms of chronic renal failure.

What are the causes of the anaemia in chronic renal failure?

562 Why are patients with chronic renal failure at risk of metastatic calcification? How can the risk be reduced?

563 In chronic renal failure gastrointestinal and neuromuscular symptoms may be prominent.

The former consist of nausea, hiccough, vomiting, abdominal pain, haematemesis and bloody diarrhoea.

What are the neuromuscular features?

564 Dietary protein restriction in chronic renal failure is not indicated until the plasma urea is above 35 mmol/l approximately. When it is indicated, would you use a Giovannetti diet?

565 A patient requiring haemodialysis may have either a vascular shunt or fistula. What is the difference between these two means of vascular access?

566 In which of the collagen vascular diseases does renal involvement occur?

567 What should a urine sediment containing the following—red cells, white cells, casts of all kinds, tubular epithelial cells, fat globules—make you think of in the presence of multisystem disease? (This is a 'telescoped' urinary sediment.)

568 Both systemic sclerosis and rheumatoid arthritis can involve the kidneys.

In the former it is often a terminal event with a sudden onset of oliguria progressing to anuria, refractory to all forms of therapy.

In rheumatoid disease, proteinuria is a common finding. What may be happening in the kidneys?

569 Haemolytic-uraemic syndrome and thrombotic thrombocytopenic purpura are two rare but serious

conditions in which disseminated intravascular coagulation (DIC) leads to renal failure by blocking small renal blood vessels with fibrin and fibrin degradation products. In TTP an amorphous eosinophilic material derived from fibrin occludes the vessels. The treatment in this condition is high dose steroids.

What is the treatment for the haemolytic-uraemic syndrome?

570 What are the four ways in which diabetes mellitus can damage the kidneys?

571 The susceptibility of diabetic patients to pyelonephritis, which may be severe and difficult to eradicate, means that they should never be catheterized if it can be at all avoided.

Under what circumstances can a diabetic become (a) oliguric and (b) anuric?

572 Both hypercalcaemia and hypokalaemia can change the sensitivity of the distal convoluted and collecting tubules to vasopressin (ADH) and cause a renal (nephrogenic) diabetes insipidus. The condition is reversible if the electrolyte abnormality is corrected early enough.

In the absence of reversible causes, what is the treatment for nephrogenic diabetes insipidus?

573 Urinary tract obstruction can cause hydronephrosis and this may interfere with distal tubular function. Benign prostatic hypertrophy is very common and some of these patients have marked nocturia because of impairment in concentrating ability of the kidneys.

What other tubular functions may be impaired in urinary tract obstruction?

574 What are the renal and urinary tract changes of normal pregnancy?

575 At 36 weeks of pregnancy, a 25-year-old woman develops hypertension, albuminuria and oedema. Investigation shows a reduction in creatinine clearance and elevation of serum uric acid.

Can all these changes be due to pre-eclampsia or is there a separate renal condition?

576 One of the many renal causes of hypertension is renal artery stenosis, although not all patients with demonstrable renal artery stenosis are hypertensive.

How could you detect renal artery stenosis on an IVP?

577 The mechanism by which renal artery stenosis and possibly other renal conditions cause hypertension is the renin–angiotensin–aldosterone system. Renin is an enzyme produced by the juxtaglomerular apparatus in response to the level of sodium in the distal convoluted tubule.

What is the rest of the system?

578 What happens to the kidneys in essential hypertension compared to accelerated or malignant hypertension?

579 Cystinuria is a disorder of the proximal tubule in which there is failure to reabsorb four amino acids for which the mnemonic is COAL (cystine, ornithine, arginine, lysine). Cystine is the least soluble of these in acid urine and forms stones, either in the renal pelvis or in the bladder.

Would you see these stones on a plain film? What is the treatment?

580 A young adult patient with bone pain unexpectedly shows radiological evidence of osteomalacia.

Would it be worthwhile checking his urine for glucose and amino acids and his blood for hypokalaemia, hypophosphataemia and hypouricaemia?

581 Renal tubular acidosis is a condition (of more than one aetiology) which can cause hypokalaemia with muscle weakness, osteomalacia due to urinary phosphate loss and nephrocalcinosis due to reduced urinary citrate.

How would you recognize a case, and what is the treatment?

582 About 30 per cent of patients with renal stones have hypercalciuria (mostly the idiopathic variety) while about 15 per cent of patients with gout develop uric acid stones, which are radiolucent.

Increased gastrointestinal absorption of calcium may underlie hypercalciuria and one treatment is oral cellulose phosphate to bind calcium in the gut.

What is the treatment for uric acid stones?

583 Polycystic kidneys are commonly asymptomatic for the first three or four decades of life, and, if renal failure supervenes, it is usually marked by a milder anaemia and slower deterioration compared with other forms of renal disease.

What symptoms can draw attention to polycystic kidneys?

584 Duplex kidney or ureter is a common anomaly, which can be responsible for complications. What are they?

585 Goodpasture's syndrome is a rare condition in which the glomerular and alveolar basement membranes are attacked by antibody.

Iron-deficiency anaemia, dyspnoea, haemoptysis, siderophages in the sputum and radiological lung opacities occur with the pulmonary disease.

What are the renal manifestations?

586 All patients with unexplained haematuria should have an IVP. Why is this?

587 How could you associate renal failure with migraine?

588 Phenacetin and possibly other analgesics have been implicated in the necrotizing papillitis and chronic pyelonephritis that comprise analgesic nephropathy.

The urine often shows a sterile pyuria (like TB) and radiologically the kidneys are shrunken with deformed calyces. In a few patients there may be ring shadows where the papillae have become necrotic.

What is the most important step in the management of these patients?

589 In the presence of renal impairment the half-life of many drugs is altered and the size and frequency of doses should always be checked, and drug levels measured where possible.

With the exception of erythromycin, the antibiotics whose names end in -mycin (including gentamicin) are nephrotoxic and their delayed excretion in renal failure enhances nephrotoxicity.

When creatinine clearance is less than 10 ml/min what would be a correct adult dose of ampicillin?

590 In renal transplantation, what are the main causes of complications and failure?

591 Major causes of water excess include acute renal failure with excessive fluid intake, the syndrome of inappropriate ADH secretion, glucocorticoid deficiency (e.g. Addison's disease), and of course inappropriate intravenous therapy or compulsive water or beer drinking.

What features may occur in 'water intoxication'?

592 Water deficiency may occur in situations where a patient is unable to drink, due for example to severe illness with impaired consciousness or severe dysphagia due to carcinoma of the oesophagus.

What conditions may cause water deficiency due to excessive fluid loss?

593 Causes of the syndrome of inappropriate ADH secretion include oat cell carcinoma of the bronchus and some other tumours, head injury and encephalitis, pulmonary infections including pneumonia and tuberculosis, acute alcoholism and myxoedema.
What are the biochemical features of the syndrome?

594 Potassium excess may be asymptomatic until sudden cardiac arrest occurs. What conditions may give rise to hyperkalaemia?

595 ECG changes found in hyperkalaemia include high peaked T waves, disappearance of P waves and widened QRS complexes.
How is hyperkalaemia treated?

596 Potassium deficiency may be due to gastrointestinal loss. If there is an associated alkalosis, one of the following is likely: vomiting, gastric suctioning, villous adenoma, colonic neoplasm or chronic laxative abuse.
In what situations may loss of potassium via the gastrointestinal tract be associated with systemic acidosis?

597 When a diagnosis of metabolic acidosis has been made the plasma 'anion gap' should be calculated from the formula $(Na^+ + K^+) - (Cl^- + HCO_3^-)$. The normal gap is 10–18 mmol/l. Metabolic acidosis with a normal gap is due to conditions such as gastrointestinal bicarbonate loss (e.g. diarrhoea), renal tubular acidosis and ingestion of some acidifying agents such as ammonium chloride.
What conditions cause metabolic acidosis with a high anion gap?

598 Lactic acidosis may be due to conditions which produce circulatory insufficiency and tissue hypoxia, for example shock or cardiac arrest.
However, lactic acidosis may also occur in the absence of circulatory insufficiency.
What conditions may cause this situation?

599 The most common cause of metabolic alkalosis is prolonged severe vomiting producing loss of hydrochloric acid from the body. This is especially likely in pyloric stenosis.

What other conditions cause metabolic alkalosis and what changes occur in plasma pH, bicarbonate and Pco_2 levels in this situation?

600 Respiratory alkalosis is due to excessive loss of carbonic acid as a result of overventilation of the lungs.

What conditions produce this situation?

Endocrine & Metabolic Disorders

601 Most patients with suspected pituitary tumours are usually unaware of any visual impairment. However, it is important to carry out full visual field assessment in every case.

Why is this and what abnormality is most frequently found?

602 Headache is the most constant symptom of pituitary tumours.

What simple radiological examination should be carried out first in cases with suspected pituitary tumours? What abnormality should be looked for on the film?

603 A large pituitary neoplasm may cause optic atrophy. Clinically in this situation there will be pallor of the optic disc. However, there is a wide variation in the colour of the normal optic disc, and there may be difficulty, especially for the inexperienced observer, in deciding whether or not there is excessive pallor of the disc in any particular case.

How may one distinguish between a pale normal optic disc and optic atrophy?

604 Acromegaly is due to excessive growth hormone production from the eosinophilic cells of the anterior pituitary. Although supraorbital ridges and jaw are frequently enlarged in this condition it is important to note that the term acromegaly implies enlargement of the extremities and one should be slow to make a diagnosis of this condition in the absence of significant enlargement of the hands and feet.

What systemic and metabolic complications may develop in this condition?

605 Hyperprolactinaemia due to an anterior pituitary microadenoma (i.e. an adenoma less than 1 cm in diameter) is an important cause of infertility and amenorrhoea in the female.

However, hyperprolactinaemia is not always due to a prolactinoma.

What other causes should be considered before embarking on extensive pituitary investigations?

606 The commonest cause of hypopituitarism is a chromophobe adenoma of the pituitary gland. Symptoms include amenorrhoea and infertility in females, and physical findings include pallor and hypotension (due to ACTH deficiency). Secondary sex characteristics may be lost.
What serious complication may occur in hypopituitarism?

607 Anterior pituitary hormonal reserve may be assessed very effectively by three stimulation tests, all of which may be carried out simultaneously, the total study lasting for one hour.
What tests are these and which hormones are stimulated by each?

608 Symptoms of cranial diabetes insipidus include thirst and polyuria. Urine output may exceed 10 litres per day and severe dehydration may occur if fluid intake fails to keep up with output.
What causes this condition?

609 In cases of cranial diabetes insipidus, the plasma osmolality will be elevated above 295 mosmol/kg and that of the urine will be low.
How is the diagnosis confirmed?

610 Hyperthyroidism due to Graves' disease is at least five times more frequent in females than in males. However, occasionally an elevated serum T_4 is found in a female patient who is in fact euthyroid.
What may cause this and how may the true thyroid status be determined?

611 In cases of hyperthyroidism where medical treatment is indicated carbimazole or thiouracil derivatives are the drugs of first choice.
What serious side-effect may occur with these drugs and what precautions should be taken in their use?

612 Important symptoms of thyrotoxicosis are sweating, heat intolerance, palpitations and weight loss.
What bowel symptom may occur in thyrotoxicosis?

613 A diagnosis of thyrotoxicosis is frequently supported by findings in the hand and wrist.
What important features should be looked for in this area?

614 Exophthalmos in Graves' disease may be unilateral or bilateral. It may be associated with ophthalmoplegia and diplopia. Frequently there is chemosis and conjunctival irritation.

What serious complications may develop with severe exophthalmos and how may they be prevented?

615 A thyroid crisis is nowadays fortunately rare due to better management of thyrotoxicosis. When it does occur the usual precipitating cause is thyroidectomy in an inadequately prepared patient, or development of a severe infection such as pneumonia in a thyrotoxic case.

What are the principal features of a thyroid crisis? What is the management?

616 Radioactive iodine is the therapy of choice for patients with thyrotoxicosis who are over 45 years of age or who appear to have a short life expectancy. In the doses used for treating thyrotoxicosis there is no evidence of increased risk of leukaemia or other malignancy. There is a theoretical risk of genetic damage and many physicians avoid this substance in patients under 45 years of age.

What is the principal complication of this form of treatment?

617 Subtotal thyroidectomy is the treatment of choice in patients during their reproductive years in whom antithyroid drugs have failed to produce a permanent remission of thyrotoxicosis, or in whom serious sensitivity reactions to the drugs have developed. A large goitre or one producing obstructive symptoms such as dysphagia should also be treated surgically.

What complications may arise following this operation?

618 Hyperthyroidism occurring during pregnancy must not be treated with radioactive iodine. Subtotal thyroidectomy may be carried out and is best done during the middle trimester. Surgery is probably the best treatment in severe cases with large goitres.

Most commonly, however, hyperthyroidism during pregnancy is treated with antithyroid drugs. What problems may arise with this form of therapy and what precautions are advisable?

619 Primary hypothyroidism has a wide variety of clinical presentations. For example the hypothyroid patient may present to the cardiologist with angina pectoris and hypercholesterolaemia, cardiac failure or pericardial effusion.

What features may cause a hypothyroid patient to present to the following specialists: gynaecologist, ENT surgeon, rheumatologist, psychiatrist?

620 Myxoedema coma is a rare and dangerous complication of untreated myxoedema. It occurs usually in winter and may be precipitated by drugs such as chlorpromazine and other sedatives and analgesics. A low reading thermometer should be used and rectal temperatures as low as 24°C may be found. Shivering is absent.

What is the management of this condition?

621 Primary hypothyroidism is due to failure of the thyroid gland and is most frequently caused by Hashimoto's thyroiditis but hypothyroidism also occurs as a sequel to radioactive iodine therapy for thyrotoxicosis.

What biochemical tests should be done to confirm the diagnosis of primary hypothyroidism?

622 Carcinoma of the thyroid gland is a relatively uncommon form of cancer. Clinically, it may present as a solitary painless thyroid nodule which appears as a cold area on isotope scanning of the gland.

What other clinical features would suggest malignancy?

623 Medullary carcinoma of the thyroid is a rare tumour which arises from the parafollicular cells. It may be associated with neuromas on tongue, lips or eyelids.

What biochemical abnormalities may be found in the plasma in this condition?

624 Cushing's disease (pituitary dependent) with bilateral adrenal hyperplasia may be treated by either pituitary ablation or bilateral adrenalectomy.

What pituitary complication may follow the latter procedure?

625 The commonest cause of Cushing's syndrome is administration of steroids or ACTH. Spontaneous Cushing's syndrome is due to one of three possible causes:

(a) Cushing's disease (pituitary dependent adrenal hyperplasia);
(b) adrenal carcinoma or adenoma;
(c) the ectopic ACTH syndrome (secretion of ACTH by tumours of non-endocrine origin).

Assuming the diagnosis of spontaneous Cushing's syndrome is confirmed biochemically, what is the single most useful biochemical estimation in distinguishing these three disorders?

626 Among the conditions which should be considered in the differential diagnosis of a case of suspected Cushing's syndrome are simple obesity and the polycystic ovarian syndrome.
What clinical features may be useful in differentiating these conditions?

627 The confirmation of a diagnosis of Cushing's syndrome can be a protracted and expensive process.
What tests are most useful for outruling this condition on an outpatient basis?

628 Pituitary dependent adrenal hyperplasia (Cushing's disease) is commoner in females, is usually of gradual onset and is associated with weight gain and truncal obesity. Skin pigmentation is usually of moderate degree.
How does this picture contrast with that of Cushing's syndrome due to production of ACTH from an ectopic site?

629 The commonest cause of Addison's disease in developed countries is autoimmune adrenal failure (approximately 75 per cent), whereas tuberculosis now accounts for only about 20 per cent of cases.
Hyperpigmentation of the skin is a major feature of this condition.
What areas in particular should be examined for hyperpigmentation?

630 Features of autoimmune adrenal failure (Addison's disease) include a female predominance, the finding of antibodies to the adrenal cortex in the plasma, and a high incidence of other organ-specific autoimmune disease such as Grave's disease and Hashimoto's thyroiditis, pernicious anaemia, premature ovarian failure and insulin dependent diabetes mellitis.
What features would suggest tuberculosis as a cause of Addison's disease?

631 Hypotension is a major feature of Addison's disease and in fact a systolic blood pressure exceeding 110 mmHg before replacement therapy makes this diagnosis unlikely. Postural hypotension is common and syncopal attacks may occur.
What routine biochemical findings would tend to support a diagnosis of Addison's disease?

632 In Addison's disease the normal daily steroid replacement dose is 10–20 mg of hydrocortisone

(cortisol) in the morning and 10 mg in the evening. Patients should be advised to double this dose in case of a minor illness, e.g. coryza. In addition patients should receive mineralocorticoid replacement in the form of fludrocortisone 0.05–0.1 mg daily. All patients should wear a Medic Alert bracelet and carry a steroid card in case of accidents.

What is the management of an acute adrenal crisis?

633 A small proportion of young patients developing hypertension may have an underlying cause. Possible causes include renal artery stenosis, coarctation of the aorta, phaeochromocytoma and Conn's syndrome.

What biochemical abnormalities would be expected in a patient with Conn's syndrome? Is oedema a feature of Conn's syndrome?

634 Phaeochromocytoma is due to increased production of adrenaline and noradrenaline by a tumour originating in sympathetic nervous tissue. Ninety per cent of these tumours are in the adrenal medulla.

How is a diagnosis of phaeochromocytoma confirmed and what drugs may interfere with the diagnostic test?

635 Major symptoms of phaeochromocytoma include attacks of apprehension, sweating, flushing, headache and palpitations, frequently preceded by an aura. Angina, abdominal pain and vomiting may also occur.

What physical findings may be present during attacks?

636 An associated feature of some cases of phaeochromocytoma is glycosuria with mild hyperglycaemia.

What precautions should be taken during the examination of a suspected case of phaeochromocytoma?

637 The majority of cases of impotence are due to psychological causes. However, occasionally it may be an early symptom of organic disease.

What organic conditions may be associated with impotence?

638 A frequent problem in casualty work is the unconscious diabetic. Coma may be due to hypoglycaemia or hyperglycaemia in this situation. A history of sudden onset, missing a meal, excess insulin and unaccustomed exercise suggests hypoglycaemia. On the other hand, gradual onset of illness over several days, with vomiting and possibly omission of insulin suggests hyperglycaemia.

What features further distinguish these conditions on physical examination?

639 A minority of cases of diabetes follow damage to the pancreas from pathological processes such as pancreatitis, haemochromatosis and carcinoma of the pancreas. Drugs such as steroids and thiazides may precipitate diabetes in genetically susceptible individuals.

Certain conditions are associated with excess production of hormones which are insulin antagonists. This leads to the development of diabetes mellitus.

What conditions may produce this situation?

640 Persons with a normal glucose tolerance test may have an increased liability to develop diabetes for genetic reasons. For example, the risk of developing diabetes to an individual with one diabetic parent is about 5 per cent and with two diabetic parents is about 10 per cent. Such individuals with increased risk are known as potential diabetics.

What are latent diabetics?

641 Juvenile onset diabetes usually starts acutely under the age of 40 years. Weight loss and ketosis are usual. There is marked reduction in beta-cell mass and strong evidence of cell mediated immunity to beta-cells. Islet cell antibodies are present in about 75 per cent of cases. Concordance in identical twins is not absolute (50 per cent) and there is an association with HLA B8. Other autoimmune disorders are frequently associated. There is usually an absolute insulin deficiency and these cases require insulin therapy permanently.

How does this picture compare with maturity onset diabetes?

642 Autonomic neuropathy due to diabetes mellitus may cause denervation of the cardiovascular system.

What clinical features may this denervation produce?

643 Retinopathy is the most frequent long-term complication of diabetes. Diabetic retinopathy is the commonest cause of blindness in persons aged 30–64 years in Britain.

Patients with only microaneurysms, retinal haemorrhages and exudates have simple or background retinopathy and in general have a good visual prognosis.

What are the features and prognosis of proliferative retinopathy?

644 Diabetic nephropathy is a more common cause of death in juvenile onset than in maturity onset diabetes. The earliest sign of nephropathy is proteinuria, which may be intermittent initially. Most young diabetics are dead within 15 years of the onset of proteinuria.

What are the later features of diabetic nephropathy? How may the severity of the nephropathy be assessed?

645 Sulphonylurea therapy is indicated mainly in maturity onset diabetics of normal weight who have failed to respond to dietary treatment alone.

Sulphonylureas are not suitable in general for use in juvenile onset diabetics. Why is this?

646 Biguanides reduce intestinal glucose absorption and increase its peripheral utilization. They are useful in obese, maturity onset diabetics who are not adequately controlled by diet alone.

What important side-effects may occur with biguanides?

647 As pregnancy advances, the renal threshold for glucose falls and measurement of glycosuria may cease to be an accurate index of diabetic control.

How should diabetic control be monitored in pregnancy?

648 Problems occurring during pregnancy in a diabetic include an increased incidence of polyhydramnios and pre-eclamptic toxaemia. The fetus may be excessively large for dates leading to difficulties with delivery. There is an increased incidence of stillbirth, neonatal death and congenital malformation in babies of diabetic mothers.

Strict control of diabetes during pregnancy will improve the chances of fetal survival. What degree of control should be aimed for?

649 Diabetic patients should have their retinae examined every 6–12 months by a competent observer, following dilation of the pupils with a mydriatic. Simple background retinopathy without macular involvement requires no specific treatment but the diabetes and any associated hypertension must be well controlled.

How should simple retinopathy involving the perimacular area, or proliferative retinopathy be managed?

650 Poor diabetic control is associated with reduced resistance to infection. The development of a skin carbuncle may unmask latent diabetes or may precipitate diabetic ketoacidosis and coma.

What other infections are increased in frequency in diabetes?

651 A characteristic symptom of diabetic polyneuropathy is the complaint of 'burning feet' which is characteristically worse at night.
What physical signs would support a diagnosis of diabetic polyneuropathy?

652 Refractive errors are common during commencement of treatment for diabetes mellitus. These are due to alteration in the water content of the eye and lens.
Of what may the patient complain, and what advice should be given to such individuals?

653 The primary presentation of diabetes mellitus in some elderly individuals may be with hyperosmolar non-ketotic diabetic coma.
What factors may precipitate this state?

654 In the majority of cases of diabetic ketoacidosis, acidosis will gradually be reversed by rehydration and control of blood sugar with insulin. Bicarbonate should not be given unless pH is below 7.1.
What problems may arise from administration of bicarbonate?

655 Haemochromatosis (or bronze diabetes) is a disorder of iron metabolism characterized by excessive iron absorption. It is 10 times more common in males, females being protected by menstrual loss of iron. The major features include diabetes mellitus, hepatic cirrhosis and cardiomyopathy, with generalized skin pigmentation.
How is this condition diagnosed?

656 Anorexia nervosa is almost invariably associated with amenorrhoea when body weight falls to 45 kg or less.
What hormonal changes are found in this situation?

657 Hirsutism may be a normal feature in some menopausal women and in certain races. Hirsutism may be due to ovarian diseases, the commonest of which is the polycystic ovarian syndrome.
What adrenal disorders may produce hirsutism?

658 Enlargement of breast tissue in the male (gynaecomastia) may be physiological in the neonate, at puberty (in 50 per cent or more of all males) and possibly in the elderly.
What commonly used drugs apart from oestrogens and androgens may cause gynaecomastia?

659 Symptoms attributed to the menopause include depression and anxiety, insomnia and hot flushes. Obesity, hirsutism and osteoarthrosis may also appear. Osteoporosis frequently presents shortly after the menopause, and pruritis vulvae due to senile vaginitis may be troublesome.

What hormonal changes occur in the menopause?

660 40–50 per cent of carcinomas of the breast possess cytoplasmic oestrogen receptors. These receptors are more commonly found in tumours of older postmenopausal patients than in those of younger women.

Of what relevance is this finding to prognosis and treatment of breast cancer?

661 Phenylketonuria (PKU), if untreated, causes severe mental retardation with athetosis, psychosis and convulsions. Children with PKU frequently have fair hair, blue eyes and eczema.

How is this disorder inherited and what are the chances of further siblings being affected in families with an affected child?

662 Acute intermittent porphyria is the most severe form of hepatic porphyria. Gastrointestinal symptoms occur in 95 per cent of attacks, and include abdominal pain, vomiting and constipation.

What signs may be found in the cardiovascular system in an attack of acute intermittent porphyria?

663 The majority of attacks of acute intermittent porphyria are associated with neurological features. A peripheral neuropathy which is both motor and sensory is common. Foot drop, wrist drop and paraesthesiae of shoulders and hips are often present. Respiratory paralysis may occur.

What central nervous system and psychiatric features may develop?

664 Drugs which may precipitate an attack of acute intermittent porphyria include barbiturates, especially intravenous anaesthetics, oral contraceptives, sulphonamides and alcohol.

How may the diagnosis of acute intermittent porphyria be confirmed?

665 Primary gout is a hereditary condition and the majority of cases have a family history of the disorder. It is infrequent before the age of 40 and in women. It is most unusual in premenopausal women.

What factors may precipitate an acute attack of primary gout?

666 Hyperuricaemia may be induced by certain drugs, including thiazides and frusemide, and small doses of salicylates.

Secondary gout may also be caused by a particular group of diseases. What are these?

667 In 90 per cent of cases of gout, the metatarsophalangeal joint of the big toe is the first joint to be affected in an acute attack. The onset is sudden with severe pain and the joint becomes swollen, hot, red and very tender, features which may suggest pyogenic arthritis or cellulitis. Pyrexia is frequent.

What haematological and biochemical abnormalities may occur during an acute attack of gout?

668 Patients suspected of having gout should always be examined for gouty tophi which may be found in periarticular tissues and in the cartilages of the ear.

What changes in the composition of synovial fluid are typically found in gouty arthritis?

669 A serious complication of gout is the development of uric acid kidney stones which may produce renal colic and chronic renal failure.

What other disorders may accompany untreated chronic gout?

670 Uric acid renal calculi are radiolucent, and therefore do not appear on radiographs.

What radiological changes do occur in gout?

671 Chondrocalcinosis (pseudogout) is a rare familial condition producing intermittent arthritis and effusions in large joints. The effusions contain calcium pyrophosphate crystals which, unlike urate crystals of gout, are positively refractile under polarized light.

What radiological features may be seen in this condition?

672 Severe hypertriglyceridaemia may occur when overproduction and reduced removal of triglycerides coincide.

Such a situation may arise where familial hypertriglyceridaemia coincides with diabetes mellitus and/or heavy consumption of alcohol.

What clinical features may occur with very high serum triglyceride levels (i.e. over 20–25 mmol/l)?

673 Type I glycogen storage disease (von Gierke's disease) is due to deficient glucose-6-phosphatase activity. This leads to accumulation of glycogen in the liver.

Symptoms develop during the first 2 years of life and include failure to thrive, abdominal pain and progressive abdominal enlargement.

What metabolic and haematological features may develop in this disorder?

674 Major complications of galactosaemia include mental retardation, Gram-negative septicaemia and meningitis.

What screening tests are available for this disorder?

675 Galactosaemia is due to absence of galactose-1-phosphate uridyltransferase activity. Early features in the untreated case include neonatal hypoglycaemia, vomiting, failure to thrive, jaundice and hepatomegaly.

What abnormalities may occur in the urine and in the eye?

676 Homocystinuria is an autosomal recessive disorder due to deficiency of the enzyme cystathionine synthetase, leading to accumulation of homocystine and methionine in the tissues and to deficiency of cysteine. This results in impairment of the strength of collagen and elastic tissues.

What skeletal abnormalities are seen in this condition?

677 In homocystinuria downward dislocation of the lens of the eye may occur. This may lead to glaucoma, optic atrophy and blindness. Mental retardation and epilepsy also occur in some cases.

What other inherited condition causing dislocation of the lens of the eye should be distinguished from homocystinuria?

678 Fasting hypoglycaemia usually indicates a definite underlying disease, whereas reactive postprandial hypoglycaemia often occurs in the absence of significant organic disease.

What are the causes of reactive hypoglycaemia and when does it occur?

679 One of the commonest causes of fasting hypoglycaemia is insulinoma.

What other conditions may be associated with fasting hypoglycaemia?

680 Patients with insulinomas characteristically present with drowsiness on waking, which is relieved by food. Symptoms may also occur after exercise. Other features include paraesthesiae and incoordination,

seizures and macropsia (which is an illusion that objects are markedly enlarged). Obesity may occur.
How is the diagnosis confirmed?

681 In McArdle's disease (type V glycogen storage disease), muscle lacks myophosphorylase and there is failure of anaerobic glucose metabolism. After exercise, particularly under ischaemic conditions, pain and cramps usually develop.
What are the biochemical findings apart from abnormal muscle biopsy enzyme assays?

682 The carcinoid syndrome comprises episodic flushing, diarrhoea and bronchospasm due to liberation of serotonin and other humoral agents from carcinoid tumours. Most of these tumours occur in the gut and do not cause symptoms until hepatic metastasis has taken place.
What is the diagnostic laboratory test, and consumption of what foodstuffs can give false positive results?

683 Lactic acidosis can occur in states of severe hypoxaemia but is sometimes due to non-hypoxic causes such as alcoholism. Treatment is with sodium bicarbonate, and large quantities may be necessary.
What risk attaches to infusing large quantities of sodium bicarbonate in the elderly or in the presence of heart failure?

684 Accidental hypothermia due to inadvertent exposure to cold is common in the elderly and in vagrants. Rewarming should be accompanied by intravenous fluids to offset the tendency to peripheral pooling that results from external rewarming.
How may the diagnosis of hypothermia be missed and how may blood gas results be misinterpreted?

685 Hypothermia may occur in normal ambient temperatures when the body's mechanisms for temperature regulation are impaired by disease or by drugs. Examples of disease are congestive cardiac failure, diabetes mellitus, myxoedema and Addison's disease. Drugs include chlorpromazine which has an alpha-blocking action which causes peripheral vasodilation.
What ECG changes may be found in hypothermia?

686 Wilson's disease is an inherited but treatable abnormality of copper metabolism. The main defect appears to be a failure of hepatocytes to excrete copper into bile. Two consequences of this are that plasma

caeruloplasmin levels are low and urinary copper excretion is increased.

What other features are diagnostic?

687 The occurrence of cirrhosis of the liver in a patient under the age of 30 should bring Wilson's disease to mind.

The same also applies to some neurological symptoms and signs. What are they?

688 Estimations of serum total cholesterol and triglycerides may suggest the presence of risk factors for atherosclerotic arterial disease but do not show in what form the lipids are present. For this lipoprotein electrophoresis is necessary. High density lipoprotein (HDL) is high in cholesterol but statistically confers a reduced risk of disease.

What is the composition of the other forms of lipoprotein?

689 Hyperlipoproteinaemia, of which six different patterns have been recognized, may be due to a primary and inherited defect. Much more commonly, however, it is secondary to other conditions. Diabetes mellitus, alcoholism and the oral contraceptive are the most frequent offenders.

What lipoprotein abnormalities occur in these three conditions?

690 Management of secondary hyperlipoproteinaemias consists of removal or vigorous treatment of the provoking condition.

Treatment of primary type 4 hyperlipoproteinaemia, where the predominant abnormality is an increase of very low density lipoproteins (VLDL), initially consists of reducing obesity, reducing carbohydrate consumption and increasing polyunsaturated fats in the diet. Patients who do not improve on these measures may respond to clofibrate.

What is the treatment for type 2 hyperlipoproteinaemia, where the predominant abnormality is an increase of low density lipoproteins (LDL)?

Bone & Calcium Metabolism

691 Vitamin D is ingested in the form of cholecalciferol (or vitamin D_3). This is not the active form of the vitamin and it must undergo hydroxylation in the liver to 25-hydroxycholecalciferol, and further hydroxylation in the kidney before becoming

1,25-dihydroxycholecalciferol which is probably the most active metabolite.

How is 1,25-dihydroxycholecalciferol (1,25-DHCC) thought to affect calcium and bone metabolism?

692 Early clinical features of rickets in an infant include enlarged epiphyses at the lower end of the radius and costochondral junctions (rickety rosary). Areas of softening of the skull (craniotabes) may occur even earlier.

What biochemical features are expected in rickets?

693 If infantile rickets continues into the second or third year of life, bending of bones tends to occur leading to kyphosis, 'bow legs' and knock knees. Pelvic deformities may lead to problems later with childbirth.

What radiological abnormalities may occur in rickets?

694 The earliest evidence of healing in rickets is radiological improvement of the growing ends of bones. Levels of calcium or phosphate in the serum are an unreliable guide to healing.

How is the effect of vitamin D therapy of rickets best monitored?

695 Bone pain, muscular weakness, waddling gait and spontaneous fractures are all features of osteomalacia.

What are the usual causes of osteomalacia in Britain?

696 The major radiological feature of ostomalacia is the finding of Looser's zones or pseudo-fractures which are tongues of radiotranslucency extending about 1 cm into the bone from the surface.

Where are Looser's zones commonly seen?

697 The diagnosis of osteomalacia may be suggested by biochemical findings such as elevated serum alkaline phosphatase, hypocalcaemia or hypophosphataemia.

How may the diagnosis be confirmed?

698 Free access to sunshine with an adequate intake of dairy produce plus administration of fish liver oil when necessary will prevent osteomalacia.

Who should receive particular attention with regard to prophylaxis?

699 Osteoporosis is the commonest metabolic disease of bone and occurs most frequently in elderly women, in whom it is known as postmenopausal osteoporosis. In

these individuals decreased oestrogen production is thought to contribute to development of osteoporosis.
With what other endocrine conditions is osteoporosis associated?

700 In osteoporosis serum calcium, phosphorus and alkaline phosphatase are all within normal limits.
What are the histological appearances of osteoporosis?

701 Fractures following slight trauma are common in patients with generalized osteoporosis. Sites frequently affected are the lumbar and thoracic vertebrae, the femoral neck and the lower end of the radius.
What other conditions may cause painful vertebral deformities?

702 Radiological features of osteoporosis are more marked in the axial skeleton than in the limbs.
What radiological features in the vertebral column suggest osteoporosis?

703 Paget's disease of bone is rare under the age of 50 years but thereafter the incidence increases progressively with age.
What are the biochemical features of Paget's disease?

704 Paget's disease is often asymptomatic and may be found incidentally during radiological examination carried out for some other reason.
What radiological changes suggest Paget's disease?

705 Paget's disease most commonly involves the lumbar spine and pelvis. However femora, tibiae, clavicles and skull may also be involved.
What problems may skull involvement produce?

706 In Paget's disease, incomplete fissure fractures may be found on bowed Pagetic bones. These usually occur on the convex side, and unlike Looser's zones in osteomalacia, they are true fractures which may progress to complete fractures.
What bones are typically the site of pathological fractures in Paget's disease?

707 A rare but definite complication of Paget's disease is osteogenic sarcoma.
What features would suggest this development?

708 In Paget's disease, the skin over affected bones may be unusually warm on palpation.
Why is this? What complication may result?

709 Most cases of hypercalcaemia are asymptomatic and detected on routine estimation of serum calcium. Physical signs of hypercalcaemia are minimal, but one specific sign of hypercalcaemia should be looked for in the eye.

What is this?

710 The commonest cause of hypercalcaemia in a hospital population is malignant disease. In this situation, hypercalcaemia may be due either to bony involvement or to humoral hypercalcaemia of malignancy.

What tumours are commonly responsible for these two types of hypercalcaemia?

711 Hypercalcaemia may produce various symptoms, including generalized weakness, thirst and polyuria. Gastrointestinal symptoms include anorexia, vomiting and constipation.

What symptoms may arise due to the effect of hypercalcaemia on the central nervous system?

712 In both primary hyperparathyroidism and humoral hypercalcaemia of malignancy the serum calcium is elevated and serum phosphorus is low.

How may estimation of serum electrolytes and acid–base status help to distinguish these two conditions?

713 Hyperparathyroidism may present with renal colic due to calculus formation, or with abdominal pain due to peptic ulceration. It may also cause osteitis fibrosa cystica.

What radiological features should be looked for in hyperparathyroidism?

714 The steroid suppression test may be useful in distinguishing hyperparathyroidism from other causes of hypercalcaemia. This test involves comparison of serum calcium before and after a 10 day course of approximately 30 mg of prednisolone daily.

What effect may steroids have on elevated serum calcium in the various conditions causing hypercalcaemia?

715 Vitamin D intoxication produces hypercalcaemia which may be sufficiently severe to cause confusion and coma. The diagnosis may be confirmed by finding very high plasma levels of 25-hydroxyvitamin D and undetectable parathyroid hormone levels.

Does stopping vitamin D administration reverse hypercalcaemia quickly in this situation?

716 Severe hypercalcaemia may be a life-threatening emergency. Correction of dehydration is the single most important measure in management, and large volumes of fluid may be required. Steroids should also be commenced but will take several days to be effective.

What other forms of therapy may be useful in the acute hypercalcaemia?

717 The finding of an abnormal serum calcium level should always be checked by repeating the estimation with the patient fasting, and by omitting a tourniquet, the use of which may produce a falsely elevated value.

What other precaution should be taken when assessing serum calcium?

718 Most patients with chronic renal failure have histological evidence of bone disease which includes osteomalacia, osteitis fibrosa cystica and osteosclerosis.

What biochemical findings in the serum are to be expected in this situation?

719 Idiopathic hypoparathyroidism may occur at any age. It may be associated with antibodies to parathyroid, adrenocortical, thyroid and ovarian tissue, and with endocrine failure of any of these organs.

What clinical, radiological and biochemical features occur in idiopathic hypoparathyroidism?

720 Tetany is due to increased excitability of peripheral nerves as a result of hypocalcaemia or alkalosis.

Symptoms of tetany include cramps in the limbs and paraesthesiae of the extremities. Carpopedal spasm is the usual finding in the adult. Children, in addition, may develop convulsions and laryngismus stridulus.

What are the principal causes of tetany?

Infectious Diseases & Immunization

721 Major causes of pyrexia of unknown origin include tumours (e.g. Hodgkin's disease or hypernephroma), infectious and parasitic disorders (e.g. tuberculosis, typhoid and malaria), connective tissue disorders (e.g. SLE) and drug hypersensitivity (e.g. penicillin). One of the single most useful diagnostic tests in determining the cause of pyrexia of unknown origin is the differential white cell count. Why is this?

722 Important early features of typhoid fever are severe headache and increasing fever. Constipation is usually present in the early stages and there is a relative bradycardia.

The Widal reaction is not the best test with which to confirm a diagnosis of typhoid fever. What is?

723 The rash of typhoid fever usually appears in the second week of illness. It consists of rose spots which usually appear on the upper abdomen and back and which fade on pressure.

What dangerous complications may appear in the third week?

724 Tetanus is caused by the Gram-positive organism *Clostridium tetani* which is a commensal of the human gut and which multiplies under conditions of low oxygen tension such as are found in necrotic wounds.

Tetanus may have to be distinguished from conditions such as perforated peptic ulcer. Why is this?

725 The first symptom of tetanus is trismus, which is a painless spasm of the masseter muscles causing difficulty in opening the mouth. This should be distinguished from the trismus of mumps which is associated with enlarged, tender parotid glands.

Tetanus also causes neck stiffness. How may this be distinguished from the neck stiffness of meningitis?

726 Acute bacterial meningitis usually presents with headache, fever and vomiting. Neck stiffness is the most important physical finding.

The diagnosis is confirmed by finding purulent CSF following lumbar puncture. How may the three common causative organisms be distinguished on examination of a Gram-stained preparation of CSF?

727 Major causative organisms of acute bacterial meningitis are meningococcus, pneumococcus and *Haemophilus influenzae*.

What features would help to distinguish between these on clinical examination?

728 Among the major causes of bacterial food poisoning in the UK are *Salmonella typhimurium* and staphylococci.

How does the pathogenesis of the illness due to these organisms differ?

729 Staphylococcal food poisoning usually produces symptoms within 1–6 hours of ingestion of the toxin. Vomiting is the major symptom. There is no fever and symptoms usually clear within 24 hours.

How does this clinical picture differ from that due to *Salmonella* gastroenteritis?

730 Would you make a diagnosis of plague in a man with a large painless mass of lymph nodes in one axilla and low-grade fever occurring one month after returning from Vietnam?
What is the treatment for plague?

731 Bacillary dysentery has an incubation period of 1–4 days. Diarrhoea is usually the main feature with *Shigella sonnei* and *Campylobacter*, but other organisms such as *Shigella shigae* may produce more severe illness with fever, vomiting, abdominal pain and bloody diarrhoea.
How does this clinical picture differ from that due to amoebic dysentery?

732 The diagnosis of bacillary dysentery is confirmed by cultivating the causative *Shigella* organism from the stool.
How is the diagnosis of amoebic dysentery confirmed?

733 The most frequent and important complication of amoebiasis is the formation of an amoebic abscess in the liver.
What are the major clinical features of this complication?

734 In cases of suspected amoebic liver abscess, the chest should be X-rayed as it may show an immobile, raised right hemidiaphragm. The blood usually shows a polymorphonuclear leucocytosis and a raised ESR.
How may the diagnosis be confirmed?

735 Measles is a highly infectious viral disease. It commences with fever, rhinitis, cough and redness of the conjunctivae (the catarrhal stage). The characteristic rash appears on the fourth day.
What changes may be seen in the mouth prior to the appearance of the rash?

736 Measles is associated with a rash which usually appears four days after the onset of the catarrhal stage. It usually starts behind the ears and at the hairline, spreading to involve the entire skin, including the face.
In a child with such a rash, what other conditions should be considered?

737 Diphtheria is an acute infectious disease due to *Corynebacterium diphtheriae*. The clinical picture

consists of a throat infection and the effects of an exotoxin.

What is seen in the throat and which tissues may be affected by the toxin?

738 Scarlet fever is associated with a punctate erythematous rash which appears 2 days after the onset of fever. The face is characteristically spared, although it may be flushed. This is useful in distinguishing scarlet fever from measles. In addition, Koplik's spots are absent in scarlet fever, but there is usually a follicular tonsillitis and cervical lymphadenopathy present. The tongue has a characteristic strawberry appearance.

How may scarlet fever be distinguished from infectious mononucleosis?

739 The initial catarrhal stage of whooping-cough is associated with conjunctivitis, rhinitis and cough. This is followed by the paroxysmal stage with severe bouts of coughing followed by the characteristic whoop. Cyanosis may occur during cough spasms.

What is the other characteristic feature of these paroxysms, and when are they worst?

740 In whooping-cough the white cell count usually reveals a lymphocytosis.

What are the complications of whooping-cough?

741 Mumps is a viral disease of low infectivity. Thirty per cent of cases are probably asymptomatic and the incubation period is long—18 days. Symptoms include painful trismus, and this may be associated with fever followed by enlargement of one or both parotid glands and possibly the submandibular glands.

What complications may occur? What changes may occur in the CSF?

742 Among the conditions which should be distinguished from mumps is suppurative parotitis. This usually occurs in elderly, ill, febrile or dehydrated patients with poor oral hygiene.

What other conditions cause parotid enlargement?

743 Chickenpox is a highly infectious viral disease, usually affecting children. The rash usually appears on the first day of the illness. There are frequently ulcerative lesions on the palate, and the rash which is maximal on the trunk spreads to involve face and limbs.

What are the complications of chickenpox?

744 The rash of chickenpox is characteristically maximal on the trunk and more sparse peripherally. The axillae are almost always involved. The lesions are superficial, elliptical, thin-walled and unilocular. Later they become pustular. Characteristically they occur in crops at different stages of development.

How may the distribution of the spots help to distinguish the rash of chickenpox from that of smallpox?

745 Malaria is a protozoal infection transmitted from humans to humans by bites from the female anopheline mosquito. Clinical features include fever, seizures, headache, vomiting and joint pains. Splenomegaly, hepatomegaly, and haemolytic anaemia are commonly present.

The most serious form of malaria is that due to *Plasmodium falciparum* in non-immune people. What are the serious complications of *P. falciparum* malaria?

746 The only proof of malaria infection is the finding of malaria parasites in a thin or thick blood film. Parasites may be very scanty in patients who have taken small doses of antimalarial drugs.

What factors are of importance in the therapy of malaria and how long should prophylaxis be continued after leaving a malarious area?

747 Vivax, ovale and malariae malaria differ from falciparum malaria in that they are associated with a persistent form of the parasite in the liver and a tendency to relapse after chloroquine treatment of the acute attack.

How may these relapses be prevented and what precaution should be taken in this situation?

748 Visceral leishmaniasis (kala azar) is a disease of the tropics and subtropics due to infection with the protozoon *Leishmania donovani* which is transmitted by female sandflies, and which multiplies in the reticuloendothelial system.

What changes may be found in the blood in this disease? How may the diagnosis be confirmed?

749 Clinical features of visceral leishmaniasis include fever, wasting and hyperpigmentation. There may be massive splenomegaly, with hepatomegaly to a lesser extent. The patient is frequently anaemic, due largely to hypersplenism.

What other conditions cause massive splenomegaly?

750 Sleeping sickness is due to infection with either *Trypanosoma gambiense* which is a protozoal organism occurring in West and Central Africa, or *Trypanosoma rhodesiense* which occurs in East and Central Africa.

How does the course of the illness vary depending on which of these organisms is responsible? How is the disease transmitted?

751 Following the bite of a tsetse fly infected with the causative trypanosomes of sleeping sickness, a chancre develops 5 or more days later at the site of the bite. About 3 weeks afterwards fever develops and is associated with lymphadenopathy, especially of the posterior triangle of the neck. A circinate rash may appear on the chest and hepatosplenomegaly with myocarditis and tachycardia may develop.

What neurological features may develop? When do they occur?

752 Chagas' disease is due to infection with the protozoal organism *Trypanosoma cruzi*. It is found in South and Central America.

What pathological effects occur in chronic Chagas' disease?

753 Chagas' disease (American trypanosomiasis) is spread to man from cats, dogs and armadillos by reduviid triatomine bugs. Infection develops when the faeces of these bugs is scratched into the skin or rubbed into conjunctiva or mucosa.

How may the diagnosis of Chagas' disease be confirmed?

754 The incubation period of rabies depends on the distance between the site of virus entry and the central nervous system, and also on the amount of virus introduced and on host factors. It ranges from 10 days to 1 year.

What is the treatment for the disease and how may it be prevented?

755 Many cases of acquired toxoplasmosis are asymptomatic. Some cases may suffer an acute febrile illness with pneumonia, myalgia and occasionally a maculopapular rash. Choroidoretinitis and uveitis are recognized features.

What features may be found in more chronic infections?

756 Lepromatous leprosy is the infectious form of the disease. There is no cell-mediated immunity to *Mycobacterium leprae*, and organisms are present in

huge numbers in skin and the reticuloendothelial system.

How does tuberculoid leprosy differ from lepromatous leprosy with respect to immunity?

757 The skin lesions of tuberculoid leprosy are anaesthetic plaques which are hypopigmented in dark skins.

What changes occur in the peripheral nerves in tuberculoid leprosy, and what complications may result from these changes?

758 Tuberculoid leprosy may cause paralysis of the facial nerve. One result of this is a tendency to exposure keratitis due to the inability to blink or close the eye.

What other mechanism may lead to eye damage in tuberculoid leprosy?

759 In contrast to the skin lesions of tuberculoid leprosy, skin macules found in early lepromatous leprosy are not anaesthetic and are smaller, more widely scattered and altogether less conspicuous. They may be hypopigmented.

What changes may appear on the face in lepromatous leprosy?

760 Late complications of lepromatous leprosy include amyloidosis, nephritis and renal failure. Testicular destruction may cause gynaecomastia.

How may the diagnosis of lepromatous leprosy be confirmed?

761 Cholera is a severe diarrhoeal disease due to infection of the small intestine with *Vibrio cholerae*. This organism produces a powerful exotoxin which stimulates adenyl cyclase in the mucosal cells, increasing intracellular cyclic adenosine 3,5-monophosphate which causes a massive outpouring of alkaline small bowel fluid.

What is the clinical course of cholera?

762 Severe cholera is distinguished clinically from other forms of gastroenteritis by the severity of the diarrhoea and the absence of fever, abdominal pain or blood in the stool.

How is the diagnosis of cholera confirmed?

763 Biochemical findings in cholera include hyponatraemia, hypokalaemia and bicarbonate loss in the stool, leading to metabolic acidosis. Acute renal failure may develop as a result of acute circulatory failure.

What is the treatment of severe cholera?

764 Anthrax is spread to man from farm animals. It is an occupational hazard of farmers, butchers and handlers of hide and bone meal.

The primary lesion may be in the skin, upper respiratory tract, lung or intestinal tract.

What complications may occur?

What is the drug of choice in the treatment of anthrax?

765 Infectious mononucleosis or glandular fever is caused by the Epstein–Barr virus. While infection in children is usually asymptomatic, a common picture in adults is pharyngitis and lymphadenopathy. There is a high incidence of ampicillin hypersensitivity.

What are the diagnostic tests and the possible complications of this infection?

766 *Schistosoma haematobium* is a trematode fluke found in Africa and the Middle East. It's life cycle includes a developmental stage inside a fresh water snail. From this snail infectious cercariae are released into water from whence they can penetrate intact human skin.

What is the cardinal symptom of infection with this organism?

767 In schistosomiasis due to *S. haematobium*, inflammation and granuloma formation in the bladder wall may lead to contraction and calcification of the bladder. This may be followed by hydronephrosis, pyelonephritis and renal failure. Bladder calculi may form also.

How is the diagnosis of *S. haematobium* confirmed?

768 Disease caused by *Schistosoma mansoni* is usually more serious than that due to *S. haematobium*. The adult worm of *S. mansoni* makes for the inferior mesenteric vein, and eggs are deposited in the submucosa of the large bowel.

What are the features of the early stage of this infection?

769 Localizing features of *S. mansoni* infection which occur when the adult worms mature include abdominal pain and diarrhoea with blood and mucus in the stool (a form of dysentery). Rectal polyps may form and prolapse during defaecation.

How is the diagnosis confirmed?

770 *Schistosoma japonicum* is found in the Far East and causes a more serious illness than *S. haematobium* or *S. mansoni*. Diagnosis is made by finding the characteristic egg with a lateral knob in the stool.

What major complications occur in this type of schistosomiasis?

771 The Weil–Felix reaction is a serological test for rickettsial antibodies which uses antigens derived from *Proteus* species. The main antigens are OX-19, OX-2 and OX-K.

What are the results of this test in Q fever and in other rickettsioses?

772 Coxsackie and ECHO viruses both belong with polioviruses in the family of enteric viruses because they multiply in the gastrointestinal tract.

Apart from non-specific upper respiratory tract infections and gastroenteritis what other infections do coxsackie and ECHO viruses cause?

773 Epidemic typhus fever is due to infection with *Rickettsia prowazeki*. This is transmitted from man to man by lice. There may be a reservoir of infection in rats.

What are the features of epidemic typhus fever?

774 *Dracunculus medinensis* (Guinea worm) is a nematode which is widespread in the tropics. The adult female inhabits the tissues of the human leg, and discharges larvae from a ruptured vesicle on the skin into fresh water while the host is wading.

How does man contract this infection?

775 Ancylostomiasis or hookworm disease is due to infection with either *Necator americanus* or *Ancylostoma duodenale*.

How is the infection contracted?

776 The main pathological effect of hookworm infestation is the development of iron deficiency anaemia, which may be very severe, especially in malnourished children.

How is a diagnosis of hookworm infestation confirmed?

777 Dengue is a disease widespread in the tropics, especially in coastal areas. It is due to an arbovirus and is transmitted by the mosquito *Aedes aegypti*.

What are the major features of this infection?

778 *Mycoplasma pneumoniae* causes a specific pneumonia which is frequently accompanied by considerable systemic illness. Physical signs in the chest may be slight despite extensive radiological changes.

What complication may develop 2–3 weeks following the respiratory illness?

779 Trachoma is a specific infection of the eyes due to an organism of the *Chlamydia* group known as the 'TRIC' agent (trachoma and inclusion conjunctivitis agent).

Where would one look for early signs of this infection, and how does it cause blindness?

780 Lassa fever is caused by an RNA containing arbovirus and occurs in West Africa where the vector and reservoir is the multimammate rat.

Fever is a major feature of the illness, but obviously in a patient coming from West Africa one should also consider commonplace conditions such as malaria and typhoid fever as a cause of pyrexia.

What features should make one consider the possibility of Lassa fever?

781 Yellow fever is caused by an arbovirus spread to man by bites of infected *Aedes aegypti* mosquitoes. It is endemic in West and Central Africa, and Central and South America. It is rare among indigenous people of endemic areas, suggesting acquired immunity from subclinical infections.

There are four major features which should suggest the diagnosis in non-immune individuals who have been resident in an endemic area.

What are they?

782 *Taenia saginata*, the beef tape worm, is contracted by eating undercooked infected beef. Man is the definitive host.

What is meant by this term? How may this worm be identified in man? In what important respect does this worm differ from *Taenia solium?*

783 Hydatid disease in man is caused by ingestion of ova of *Taenia echinococcus*. These are excreted in the stool of the definitive host which is the dog.

What clinical features are found in hydatid disease of the liver? What investigations are helpful?

784 *Enterobius vermicularis* (the threadworm) is a helminth with a worldwide distribution and it affects mainly children. The female lays ova around the anal orifice and these may reinfect the host or other children, being carried to the mouth on the fingers.

What symptoms may occur? How may the diagnosis be confirmed?

785 Human toxocariasis is due to ingestion of eggs of *Toxocara canis* which are excreted by the definitive host, the dog. Children aged 3–5 years are most commonly affected, due to their habit of eating earth—pica.

What serious problem may arise from this infection?

786 Clinical features of *Strongyloides stercoralis* infection include larva currens which is a creeping, reddish, serpiginous skin eruption. Intestinal symptoms including epigastric pain and intermittent diarrhoea may occur and in severe cases malabsorption and anaemia may develop.

How does the diagnosis of this condition differ from that of intestinal nematode infections?

What iatrogenic complication may arise during treatment of this infection?

787 Trichinosis is due to infection with larvae of *Trichinella spiralis* acquired by eating undercooked pork.

What features may develop?

788 Bancroftian filariasis is due to infection with the nematode *Wuchereria bancrofti*. The adult worms usually reside in the lymphatics and lymph nodes of the inguinal area.

How is the disease transmitted and what is the relevance of the method of transmission to diagnosis?

789 Early features of bancroftian filariasis are recurrent lymphangitis, funiculitis, epididymitis and orchitis with tender, swollen inguinal lymph nodes. Eosinophilia is characteristic.

What are the main late complications?

790 Onchocerciasis, or river blindness, is due to infection with the filarial parasite *Onchocerca volvulus*, which is spread by biting flies of the genus *Simulium*. The most serious complication is blindness due to a combination of keratitis, choroidoretinitis and optic atrophy.

What investigations may be useful in the diagnosis of this condition?

791 In what setting would you think of actinomycosis and to which antibiotic is the causative organism sensitive?

792 There are three main types of poisonous snakes.

Elapids (e.g. cobras, mambas) may produce local skin necrosis or systemic neurotoxicity with ptosis and respiratory paralysis.

Vipers (e.g. European viper, rattlesnake) also produce local skin damage but systemic toxicity includes hypotension and haemorrhagic features.

Sea snakes do not cause local damage but may produce generalized muscle necrosis with myalgia and myoglobinuria.

What are the indications for giving antivenom? What side-effects may occur from its use?

793 Giardiasis is an infection of the upper bowel with the flagellated protozoon *Giardia lamblia*. Most infections are asymptomatic but explosive diarrhoea, abdominal pain, vomiting and weight loss may occur due to malabsorption.

How is the disease transmitted? How is the diagnosis confirmed? What treatment is recommended?

794 It is well known that hepatitis B and hepatitis non-A, non-B may be transmitted by blood transfusion or contaminated needles. Cytomegalovirus and Epstein–Barr virus may also be transmitted by this means.

What non-viral infections are transmitted by this route?

795 The combination of fever, excessive sweating and backache with a history of occupational exposure to cattle, or of drinking raw sour milk, are suggestive of acute brucellosis due to *Brucella abortus*.

What blood picture is commonly found in acute brucellosis?

796 Legionnaires' disease is a form of pneumonia caused by the Gram-negative bacterium *Legionella pneumophila*. Important clinical features are fever, cough, confusion and diarrhoea.

What radiological features occur?

797 In Legionnaires' disease there is usually a polymorphonuclear leucocytosis and frequently a lymphopenia. The ESR is usually raised and hyponatraemia is common.

What treatment is recommended in Legionnaires' disease?

798 Bone pain is the major symptom of acute osteomyelitis. The major sign is bone tenderness. Fever, polymorphonuclear leucocytosis and raised ESR are usual.

What value are X-rays for early confirmation of acute osteomyelitis?

799 Leptospirosis is a cause of infectious jaundice, and in addition may cause renal tubular necrosis (proteinuria, red cells and granular casts in the urine),

meningitis (headache, neck stiffness and an increased number of lymphocytes in the CSF), and myocarditis (tachycardia, hypotension, cardiac failure and cardiomegaly on chest X-ray).

However leptospirosis may present only with features of hepatitis. In this situation, how may it be distinguished from viral hepatitis, and why is it important to make this distinction?

800 Pinta is seen in the United Kingdom in the tertiary stage of the disease as depigmented or atrophic lesions of the skin, often of the legs, accompanied by hyperkeratosis of the soles.

What is the causative organism? In which patients may it be present and what is the clinical significance of the infection?

801 Anti-hepatitis B immunoglobulin is prepared from blood donations and is available only in limited quantities. A major indication for its use is for protection of hospital staff who suffer skin pricks with contaminated needles or instruments. The first dose should be given as soon after the injury as possible—preferably within 48 hours; the second 1 month later.

What other indications exist for use of this immunoglobulin?

802 Whooping-cough is caused by *Bordetella pertussis*. It is a very infectious disease which is spread by droplet infection. Ninety per cent of cases occur under the age of 5 years and there is a significant mortality—mainly in infants under 3 months of age.

Why, then, is it recommended that immunization should commence at 3 months of age?

803 There should be an interval of at least 3 weeks between injection of any two live vaccines. The reason for this is that administration of two live vaccines at shorter intervals, or simultaneously, may impair antibody response to one or both of the vaccines.

What live vaccines are commonly used at present?

804 There is some evidence that pertussis immunization may, on rare occasions, be associated with convulsions, and possibly with brain damage. However, the benefits of pertussis immunization outweigh the dangers.

What conditions contraindicate use of this vaccine?

805 Rubella vaccine is a live attenuated vaccine used in order to prevent the disaster of congenital rubella.

To whom is this vaccine normally offered?

Venereal Diseases

806 Serological tests for syphilis may be positive from the fourth week following infection in untreated cases and are invariably positive by the end of the third month.

What conditions may cause false positive serological tests for syphilis?

807 Syphilis is classified as either early or late. Early syphilis refers to a period of 2 years following infection, or, in the case of congenital syphilis, to the first 2 years of life.

What is the importance of this distinction?

808 Whenever a genital ulcer is discovered, the diagnosis of primary syphilis must be established or excluded.

How may the diagnosis be confirmed in the early stages, before serological tests become positive?

809 Non-specific or lipoidal tests for syphilis include the Wasserman reaction, the Kahn test, the rapid plasma reagin (RPR) test and the automated reagin test (ART).

What are the specific tests for syphilis?

810 Primary syphilis has an incubation period of 10 days to 10 weeks and usually produces a primary chancre on the genitals associated with enlargement of the inguinal lymph nodes. It is essential to note that the chancre is indurated and that both the chancre and the regional lymph nodes are painless.

What are the four cardinal features that may occur in secondary syphilis?

811 Chlamydial organisms are isolated in about 40 per cent of cases of non-specific urethritis (NSU) in the male, and may well be the causative organism.

What are the main features of NSU? What drug is most effective in treatment?

812 The classical description of Reiter's disease comprises a triad of non-specific urethritis, arthritis and conjunctivitis. It is now the commonest cause of acute arthritis in young men.

What changes may be seen in the feet in this condition?

813 Gonorrhoea is caused by a Gram-negative intracellular diplococcus—*Neisseria gonorrhoea*.

Incubation period is 3–10 days. Symptoms in the female include dysuria and vaginal discharge. However, the condition may be virtually asymptomatic in the female. It is important to note that inguinal lymph nodes are not enlarged in this venereal disease.

What complications may occur in females? Is follow-up necessary after treatment?

814 Chancroid or 'soft sore' is a common venereal disease of the tropics. It is caused by the Gram-negative bacillus *Haemophilus ducreyi*.

How does this condition differ clinically from primary syphilis?

815 Infection of the cervix with a herpes virus is a suspected but not proven factor in the development of cervical cancer. Women who have promiscuous sexual contact from an early age are at increased risk of developing cervical cancer.

What advice should one give to such individuals?

Haematology

816 The commonest form of anaemia in the world is iron deficiency anaemia occurring in women of child-bearing age.

Why is this?

817 Iron deficiency anaemia in a middle-aged male is evidence of a serious underlying lesion.

What line of investigation, starting with the simplest tests, should one adopt in such a case, assuming there are no clinical pointers to the location of the underlying lesion?

818 In an anaemic patient, one of the most useful indices for identifying the cause of the anaemia is the mean corpuscular volume (MCV).

Why is this?

819 The commonest cause of microcytic anaemia is iron deficiency. Thalassaemia may also cause a microcytic anaemia.

What are the major causes of normocytic anaemia?

820 Having determined from the MCV that a particular case of anaemia is normocytic, it is useful to look at the white cell and platelet count.

Why is this?

821 The terms megaloblastic anaemia and macrocytic anaemia are not synonymous. Megaloblastic anaemia

implies the finding of megaloblasts in the bone marrow, and is usually due to vitamin B_{12} or folate deficiency.

What does the term macrocytic anaemia mean, and which conditions may cause it?

822 Leucopenia and thrombocytopenia may occur in Addisonian pernicious anaemia. The granulocytes are mature, but their nuclei may be hypersegmented with more than five lobes.

How soon after commencement of therapy may signs of recovery appear in marrow and peripheral blood?

823 Megaloblastic anaemia due to folic acid deficiency is usually due to poor dietary intake possibly combined with conditions causing increased utilization of folate. It is common in tropical countries, in inmates of institutions and in elderly individuals living alone. Pregnancy, lactation and alcoholism may also be associated with folate deficiency.

Which gastrointestinal disorders may be associated with folic acid deficiency?

824 Neutrophil leucocytosis is usually due to infection. However it may also be due to non-infectious factors. What are these?

825 Neutropenia is usually due to viral infection (e.g. influenza, infectious hepatitis, infectious mononucleosis). Some bacterial conditions may also cause it (typhoid fever, brucellosis and staphylococcal or Gram-negative septicaemia).

Which non-infectious factors may cause neutropenia?

826 A raised eosinophil count is always of significance. It may be due to parasitic infections (e.g. *Ascaris lumbricoides, Ancylostoma, Toxocara canis*). Other common causes include drug reactions, extrinsic asthma, atopic eczema and scabies.

Which more serious systemic disorders may cause eosinophilia?

827 Many individuals, especially females, complain of easy bruising. When should these cases be investigated?

828 Henoch–Schönlein purpura occurs in children and young adults. Characteristic features include purpura which usually involves buttocks and extensor surfaces of limbs, abdominal pain with melaena, and joint pains.

What abnormalities may be detected in coagulation studies and platelet count in this condition?

829 The normal platelet count is 150–400 × $10^3/\mu l$. Spontaneous haemorrhage is unusual when the platelet count exceeds 40 × $10^3/\mu l$. It frequently occurs when the count is less than 40 × $10^3/\mu l$, and is usually severe at levels under 10 × $10^3/\mu l$.

What results are expected when bleeding time or coagulation time are tested in cases of thrombocytopenia?

830 In patients with thrombocytopenia or vascular defects, bleeding manifestations tend to occur in the form of spontaneous cutaneous haemorrhage, mucosal haemorrhage and petechiae. Bleeding starts immediately after injury and may continue for several hours but it does not usually recur once it has ceased.

How does bleeding due to coagulation defects differ from the above picture?

831 The occurrence of recurrent bleeding in a male with a family history of haemorrhage in male relatives should lead to consideration of a diagnosis of haemophilia A or haemophilia B (Christmas disease).

Which tests are useful in confirming a diagnosis of haemophilia A?

832 Liver disease may cause bleeding disorders due to coagulation defects. Prolongation of the prothrombin time is the most useful finding in establishing the existence of a coagulation defect in a case of liver disease. What treatment is useful in treating bleeding due to liver disease?

833 The majority of cases of disseminated intravascular coagulation (DIC) are due to either septicaemia, (e.g. Gram-negative or meningococcal), malignancy (e.g. acute promyelocytic leukaemia or prostatic carcinoma) or obstetrical complications (abruptio placentae, amniotic fluid embolism).

What haematological investigations are useful in confirming a diagnosis of DIC?

834 Major indications for splenectomy include idiopathic thrombocytopenic purpura, hereditary spherocytosis, traumatic rupture of the spleen, staging of Hodgkin's disease and some cases of massive splenomegaly causing hypersplenism or severe discomfort.

What complications may follow splenectomy?

835 Beta-thalassaemia is a genetic disorder causing failure to synthesize the β-chains of haemoglobin. It is common in individuals originating in the Mediterranean area, especially Cyprus. Individuals

who are homozygous for β-thalassaemia develop thalassaemia major.

What is the blood picture of thalassaemia major and what findings are expected on haemoglobin electrophoresis?

836 In sickle cell disease, anaemia is treated by regular folic acid supplements. Transfusion should be withheld if possible, unless haemoglobin levels fall below 5 g/dl, due to the problem of iron overload. Obviously iron supplements are strongly contraindicated.

How should painful infarction crises be managed?

837 Acute lymphoblastic leukaemia is a common cause of death from malignant disease in children in Britain. The diagnosis of acute leukaemia should be considered in any child presenting with anaemia, bruising and lymphadenopathy.

What blood picture may be expected in acute lymphoblastic leukaemia?

838 The differential diagnosis of acute leukaemia includes infectious mononucleosis. However, in infectious mononucleosis haemoglobin level and platelet count are usually normal despite the presence of atypical mononuclear cells. In addition the Paul–Bunnell reaction is positive in infectious mononucleosis, but not in leukaemia.

How may another major differential diagnosis, idiopathic thrombocytopenic purpura (ITP), be distinguished from acute leukaemia?

839 One important distinguishing feature of chronic myeloid leukaemia is the finding of the Philadelphia chromosome in the myelocytes. There is a staining reaction of developing granulocytes which helps to distinguish those of chronic myeloid leukaemia from normal granulocytes. What is this?

840 The treatment of choice for patients with aplastic anaemia who are aged less than 30 years is bone marrow transplantation from a histocompatible donor, usually a sibling.

What problems may follow this procedure?

841 Leucoerythroblastic anaemia describes the blood picture in which both normoblasts (immature red cells) and myelocytes (immature white cells) are present in the peripheral blood of an anaemic patient.

Which conditions may cause this appearance?

842 Polycythaemia rubra vera is a rare disease. Seventy-five per cent of cases have palpable splenomegaly. Occasionally it progresses to chronic myeloid leukaemia or myelofibrosis.

What thrombotic and haemorrhagic complications may occur?

843 Secondary polycythaemia (erythrocytosis) is much commoner than polycythaemia rubra vera. It is usually due to hypoxia, e.g. high altitude, or cyanotic congenital heart disease. Occasionally it is associated with tumours (renal, hepatic or cerebellar).

How does the blood picture of secondary erythrocytosis differ from that of polycythaemia rubra vera?

844 The treatment for both polycythaemia rubra vera and secondary polycythaemia is repeated venesection.

An additional treatment for polycythaemia rubra vera is radioactive phosphorus, ^{32}P.

What theoretical risk is associated with ^{32}P?

845 Acute myeloblastic leukaemia predominantly affects adults. It may occur as a fresh disease or may develop as a blast crisis in chronic myeloid leukaemia.

What are the main principles of treatment?

Immunology, Autoimmune Disease & Rheumatology

846 There are two populations of lymphocytes known as B cells and T cells. They are distinguished by their different function and cell membrane receptors.

What are these?

847 Macrophages are an important part of the immune response. They are present in the peripheral blood as monocytes, but also line endothelial surfaces and reside in the liver, lungs, spleen and elsewhere.

What receptors do macrophages carry on their surface and what are their two main functions?

848 There are five classes of immunoglobulin, IgG, IgM, IgE, IgA and IgD. On plasma protein electrophoresis, most of the immunoglobulin is in the gamma band but some may be in the beta band.

What is the basic structure of an immunoglobulin and what role does each part of the molecule play?

849 The main properties of IgG are ability to activate complement, cross the placenta and bind to macrophages. IgG is the most plentiful

immunoglobulin in the blood, the normal level being about 10 g per litre.

What are the main properties of the other classes of immunoglobulin?

850 T lymphocytes, acting together with macrophages, are responsible for cell-mediated immunity. This form of immune response occurs in the delayed hypersensitivity reaction of a positive tuberculin (Mantoux) test.

In which infections and conditions are T cells active?

851 The binding of a lymphocyte with an antigen to which it has previously been sensitized results in the release of a number of substances. What is the nature and function of these?

852 The absence of autoimmunity in the normal individual is the result of immunological tolerance. Autoantibodies can be found in the elderly, however, suggesting that the active mechanisms providing tolerance weaken with time.

How is immunological tolerance maintained and how may it break down?

853 Complement is the name for a group of proteins, which interact in set sequence to produce factors capable of lysing cells, triggering an inflammatory response or initiating the coagulation or fibrinolytic pathways. Complement comprises about 10 per cent of normal plasma proteins.

What is the clinical significance of complement?

854 Complement can be activated either by immune complexes via the classic pathway or by endotoxin (and some other substances) via the alternate pathway. These two pathways differ only in the initial steps but are the same from C3 onwards.

The finding of low levels of complement may mean reduced synthesis but it is more often interpreted as increased consumption. Why are C3 and C4 routinely measured and how would you distinguish between classic and alternate pathway activation?

855 Hereditary angio-oedema has been shown to be due to a deficiency of C1 esterase inhibitor. This permits the inappropriate activation of complement. One of the early products of this process has kinin-like properties and can initiate an episode of oedema.

How is the diagnosis confirmed and what treatment may be effective?

856 Type I or immediate hypersensitivity reactions are mediated by IgE. This antibody is mostly bound to mast cells and its combination with specific antigens triggers mast cell degranulation with release of histamine, serotonin, kinins and slow reacting substance-A. The presence of this form of response can be tested for by controlled exposure to antigens. Inhalation and parenteral testing may be dangerous, but intradermal skin prick testing is safe.

What clinical conditions result from type I reactions?

857 Type II or cytotoxic immune reactions comprise those situations where antibodies combine directly with cells and cause lysis by complement activation. IgG or IgM antibodies are involved. Clinical examples of this are autoimmune haemolytic anaemia, transfusion reactions and Goodpasture's syndrome.

What laboratory test can demonstrate the presence of antibodies to red cells?

858 Type III immune complex-mediated reactions (Arthus type) result from the deposition of immune complexes in vessel walls. Vasculitis is a central feature of the resulting inflammation. Complement activation and macrophage activity both liberate inflammatory mediators.

In what clinical conditions does this form of reaction occur?

859 Type IV cell-mediated immune reactions do not require the presence of antibody. The inflammation and injury result from the liberation of lymphokines following binding of antigen with sensitized T lymphocytes. Apart from tuberculosis, the tuberculin test, transplant rejection and tumour cytotoxicity, what other clinical conditions feature cell-mediated immunity?

860 Antibodies can cause disease or complications by combining with hormones or their receptors.

In Graves' disease antibodies to the thyroid TSH receptor occur and their effect is to stimulate the gland, hence the name long-acting thyroid stimulator or LATS. This situation is unique to Graves' disease. Usually autoantibodies block their target receptors. Can you give an example of this?

861 Immune reactions occur in which both antibody and lymphocyte are involved. Antibody-dependent cell-mediated cytotoxicity (ADCC) is the name for cell lysis brought about by specific IgG combining with cell surface antigens.

What happens next in this type of immune reaction?

862 Immunodeficiency syndromes may be congenital, acquired or iatrogenic. What features do they have in common?

863 IgA deficiency occurs in 1 in 600 people and is the commonest immunodeficiency syndrome. The main features of the syndrome include a high incidence of atopy, severe blood transfusion reactions, chronic respiratory infection and autoimmune disorders.

What is the cause of the severe transfusion reactions?

864 Multiple myeloma is a malignant condition involving plasma cells. It is commonest in the elderly.

What symptoms would suggest this diagnosis?

865 In multiple myeloma, there is often bone tenderness, and fundoscopy may reveal a florid picture of retinal haemorrhages, exudates and dilated retinal veins. Physical examination may be otherwise unremarkable.

What are the distinctive laboratory findings?

866 Radiological changes are of considerable diagnostic importance in multiple myeloma and include punched-out lytic lesions in the skull, vertebrae, pelvis or long bones, pathological fractures, particularly compression fractures of the vertebrae, and generalized osteoporosis.

How can multiple myeloma damage the kidneys?

867 The prognosis in multiple myeloma depends on the tumour cell mass at the time of initiating chemotherapy and on the presence of renal impairment. Response to chemotherapy is variable and also affects prognosis. Survival ranges from a few months to several years.

What forms of treatment are given?

868 Waldenström's macroglobulinaemia commonly presents with anaemia, hyperviscosity symptoms, lymphadenopathy and chronic lymphocytic leukaemia. Renal failure does not occur but a bleeding tendency is often present, due to interference with clotting factors and platelets by the high levels of IgM.

What would you expect to see on fundoscopy? What is the treatment for this condition?

869 Heavy chain diseases are rare abnormalities of immunoglobulin production in which only the Fc portion of the antibody is formed. In gamma heavy

chain disease, in which the abnormality affects IgG, electrophoresis of serum and urine proteins will show a monoclonal band of abnormal protein corresponding to the abnormal heavy chains.

What are the features of alpha heavy chain disease?

870 Amyloidosis should come to mind when a patient with rheumatoid disease, tuberculosis, chronic osteomyelitis or other chronic inflammatory condition develops proteinuria, hepatosplenomegaly, malabsorption or cardiac disease.

What is amyloid?

871 Immune complex diseases tend to have vasculitic skin lesions, arthritis and glomerulonephritis in common, although the size of blood vessel affected by deposition of immune complexes depends on the antigen involved.

What laboratory findings are shared by immune complex diseases?

872 Polyarteritis nodosa is an immune complex disease in which the antigen is often the hepatitis B surface antigen (Australia antigen) and the vessels involved are medium and small arteries.

A variety of clinical features can occur.

Which arteries are commonly involved?

873 There is a variety of small artery and arteriole vasculitis which commonly affects the lungs as well as other parts of the body. Regarded as a form of polyarteritis nodosa, it is also called allergic granulomatosis since the arteritic lesions show granulomas containing giant cells. Eosinophils are found in the lesions and circulating in the peripheral blood.

What are the lung symptoms?

874 Temporal or giant-cell arteritis is a vasculitis affecting medium and large arteries, particularly the temporal arteries. It affects the elderly and making the diagnosis is a matter of some urgency since involvement of the retinal arteries may cause sudden and irreversible blindness. Intracranial arteries may be involved.

What are the characteristic symptoms, signs and laboratory findings?

875 Polymyalgia rheumatica is a disorder of the elderly characterized by aching pain in the muscles of the neck, shoulders, upper arms, hips and thighs. Morning stiffness is very common but joints are not objectively involved. Arterial histology shows a giant-cell

arteritis and the condition is closely related to temporal arteritis.

What laboratory finding is essential to the diagnosis and what is the treatment?

876 Hypersensitivity vasculitis, or small vessel vasculitis, is the commonest form of vasculitis. It affects arterioles, capillaries and venules and lesions of the skin may predominate. Maculopapular lesions, nodules, purpura, erythema multiforme or urticaria may occur. Serosal surfaces may be involved. Henoch–Schönlein purpura is one form of this condition in which skin lesions are recognized but in which systemic disease also occurs.

What do the skin lesions tend to appear and what are the important aetiological factors?

877 In SLE antibodies to several components of cell nuclei are present. These antibodies cause damage by forming immune complexes with their antigens. These complexes are responsible for the disseminated lesions of this disease.

What other immunological abnormalities are present in SLE and what complications result?

878 There is evidence to suggest that all patients with SLE have renal deposition of immune complexes and complement, despite the fact that not all develop signs of renal involvement.

What histological lesion accounts for joint, brain and heart manifestations of SLE?

879 SLE is predominantly a disease of women in their child-bearing years. The alternative name, disseminated lupus erythematosus, draws attention to the intermittent, multisystem nature of the disease.

The five commonest manifestations are arthritis and arthralgias, fever, skin lesions (butterfly rash), lymphadenopathy and renal involvement.

What features distinguish SLE from other causes of arthritis and nephritis?

880 In SLE arthritis may respond to non-steroidal anti-inflammatory drugs, including aspirin.

For what features of SLE are steroids indicated?

881 The HLA system of surface antigens appears to be the main determinant of histocompatibility. It is customary to try to match as many antigens as possible in organ transplantation.

In what other way is the HLA system of clinical interest?

882 In joint diseases much diagnostic information can be obtained from examining the synovial fluid. After noting the appearance of the fluid and the occurrence of any clot, the main laboratory tests on the synovial fluid are microscopy for cell count, microscopy with polarized light for crystals and glucose estimation. A simultaneous blood glucose estimation should be obtained.

What findings indicate septic arthritis?

883 In rheumatoid arthritis, the most commonly involved joints in the upper limbs are the metacarpophalangeal, proximal interphalangeal and the wrist joints. Symmetrical involvement with morning stiffness is a common presentation.

Would you consider rheumatoid disease in a patient presenting with arthritis of one knee?

884 Rheumatoid factor is an antibody against IgG immunoglobulin. It may consist of IgM, IgG or IgA, but routine laboratory assay usually estimates IgM rheumatoid factor. This factor is not specific for rheumatoid disease, nor does it correlate with the activity of the disease. Nevertheless it is usually present at some stage of the illness.

With which two extra-articular manifestations of rheumatoid disease is the presence of rheumatoid factor closely associated?

885 In the treatment of rheumatoid disease, corticosteroids are contraindicated with the possible exception of temporarily tiding a patient over a severe exacerbation of the illness.

What are the main forms of treatment available for rheumatoid disease?

886 Ankylosing spondylitis mainly affects young men and usually involves the sacroiliac joints. The common presenting symptom is low back pain which may be worse at night.

What are the radiological changes of sacroiliitis?

887 Patients with ankylosing spondylitis are seronegative, i.e. rheumatoid factor is not present. The majority of patients with ankylosing spondylitis carry the HLA B27 histocombatibility antigen, as do many patients with Reiter's syndrome, psoriatic spondylitis and the arthritis that accompanies inflammatory bowel disease.

What ocular, cardiovascular and renal conditions may occur in ankylosing spondylitis?

888 The sicca syndrome consists of the combination of keratoconjunctivitis sicca with xerostomia, i.e. loss of tears and saliva. It may occur in sarcoidosis. The combination of the sicca syndrome with an autoimmune or collagen vascular disease (most commonly rheumatoid disease) is known as Sjogren's syndrome.

What does labial gland histology reveal in Sjogren's syndrome and what are the possible consequences of the sicca syndrome?

889 Like ankylosing spondylitis, Reiter's syndrome typically affects young men who carry HLA B27. It tends to occur either following sexual exposure or after a dysentric infection with *Shigella* or *Salmonella* bacteria.

What are the features of the syndrome?

890 A small minority of patients with psoriasis develop arthritis. There are several different variants of psoriatic arthritis. In one form, arthritis of the distal interphalangeal joints accompanies psoriasis of the nails. In another, acute inflammation of a toe joint may mimic acute gout, with hyperuricaemia as a further point of similarity.

What other forms of psoriatic arthropathy are there?

891 Arthritis of the knees or ankles or spondylitis can accompany ulcerative colitis and Crohn's disease, particularly when other extra-intestinal features are present.

The spondylitis is indistinguishable from ankylosing spondylitis except in one respect.

What is this?

892 Behçet's syndrome consists of orogenital aphthous ulceration with uveitis or other ocular inflammatory lesions. It can occur at any age and is commoner in men.

What other features occur in Behçet's syndrome?

893 Scleroderma, also known as progressive systemic sclerosis, is characterized histologically by inflammation of small arteries and diffuse fibrosis.

A common presentation is the CRST syndrome.

What do these letters stand for?

894 Death from scleroderma usually results from renal involvement.

Which other internal organs are commonly involved in scleroderma?

895 Osteoarthritis is a wear-and-tear phenomenon. Other factors, including heredity, play a part in its aetiology. Diabetes mellitus, acromegaly and damage to joint surfaces, especially aseptic necrosis of the femoral head, all predispose to osteoarthritis.

What are the radiological features of osteoarthritis?

Muscle Disorders

896 Pseudohypertrophic (Duchenne type) muscular dystrophy is an X-linked recessive disorder, and therefore occurs almost exclusively in males. It is usually first noticed during the first 3 years of life, starting in the pelvic girdle and legs. It is the commonest genetic myopathy and actually commences *in utero*.

What is the natural history of this disorder?

897 Children with Duchenne type muscular dystrophy have a waddling gait, and, when rising from a supine position, tend to roll into a prone position and then use their arms to push themselves up.

What blood test may provide useful diagnostic information in this disease?

898 Myotonic dystrophy is an autosomal dominant disorder of variable expression. It usually appears during the twenties. There is ptosis plus wasting and weakness of facial, sternomastoid and limb muscles, distal areas being more severely affected in the limbs. Myotonia is manifest by difficulty in relaxing the grip and also occurs on percussion of muscles.

What non-muscular features are commonly present?

899 Polymyalgia rheumatica usually occurs in the elderly and it causes muscular pain and stiffness which is usually worse on waking. Fever and weight loss may be associated.

Which blood test is useful in diagnosis? Which serious condition may be associated with polymyalgia rheumatica, and what is the treatment?

900 Polymyositis-dermatomyositis is usually a disease of insidious onset associated with progressive muscular weakness. Skin manifestations include a heliotrope violaceous periorbital rash and erythematous plaques over cheeks, trunk and extensor surface of limbs.

What serious condition may underly polymyositis-dermatomyositis?

901 Ninety per cent of cases of generalized myasthenia gravis have serum antibodies to acetylcholine

receptors. Some cases also have antistriated muscle antibody.

If this latter antibody is absent what can one infer about a case of myasthenia gravis?

902 In myasthenia gravis weakness of skeletal muscle develops following exertion. Frequently ocular muscles are involved first, and this causes diplopia or ptosis.

What other muscles may be involved?

903 Immune disorders associated with myasthenia gravis include rheumatoid arthritis, SLE, thyrotoxicosis, Hashimoto's disease, pernicious anaemia and diabetes mellitus.

Which conditions may exacerbate the symptoms of myasthenia gravis?

904 Familial periodic paralysis is characterized by attacks of severe muscular weakness and flaccidity, often occurring after heavy exercise or a heavy carbohydrate meal. Attacks usually start in adolescence and in the common variety they are associated with hypokalaemia.

What is malignant hyperthermia?

905 Endocrine disorders associated with proximal myopathy include hyperthyroidism and Cushing's syndrome. Steroid therapy may also cause a myopathy.

What metabolic bone disease may be accompanied by myopathy? How may this myopathy present and what blood test is useful in diagnosis?

Dermatology

906 A macule is a discoloured skin lesion which is not raised above the skin surface and which is not more than 1 cm in diameter. A papule is a solid raised skin lesion not more than 1 cm in diameter. A nodule is a solid raised skin lesion which exceeds 1 cm in diameter.

What is (a) a vesicle; (b) a bulla; (c) a pustule?

907 The commonest cause of bullae of the skin is burns or scalds.

What infectious conditions may cause vesicular or bullous lesions?

908 Pemphigus vulgaris is a disease characterized by a bullous skin eruption, and in 90 per cent of cases by involvement of the mucous membrane of the mouth in the bullous process.

In what age group does this disease commonly occur? How may the diagnosis be confirmed?

909 The Stevens–Johnson syndrome consists of cutaneous erythema multiforme with ulceration of the mucosae including the mouth, nose, eyes and genital orifices. Severe cases may be associated with fever and prostration.
What drugs may precipitate this condition? What treatment may be necessary in severe cases?

910 Light sensitivity occurs in albinism, pellagra and various porphyrias. Features of light sensitivity include erythema on exposure to sunlight, followed by vesiculation and bulla formation in severe cases.
What drugs may cause light sensitivity?

911 A telangiectasis is a cluster of dilated capillaries and venules. They are a common feature of liver disease, in which they occur on the face and chest.
Which collagen disorders involving the skin may be associated with telangiectases?

912 Erythema nodosum in association with bilateral hilar lymphadenopathy is virtually diagnostic of sarcoidosis. However, certain drugs and bacterial infections may cause erythema nodosum without hilar adenopathy.
What are these?

913 Both SLE and dermatomyositis may produce erythema of the dorsal aspects of the fingers.
How does the pattern of this erythema differ between the two disorders?

914 Psoriasis is a disorder in which epidermal cell turnover is increased, causing epidermal thickening and scaling. Elbows and knees are commonly involved and lesions are frequently symmetrically distributed.
Does itching usually occur? Does scalp involvement occur?

915 Pitting or more severe dystrophy of the nails is frequent in psoriasis.
What is psoriatic arthropathy?

916 Psoriasis may be associated with a pustular eruption on the palms and soles. Blackish hyperkeratosis of palms and soles may be seen in chronic inorganic arsenical poisoning.
What venereal conditions may be associated with palm and sole lesions?

917 Atopic eczema is a familial inflammatory disorder of the skin affecting 1–3 per cent of the population. Itching is severe and prolonged excoriation and exudation may be followed by lichenification.

Which areas of the skin are mainly affected? What is the natural history of this disorder?

918 Lichen planus is a skin disease of uncertain aetiology which affects the sexes equally. The individual lesions are shiny flat-topped papules which occur in groups.

Where are these lesions commonly seen? Is pruritus a feature?

919 Dermatitis herpetiformis is a fairly uncommon condition which affects young adults. It usually presents with an extremely itchy vesicular eruption involving the back, sacral area, buttocks and elbows.

What changes in the gastrointestinal tract are frequently associated with dermatitis herpetiformis?

920 Impetigo is a skin infection of children characterized by superficial blisters which rupture to produce a yellow crust overlying a lesion with a finely crenated rim.

Which skin areas are usually involved? What is the usual causative organism?

921 Tinea corporis (ringworm of the trunk or limbs) is common. The usual lesion it produces is a reddish papular circinate lesion with an advancing border and healing centre. Pruritus may be troublesome.

How should the diagnosis be confirmed?

922 A 28-year-old woman complains of an itchy papular rash affecting her hands, forearms and breasts. Itching is worse at night. Her husband and one of her children complain of similar symptoms.

What is the most likely diagnosis? What is the treatment?

923 Common causes of severe pruritus are scabies and drug allergies.

Which generalized disorders may be associated with pruritus?

924 Endocrine disorders which may cause alopecia include hypothyroidism. It may also result from SLE.

Which drugs may cause alopecia? What other iatrogenic cause of alopecia exists, apart from drugs?

925 Endocrine disorders are important causes of hyperpigmentation of the skin. These include

Addison's disease and Cushing's syndrome. Pregnancy and oral contraceptives may also cause pigmentation.
What other serious disorders may produce pigmentation?

926 Vitiligo consists of irregular sharply demarcated patches of depigmentation of the skin. It may run in families.
Which autoimmune disorders may accompany vitiligo

927 Malignant melanoma is one of the most malignant of all cancers. It may arise in a pre-existing pigmented naevus, or mole, or it may arise in apparently normal skin, or beneath the nails.
What features may suggest malignant change in a pre-existing mole?

928 Basal cell epithelioma is the most common form of skin cancer. A 'rodent ulcer' is the most frequent variety of this and appears as a crusted sore which fails to heal.
Where is this lesion usually situated? How does it spread?

929 Acanthosis nigricans is a velvety rough thickening and hyperpigmentation of the skin of flexures, palms and soles.
What is the significance of this condition in children and in adults?

930 The appearance of firm nodules on the skin, in the absence of any other skin lesion should make one consider metastatic malignant disease.
Which malignant conditions commonly metastasize to the skin?

Iatrogenic Disease

931 Following partial gastrectomy over 50 per cent of patients develop iron deficiency anaemia.
Why is this?

932 Following partial gastrectomy the incidence of megaloblastic anaemia is about 7 per cent. This is usually due to vitamin B_{12} deficiency.
What is the mechanism of this B_{12} deficiency?

933 Some time following a partial gastrectomy a patient may complain of bone pain, especially in the back or pelvis. Pseudofractures may be seen on the pubic rami and serum alkaline phosphatase may be elevated, with a low serum calcium and phosphorus.

Which sequence of events is likely to cause this situation?

934 Drugs are responsible for up to 10 per cent of all hospital cases of jaundice. The most frequent mechanism by which they cause jaundice is by a hypersensitivity reaction, which is not dose-dependent. In the majority of cases, the jaundice is obstructive (cholestasis).

What drugs cause hypersensitivity cholestasis?

935 A 60-year-old man has had treatment with clindamycin for a serious anaerobic lung abscess which had not responded to penicillin therapy. Two weeks later he complains of severe diarrhoea.

How may this development relate to the therapy used?

936 The safest antibiotics to use in pregnancy are penicillins, cephalosporins and aminoglycosides. There have been no reports of fetal abnormality following their use. Tetracyclines are contraindicated in pregnancy.

Which other antibiotics should not be used in pregnancy?

937 A 60-year-old man presents with weakness, purpura and a necrotic ulcer in the throat. Full blood count reveals pancytopenia. A full drug history is essential.

What drugs in particular should one enquire about? What is the prognosis of drug-induced pancytopenia?

938 A 21-year-old girl presents with marked facial hirsutism. On history taking she admits to being on treatment for grand mal epilepsy for the past 10 years.

How may these two facts be related?

939 A 40-year-old man whose sputum was found to be positive for tubercle bacilli 8 weeks previously, and who is now on chemotherapy, complains of difficulty in seeing television.

How may the new complaint be related to the fact that he is on treatment for tuberculosis?

940 A 30-year-old woman is finishing a course of tetracycline prescribed for mycoplasmal pneumonia. She now complains of severe vaginal itching and discharge. She has also been on anovulants for the past 2 years.

What is the likely cause of her vaginal symptoms?

941 A 35-year-old man presents at an endocrine clinic with a goitre first noted 6 months previously. Clinically he

is euthyroid. On questioning he admits to having had psychiatric treatment for the past 5 years.

How may this latter fact be related to the presenting complaint?

942 A 50-year-old man has had insulin-dependent diabetes for 20 years. His control has always been somewhat 'brittle', but he has usually managed to avoid losing consciousness as a result of hypoglycaemia by taking glucose sweets when symptoms occur. During the past month, however, he has had three hypoglycaemic blackouts, without warning. Shortly before that he started treatment for hypertension.

In what way may the antihypertensive therapy relate to his blackouts?

943 All aminoglycosides are ototoxic. Streptomycin causes more damage to the vestibular apparatus while kanamycin affects mainly the auditory component. Other commonly used aminoglycosides include gentamicin, tobramycin and amikacin.

What precautions should be taken during aminoglycoside therapy?

944 A few hours following a thyroidectomy, a patient finds that he is hoarse. He is initially reassured that some hoarseness always occurs due to endotracheal intubation. A few days later, however, the hoarseness is still present.

What is the likely cause?

945 Following a hip replacement operation for severe osteoarthritis, a patient develops pain in the leg, numbness in the foot and foot drop on the same side as the surgery.

What is the likely cause of these symptoms and signs?

946 A young adult sustains a severe head injury and is ventilated by intermittent positive pressure ventilation (IPPV) to reduce arterial $P\text{CO}_2$ and thereby diminish cerebral vasodilatation.

Inadvertently an inspired fraction of oxygen ($F_{\text{i}}\text{O}_2$) of 60 per cent is given and is not reduced despite high arterial oxygen tensions. After a few days his arterial $P\text{O}_2$ is noted to be dropping.

What is the possible cause of this fall in $P\text{O}_2$?

947 A 35-year-old woman presents with tetany and convulsions. Examination reveals a surgical scar at the base of the neck and blood tests show a low calcium, raised phosphate and no evidence of renal impairment.

What is the significance of the scar at the base of the neck?

948 Following a year-long history of gradually increasing weakness of the right leg in a 60-year-old man, a large benign intracerebral meningioma is detected and removed surgically. After surgery, weakness of the leg remains. Some months later he develops epilepsy.
Could this epilepsy be related to his neurosurgery?

949 A 50-year-old man with chronic lung disease is admitted with severe abdominal pain of sudden onset and the physical signs of a gastric perforation.
What connection could there be between the perforation and his chronic lung disease?

950 A 70-year-old woman is found to have temporal arteritis. A few months after starting steroid therapy she is admitted to hospital with a stroke.
Her stroke was probably due to cerebrovascular disease and the cerebral arteries may have been involved in the arteritic process.
Which other factor, however, may have contributed?

951 A 60-year-old woman on long-term steroid therapy for ulcerative colitis is admitted to hospital with pain and immobilization due to vertebral collapse. X-rays show severe osteoporosis which has probably resulted from steroid therapy in a postmenopausal patient.
In what way can this adverse effect of steroids be minimized?

952 Some patients on corticosteroids for longer than a few months develop a myopathy affecting the proximal musculature. Raising the arms and getting up from sitting or squatting positions becomes impossible. Steroid withdrawal leads to recovery within a few weeks.
Which blood tests are abnormal in steroid myopathy?

953 Both retropubic prostatectomy and colectomy are quite commonly followed by impotence in men.
What is the reason for this?

954 Men commonly suffer from impotence as a result of treatment for hypertension. No drug is free of this adverse effect.
What are the probable reasons why few patients actually complain of this problem?

955 At the age of 30, a businessman is advised to take a diet high in polyunsaturated fats in order to reduce a

slightly elevated serum cholesterol. Five years later he begins to develop attacks of colic in the right upper quadrant.

What is the likely cause for his attacks of pain?

956 A 55-year-old man undergoes laparotomy for a benign intra-abdominal condition. Postoperatively he develops paralytic ileus and despite careful attention to fluid and electrolyte balance, he is not able to start light oral feeding before the fifth postoperative day. On the seventh postoperative day, wound dehiscence and a general deterioration in his condition occur due to septicaemia. His oral intake becomes negligible, and fluid input is maintained throughout a protracted convalescence by the intravenous route. His wound heals very slowly.

Which iatrogenic deficiency states may have contributed to his slow progress?

957 A prerequisite for coronary artery bypass graft surgery is coronary angiography. This investigation carries a morbidity and mortality which are greater in the presence of significant coronary artery disease.

What is the mortality rate for coronary angiography, and which complications can occur?

958 Deep venous thrombosis and pulmonary embolism are complications of hospitalization.

What is the reason for this?

959 A hospital with a coronary care unit can offer myocardial infarction patients a good chance of resuscitation from arrhythmias. Conversely, patients with undiagnosed chest pain admitted for observation may be led to think that they have heart disease by the profusion of ECGs, monitoring, blood tests, observations and the special atmosphere of the coronary unit.

Even a clear statement of health on discharge may not be sufficient to over-ride the anxieties aroused by hospitalization and investigation. This anxiety may subsequently produce symptoms of heart disease.

What is the name for this condition?

960 Considerable patient anxiety and also lack of patient cooperation commonly result from a failure to explain to the patient the important essentials of what is happening to him in hospital.

Which aspect of doctors' traditional ward routine is inadvertently a frequent source of anxiety and confusion to the patient?

961 Recurrent bleeding from oesophageal varices is an indication for surgery to reduce portal hypertension. One operation for this is portocaval shunting.

What is the incidence of hepatic encephalopathy following this operation?

962 A 30-year-old woman suffers from extensive psoriasis. During a severe relapse with little response to local applications, a decision is made to give a course of methotrexate.

What question must be asked (or test performed) before this is given?

963 A patient with some degree of renal impairment develops jaundice due to common bile duct obstruction and undergoes surgery for removal of an obstructing gall stone. Postoperative wound infection and a deterioration in renal function lead to a prolonged period of hospital care. During this time, he requires intravenous fluids.

At a later date, renal function deteriorates further and haemodialysis is decided upon. The patient is found to have no patent veins in the forearms, considerably hampering vascular access and jeopardizing satisfactory dialysis.

How could these dialysis difficulties have been avoided?

964 Some months after successful abdominal surgery a patient presents with vomiting and signs of intestinal obstruction.

In what way could these symptoms and signs be related to the previous surgery?

965 Percutaneous needle biopsy of the kidneys and of the liver has become an important investigation for diagnostic purposes and for assessing response to therapy.

What is the main complication of needle biopsy?

Poisoning & Overdoses

966 Paraquat is a widely used and very effective weedkiller. It is, however, extremely toxic when ingested by mouth in its concentrated form. This has occurred accidentally when it has been inappropriately stored in lemonade bottles, but the majority of cases of fatal poisoning have been suicidal.

What are the toxic effects of paraquat?

967 Effects of severe barbiturate poisoning include coma, hypotension, anuria and respiratory depression. Artificial ventilation may be necessary.

(a) How may the need for artificial ventilation be assessed? (b) Is forced alkaline diuresis useful in barbiturate poisoning?

968 Methanol is not a particularly toxic substance intrinsically but it is metabolized in the body into extremely toxic products—formaldehyde and formic acid. As little as 25 ml of methanol may be lethal. Blindness is a sequel of sublethal doses.

What are the features of acute methanol poisoning?

969 The major toxic effect of acute paracetamol poisoning is liver damage. A dose in excess of 25 grams is likely to be fatal. There is, however, an antidote available which is effective in preventing liver damage when given early.

What is this?

970 Gastric lavage is effective in removing ingested poisons when carried out within 4 hours of ingestion of most poisons. However, in the case of salicylate, atropine or antidepressant poisoning it is worthwhile removing the stomach contents 12 hours or more after ingestion.

What precautions are necessary in the use of gastric lavage?

971 Severe salicylate poisoning is a potentially fatal condition. But mortality should be kept very low by the efficient application of the techniques of gastric lavage and forced alkaline diuresis.

What metabolic disturbances occur in severe salicylate poisoning?

972 Overdosage with narcotic or opioid drugs such as heroin, morphine, pethidine or methadone produces a triad of features, namely coma, respiratory depression and miosis (pupillary constriction).

What antidote is available for this form of poisoning?

973 Features of cyanide poisoning include an odour of bitter almonds, shock, hypoventilation, a pink colour of the skin and widely dilated pupils.

What antidote is available for cyanide poisoning?

974 Tricyclic antidepressant overdosage is a common problem. Toxic effects include dryness of the mouth, dilation of the pupils, sinus tachycardia, cardiac arrhythmias and hyper- or hypotension. Acidosis, respiratory depression and convulsions may also occur.

What are the important aspects of management of this form of poisoning?

975 Accidental poisoning with iron tablets is common in small children. It produces a haemorrhagic gastroenteritis, and in severe cases, shock. Later, coma, convulsions, liver necrosis and metabolic disturbances such as acidosis may occur.
What is the treatment for iron poisoning?

976 Carbon monoxide gas is an extremely dangerous poison. It is an odourless gas but its presence may be suspected by smelling coal gas in the breath of a comatose patient.
What are the clinical features of carbon monoxide poisoning and how may the diagnosis be confirmed?

977 Organophosphorus insecticides such as parathion may be absorbed through the skin or lungs. Their toxic effects include constriction of the pupils, bradycardia, salivation, vomiting, diarrhoea and colic and excessive bronchial secretions.
How do organophosphorus compounds cause these effects?

978 Solvent abuse is now a common and serious problem among teenagers. Substances 'sniffed' include glue, petrol, chlorinated hydrocarbons (including dry cleaning agents) and fluorinated hydrocarbons which are present in aerosol cans.
What features may suggest solvent abuse in a particular individual?

979 Most household products are of low toxicity if ingested and cause little more than some nausea, vomiting, diarrhoea or abdominal cramps. However, some such products are very toxic and may lead to fatalities.
Which are these?

980 Features of chronic lead poisoning include abdominal pain and constipation, and a blue line on the gums. Neurological problems include an encephalopathy with convulsions, plus a peripheral motor neuropathy which may cause wrist or foot drop.
What haematological and radiological changes may occur?

Genetics

981 The best known X-linked recessive condition is haemophilia. Others include Christmas disease, glucose-6-phosphate dehydrogenase deficiency and pseudohypertrophic muscular dystrophy (Duchenne).

These conditions usually affect males and are transmitted by healthy female carriers.

Why is this?

982 The commonest autosomal recessive trait in Western Europe is cystic fibrosis. It affects approximately one birth in every 2000.

What are the characteristic features of autosomal recessive inheritance?

983 A numerical abnormality of chromosomes where one or more chromosomes is lost or gained is referred to as 'aneuploidy'. Turner's syndrome is one example of aneuploidy. In this syndrome one X chromosome is missing, resulting in a total complement of 45 chromosomes and an XO sex chromosome constitution.

What are the salient features of Turner's syndrome?

984 The first sex chromosome aneuploidy described in humans was Klinefelter's syndrome. Affected individuals are males and they have an extra X chromosome which results in a total of 47 chromosomes with an XXY sex chromosome constitution.

What are the features of Klinefelter's syndrome?

985 A dominant trait is manifest in heterozygous individuals. The individual exhibiting an autosomal dominant trait may have both the normal gene and the mutant gene. The effect of the dominant mutant gene, unlike that of a recessive mutant gene is expressed in the individual despite the presence of an accompanying normal gene.

Explain the usual pattern of inheritance in autosomal dominant conditions, naming three such conditions.

986 Occasionally an individual carrying a dominant mutant gene may not manifest any of its effects. The gene is then said to be non-penetrant and may appear to 'skip' generations in certain affected families.

Describe the features of tuberous sclerosis (epiloia) which is one such condition.

987 The Philadelphia chromosome (Ph^1) is an acquired chromosomal disorder associated with chronic myeloid leukaemia.

What exactly is the Philadelphia chromosome?

988 Many disorders 'run in families' without necessarily following the Mendelian laws of dominant and recessive inheritance. These disorders, which include hypertension, coronary artery disease and diabetes

mellitus, are said to be inherited on a multifactorial basis. Both genetic and environmental factors are involved.

It is clear that different relatives may experience different environments.

Which property of genes provides an explanation for varying disease experience amongst different generations of the same family?

989 Drug metabolism is an area of clinical medicine where genetics and heredity play a role. Some adverse effects have a known genetic explanation, e.g. haemolysis in G6PD deficient individuals, due to sulphonamides, salicylates and other drugs.

Slow acetylation and pseudocholinesterase deficiency are both genetically determined by autosomal recessive inheritance.

What are the consequences of slow acetylation and pseudocholinesterase deficiency respectively?

990 When faced with the risk of passing on an inherited disorder to their children, prospective parents may request genetic counselling, amniocentesis and termination of pregnancy.

A healthy husband and wife consult you with regard to the risk to their future children having sickle-cell disease. Both have a family history of sickle-cell anaemia.

What advice and management can you offer this couple?

Nutrition

991 It is unwise to prescribe vitamin preparations widely and in high dosage without definite indications. For example an excess intake of vitamin D may cause hypercalcaemia. Some vitamin K analogues may cause hyperbilirubinaemia and kernicterus in neonates.

How may an excess of vitamin A or C be harmful?

992 Kwashiorkor is a form of protein–calorie malnutrition, the essential feature of which is deficiency of protein with a relatively adequate calorie intake. It occurs in developing countries in children aged 1–4 years following weaning, and is more frequent in rural areas.

What clinical features would suggest kwashiorkor? What is the mortality rate in this condition?

993 Epidemiological studies have shown that the addition of fluoride up to 1 part per million (p.p.m.) to drinking water in areas where it is lacking, produces a definite

reduction in dental caries in individuals who start drinking it during childhood.

However, in some areas of the world, such as parts of South Africa, the water supply contains over 10 p.p.m. of fluoride, and in these quantities it may be toxic.

What features may occur in chronic fluoride poisoning?

994 Eye changes are an important feature of vitamin A deficiency. Among these is 'night blindness' which is due to deficiency of rhodopsin (visual purple) on which vision in poor light depends.

How may the conjunctiva and cornea be affected by vitamin A deficiency?

995 Scurvy is rare nowadays in Britain but is occasionally seen in elderly men living alone in poor circumstances. The basic abnormality is defective collagen formation due to lack of vitamin C.

What are the principal features of scurvy?

996 Korsakoff's psychosis consists of an acute psychiatric state with disorientation, faulty memory, confabulation, delusions and abnormal behaviour.

What is the usual cause of this disorder and describe the features of the encephalopathy which is frequently associated with this condition?

997 Beriberi is due to vitamin B_1(thiamine) deficiency which leads to incomplete metabolism of carbohydrates with accumulation of pyruvic and lactic acid in the tissues. These metabolites cause peripheral vasodilatation which may be so marked that fluid leaks through capillaries, causing oedema.

What are the clinical features of wet beriberi?

998 In some instances of beriberi, oedema is absent and in this situation the condition is described as dry beriberi.

What features suggest this condition?

999 Pellagra is due to niacin deficiency and occurs in individuals who subsist chiefly on maize. It is occasionally seen in chronic alcoholics, patients with renal failure on very low protein diets, and in malabsorptive states.

Pellagra has been called the disease of the 'three Ds'.

What are the 'three Ds'?

1000 Causes of angular stomatitis include ill-fitting dentures with associated candidiasis. It may also be due to deficiency of iron and B vitamins including niacin, pyridoxine and riboflavin.

Which nutritional deficiencies cause glossitis?

1001 Milk has a very small vitamin D content, as does lean meat. Cereals, vegetables and fruit contain none.

What are the chief dietary sources of vitamin D?

1002 Intravenous feeding, also called total parenteral nutrition, should be considered when a patient has been unable to take food for one week.

What is the average daily calorie requirement for an afebrile patient to maintain a steady weight? How much is this requirement increased if the patient has a septicaemia or a temperature of 40 °C?

1003 Amino acids given intravenously in parenteral nutrition are not incorporated in protein synthesis unless given together with an energy supply, either sugar or fat. Potassium, magnesium and phosphate are also required to achieve protein synthesis and tissue formation.

What are the more commonly used preparations of sugar and fat for intravenous feeding and what advantages does either have?

1004 Vitamins and minerals must be included in intravenous feeding regimens. A reasonable vitamin supplementation regimen includes vitamin B complex and vitamin C given daily, vitamins A and D every second day, folic acid once weekly, and vitamin K and B_{12} every 3 weeks.

Zinc, copper and chromium are important trace elements.

What are the consequences of zinc deficiency?

1005 Unconscious or paralysed patients often need feeding by nasogastric tube. In postoperative or critically ill cases nasogastric feeding may follow a period of a week or more without food.

What happens to the gastrointestinal tract and the pancreas during even such short periods of starvation and what may be the initial result of feeding, especially if a concentrated, complete food is used?

Multisystem Disorders

1006 A 14-year-old boy suffers from arthritis of the ankles and knees. He describes a recurring pattern of pain, swelling and bruising of these joints some hours after football or other vigorous exercise. These acute signs settle within a few days.

What fact would you want to know about any tooth extractions or other minor surgery in the past, and what is the probable diagnosis?

1007 A 35-year-old ruddy-complexioned furniture store manager describes breathlessness on exertion of 3 months' duration. Whereas he could previously unload a van without pause, now he feels exhausted after 10 minutes of work.

No abnormality is found on physical examination. Chest X-ray and ECG are both normal. He is treated for exercise-induced asthma but without improvement. A few weeks later, he is admitted to hospital with blood-streaked, tarry stools, and undergoes laparotomy for resection of a carcinoma of the ascending colon.

What was the cause of his breathlessness?

1008 A 55-year-old woman investigated for epigastric pain of one year's duration is found to have a gastric ulcer on the lesser curvature. Endoscopic biopsy is not available.

Six weeks later, following a full course of treatment, her symptoms remain and the radiological appearance has not changed.

What suspicions should this case history arouse?

1009 A 30-year-old man is admitted to hospital with severe precordial chest pain and electrocardiographic and biochemical evidence of myocardial infarction.

Of which underlying disorders is his heart attack likely to be a manifestation?

1010 A 50-year-old woman is admitted to a neurosurgical unit with a diagnosis of subarachnoid haemorrhage. This diagnosis had been made correctly on the basis of headache, neck stiffness, blood-stained cerebrospinal fluid (CSF) and CSF xanthochromia.

Routine blood count, however, was abnormal.

What haematological conditions could have contributed to the subarachnoid haemorrhage?

1011 Livedo reticularis is a striking blue-brown mottling of the skin in the pattern of a net with a large mesh.

Like Raynaud's phenomenon, it occurs most commonly in a benign context (old people sitting for long periods in front of a fire, i.e. erythema ab igne) but it may also be associated with underlying diseases.

Which ones?

1012 The shoulder–hand syndrome is a painful condition in which the shoulder is immobilized by stiffness and weakness. The hand may swell and become very tender to touch.

Can this syndrome follow myocardial infarction?

1013 A patient admitted for investigation of a bruising tendency rolls over in bed and dislocates a knee.

What condition is likely to be present?

1014 A young man admitted with severe abdominal pain, hypotension and absent pulses in the left leg is noted to be thin, with long limbs, thin fingers and a high arched palate.

(a) What syndrome is present and (b) what is the condition precipitating his admission?

1015 A young adult is admitted with haematemesis. He has had haematemesis before and investigations to find a source of the bleeding have failed to demonstrate it. On the basis of skin changes in the neck, axillae and groin and abnormal fundi, he is believed to have a genetically determined disorder for which no treatment is possible.

What is the name of this disorder?

1016 When a patient presents with haematemesis, physical examination seldom distinguishes between the common causes, i.e. duodenal ulcer, gastric ulcer, oesophageal varices. Physical examination does, however, identify rare conditions which may cause haematemesis. In one of these, multiple telangiectases are present in the gastrointestinal tract and may be spotted on the lips or buccal mucosa.

What is the name of this condition?

1017 Changes in the nails may reflect non-dermatological systemic disease. Koilonychia is a spoon-shaped deformity resulting from severe iron deficiency. It is not common, but other more frequently seen changes of iron deficiency include brittleness, flattening and longitudinal ridging of the nails.

What other conditions cause brittle nails?

Addendum

1018 Most cases of myelofibrosis occur without preceding illness. However, it may accompany polycythaemia rubra vera, chronic myeloid leukaemia or marrow infiltration by lymphoma or carcinoma.

What is the main physical sign in myelofibrosis and what serious complications may occur?

1019 Brain abscess frequently presents with progressive neurological disorder and fever.
Why should lumbar puncture be avoided if this diagnosis is strongly suspected?

1020 Localized disorders predisposing to brain abscess include middle ear infection, frontal sinusitis and penetrating head injury.
What systemic disorders predispose to brain abscess?

1021 Hodgkin's disease accounts for about one-third of all lymphomas. The cell of origin is uncertain but the diagnostic finding in a lymph node biopsy is the presence of Reid–Sternberg cells.
What is the cell of origin of the non-Hodgkin's lymphomas?

1022 Lymph nodes involved by Hodgkin's disease are painless, discrete and rubbery. The patient may be asymptomatic or may have fever, night sweats and weight loss.
How is Hodgkin's disease staged?

1023 Radiotherapy and chemotherapy singly or in combination can be extremely effective in treating Hodgkin's disease. Radiotherapy is used for stage IA and IIA cases while more disseminated disease requires chemotherapy. The standard regimen is MOPP (mustine, oncovin, prednisone, procarbazine).
What factors affect the response to chemotherapy?

3 Answers

Cardiovascular System

1 Ventilation/perfusion (*V/Q*) imbalance and right-to-left intracardiac shunt. Distortion of lung tissue as in pulmonary fibrosis or chronic bronchitis, or abnormal pulmonary circulation as in pulmonary embolism or left ventricular failure, will cause mismatching of ventilation and perfusion. Right-to-left shunts can occur with atrial or ventricular septal defects or a patent ductus arteriosus (or other rare anomalies) when pressures on the right side of the defect are higher than on the left.
[A: 116; B: 16.4; C: 147; D: 49; E: 268; F: 669; H: 166–7]

2 Chronic bronchitis causes narrowing of the airways, which in turn leads to underventilation of the lungs. Blood which perfuses such underventilated lung tissue is inadequately oxygenated and therefore cyanotic. If heart failure accompanies the situation, pulmonary arterial blood is diverted to the relatively underventilated upper lobes, and is therefore inadequately oxygenated and cyanotic. An additional factor may be polycythaemia secondary to chronic hypoxia.
[A: 116; B: 16.4; C: 147; D: 49; F: 669; H: 166]

3 That the circulation is not maintaining peripheral perfusion. Attention is sometimes given to simultaneous measurements of skin temperature (of the foot) and core temperature (rectal). These can be measured continuously and a gradual widening between core and skin temperatures indicates that peripheral circulation is diminishing.
[A: 117; B: 16.20; C: 147; H: 177]

4 Pulmonary, cardiac and extrathoracic disease. When describing clubbing which is not obvious or marked, the word 'equivocal' is preferable to 'early' or 'slight'. Examples are: pulmonary: bronchiectasis, lung abscess, bronchogenic carcinoma; cardiac: cyanotic congenital heart disease, infective endocarditis; extrathoracic: hepatic cirrhosis, inflammatory bowel disease.
[A: 117; C: 147; D: 48; F: 670; H: 167]

5 Fever, bleeding and thyrotoxicosis.
[A: 117; B: 16.31; C: 156; D: 58; F: 671; G: 1243]

6 Abnormality of the pacemakers or of the conduction system, due to pathological processes (ischaemia, inflammation) or to drugs (digoxin, beta-blockers). A sinus bradycardia is a common arrhythmia in the acute stages of myocardial infarction but usually responds to atropine. When complete atrioventricular heart block has occurred, the ventricular pacemaker that takes over usually has a rate of about 40.
[A: 117; B: 16.31; C: 156; D: 58; F: 692; G: 1243]

7 As the extrasystole occurs earlier than normal, the ventricles may not have had time to fill. Between the next normal beat and the preceding extrasystole a pause will be apparent and because the ventricles have had extra time for filling, the next normal beat will be more forceful. Some patients notice the pause, 'it missed a beat', others the more forceful beat, 'a thump'.
[A: 143; B: 16.31; C: 156; D: 67–8; E: 270; F: 700–1; G: 1246–51; H: 1051–7]

8 Atrial extrasystoles characteristically have a normal QRS contour which is preceded by a P wave. The P wave is very likely to have an abnormal shape.

Ventricular extrasystoles, on the other hand, tend to have QRS complexes that are wide and often of large amplitude. The ST segment is usually missing and the T wave is written in the opposite direction to the QRS. There is no preceding P wave.
[A: 143; B: 16.31; C: 159; D: 67–8; E: 271; F: 700–1; G: 1246–51; H: 1051–7]

9 The rate is usually very regular at about 200 beats per minute. The heart sounds are very constant in quality and loudness. The arrhythmia occurs in attacks which some patients link to emotional stress, heavy exertion or sudden head movements. Fainting may occur at the outset of an attack because of an abrupt fall in cardiac output. Stimulating the vagus by carotid sinus massage or eyeball pressure may bring sudden reversion to normal sinus rhythm.
[A: 145; B: 16.31; C: 156; D: 58; E: 271; F: 704–5; G: 1249; H: 1052]

10 Inspection of the jugular venous pulse may reveal the pulsation of the right atrium at a much slower rate, and occasional cannon waves may occur when an atrial contraction coincides with ventricular systole. On auscultation, variation in intensity of the first heart sound should be listened for. It is definite if present and is due to the varying intervals between atrial and ventricular contraction.

[A: 145; B: 16.33; C: 159; D: 58; E: 272; F: 709; G: 1252; H: 1058]

11 Wolff–Parkinson–White syndrome (WPW). The commonest set of ECG appearances comprises a short PR interval and a widening of the QRS complex due to the delta wave, the slurred first part of the QRS complex. The PJ interval (measured from the onset of the P wave to the end of the QRS complex) is usually normal.

There are variations, depending on the anatomical position or functional nature of the anomalous conduction pathway.
[A: 157; B: 16.36; D: 59; E: 271; F: 707; G: 1257; H: 1062]

12 Yes. These are the two commonest situations in which this arrhythmia occurs. In the acute stages of myocardial infarction the alternating bradycardia and atrial arrhythmias may be controlled by drugs. If atrophine fails to improve the bradycardia, then a pacemaker is needed. In the chronic condition in the elderly, a pacemaker is the definitive treatment.
[A: 152; D: 60; E: 276; F: 693; G: 1244; H: 1056]

13 Lignocaine. It is used as a bolus intravenous injection of 50–100 mg followed by an infusion. Practice varies in the doses given. Some start with 1 mg per minute, increasing by 1 mg per minute up to 3 or 4 mg per minute until a response is obtained. Others start with 4 mg per minute for 30 minutes, then 2 mg per minute for 2 hours and then 1 mg per minute thereafter. Lignocaine may cause confusion and even convulsions.
[A: 150; B: 16.33; C: 160; D: 59; E: 272; F: 703; G: 1264; H: 1070]

14 Like other drugs that decrease cardiac excitability, it causes myocardial depression which may lead to heart failure. Nausea, diarrhoea and skin rashes can occur. It can also cause a drug-induced SLE-like syndrome, which remits on stopping the drug.
[A: 150; B: 16.33; C: 160; E: 273; F: 703; G: 1264; H: 1069]

15 Digoxin-induced arrhythmia. Experimental work has shown that phenytoin depresses ventricular automaticity but at the same time enhances AV conduction. In this respect it differs from other antiarrhythmic agents.
[A: 151: C: 166; F: 703; G: 1265; H: 1070]

16 All of them. The factors that predispose a patient to the toxic effects of digoxin are long-term diuretic

therapy causing intracellular potassium depletion, low serum potassium levels, old age and hepatic or renal impairment.
[A: 140; C: 171; D: 250; E: 273; F: 689; H: 1066]

17 Disopyramide and mexiletine. Both drugs are indicated particularly after myocardial infarction and both can be given intravenously or orally. These drugs may be used in place of procainamide and lignocaine and some claim that they have fewer side-effects.
[A: 150; C: 165; D: 58–9; E: 273; G: 1266; H: 1070]

18 Other indications for beta-blockers include hypertension, angina, thyrotoxicosis and somatic symptoms of anxiety. Blockade of beta-adrenergic receptors in the lungs may cause bronchospasm, precipitating an attack of asthma. The 'cardioselective' beta-blockers which are supposed not to block beta-2- receptors, are, in practice, not entirely to be trusted in this respect. In the peripheral vasculature, beta-blockade, leaving unopposed alpha activity, leads to vasoconstriction, causing or aggravating Raynaud's phenomenon and exacerbating intermittent claudication. The warning symptoms and signs of hypoglycaemia may be masked. Nightmares may be troublesome.
[A: 151; B: 16.32; C: 166; E: 272; F: 703; G: 1265; H: 393]

19 Long-term oral use causes the unpleasant oculomucocutaneous syndrome which includes conjunctival scarring, corneal opacity, psoriasis-like rash and peritoneal fibrosis (not retroperitoneal fibrosis).
[A: 151; C: 166; D: 59; E: 273]

20 By reducing the force of myocardial contraction (negative inotropic effect) they may lead to heart failure and hypotension. The attendant fall in heart rate may cause an additional reduction in cardiac output.
[A: 151; C: 166; F: 703; G: 1265; H: 393]

21 In slowing the ventricular response in cases of atrial flutter or fibrillation when rapid slowing is required, digoxin can be given intravenously in a dose of 0.5–1 mg. When the situation is not critical, oral therapy is given, starting with 0.25 mg twice a day for the first few days, adjusting the dose thereafter according to the ventricular rate.
[A: 147; C: 171; E: 272–3; F: 705]

22 Supraventricular, nodal and Wolff–Parkinson–White tachycardias, in which the tachycardia may be maintained by retrograde conduction of the impulse back up to the atria along an abnormal pathway. Delaying conduction in the abnormal pathway will interrupt the tachycardia.
[A: 151; C: 166; D: 58–9; F: 703; G: 1257; H: 1062]

23 Atrial flutter: 300 beats per minute is the typical atrial rate, but there is usually some degree of atrioventricular block, in this case 2:1. Carotid sinus stimulation nearly always slows the ventricular rate by increasing the block to 4:1 or more. When stimulation is stopped the faster rate usually returns. Treatment is usually with dixogin, beta-blockade or d.c. cardioversion.
[A: 147; B: 16.32; C: 157; D: 58–9; E: 275; F: 704; G: 1248; H: 1054]

24 Mitral stenosis and thyrotoxicosis. In mitral valve disease, the onset of atrial fibrillation may be followed by clot formation in the left atrial appendage leading to systemic embolization. Digoxin to control the arrhythmia and heparin (followed by oral anticoagulation) are urgently indicated.
[A: 148; B: 16.32; C: 158; D: 58–9; E: 273; F: 704; G: 1247; H: 1055]

25 Cardiac function is always impaired by losing atrial contraction. Whether or not the patient notices this depends on the presence of underlying heart disease.

Once atrial fibrillation becomes established in mitral valve disease, disability is nearly always increased. The deterioration in the patient's condition may mean that surgery becomes necessary.
[A: 148–9; B: 16.32; C: 158–9; E: 273; F: 704; G: 1247 H: 1055]

26 'Lone' atrial fibrillation, usually an accidental finding, occurs predominantly in males. Care must be taken to exclude minimal mitral stenosis, both in the physical examination (by listening in the left lateral position after exercise) and on investigation (echocardiography) before deciding not to attempt treatment since this arrhythmia is very resistant to both drug and electrical treatment.
[A: 149; C: 158; H: 1055]

27 D.c. conversion (direct current conversion) in which a shock, often of low voltage and timed to coincide with an R wave of the patient's rhythm, depolarizes the whole myocardium and allows the sinoatrial node to resume as the pacemaker. The procedure is performed

under a light general anaesthetic or intravenous diazepam and should not be carried out within 24 hours of digoxin therapy, nor where there is the likelihood of dislodging an embolus, i.e. mitral valve disease (without prior anticoagulation).
[A: 152; B: 16.36; C: 166; D: 249; E: 273–4; F: 710; G: 1266; H: 1073]

28 Sinoatrial block (with 5 : 4 conduction). This form of heart block is much less common than atrioventricular block and is due to a normal sinus impulse failing to reach and excite the atrial musculature. The evidence for this is necessarily indirect since the P wave is only the wave of atrial depolarization and the sinus impulse itself cannot be recorded. But the existence of SA block can be deduced from the time relationship of successive P waves. The condition may be asymptomatic or there may be dizziness or syncope occurring when the patient is lying down. This is probably because of the increased vagal activity that occurs on lying down.
[A: 152; B: 16.33; C: 162; E: 276; F: 692–3; G: 1244; H: 1051]

29 A diagnosis of first degree heart block cannot be made without an ECG, but it may be suspected clinically on two grounds: if the first heart sound is soft and secondly if there is apparent delay between the 'a' and 'v' waves in the jugular venous pulse.

The loudness of the first heart sound is determined by the position of the valve cusps at the end of ventricular diastole. If the cusps have had time to float towards a closed position, as is possible when atrioventricular conduction is prolonged, then they have a shorter distance to move at the onset of systole and the sound of the valves shutting is softer.
[A: 153; B: 16.33; C: 162; D: 64–5; F: 693; G: 1260; H: 1060]

30 In Mobitz type 2 block, there is no lengthening of the PR interval prior to the blocked impulse and the number of blocked beats (i.e. the degree of block) increases the faster the atrial rate. Progression to complete block can be expected.
[A: 153; B: 16.35; C: 163; D: 64–5; F: 694; G: 1261; H: 1060]

31 Prolongation of the relative refractory period of the AV node as a result of damage (ischaemic, inflammatory etc.)
[A: 153; B: 16.35; C: 163; D: 64–5; F: 694; G: 1261; H: 1060]

32 Complete (or third degree) heart block. The ECG shows slow, regular ventricular rhythm with more frequent P waves which show a continually varying time relationship to the QRS complexes.
[A: 153; B: 16.35; C: 163; D: 64–5; E: 275; F: 694–5; G: 1263; H: 1061]

33 With the onset of circulatory arrest, the face suddenly becomes deathly pale. After five seconds, consciousness is usually lost and after fifteen seconds convulsions may occur with heavy respiratory efforts. Thereafter, the patient may appear to be dead. The return of the circulation is marked by a vivid facial flush.
[A: 154; B: 16.35; C: 164; E: 275; F: 695; G: 743; H: 1060–1]

34 The immediate objective in resuscitation is to maintain a circulation of oxygenated blood to the brain until such time as acidosis can be corrected and the underlying cardiac arrhythmia treated.

The first thing to be done, therefore, is to give external cardiac massage and the second person on the scene should provide ventilation. Once these are in progress one or more drips must be put up to give sodium bicarbonate and provide a route for administration of drugs. The fourth thing to be done (if these steps can only be taken in sequence) is to attach the cardiac monitor.
[A: 155; B: 16.20; C: 161; D: 58; F: 710; G: 1053; H: 182–6]

35 Direct current. The first defibrillators used alternating current but direct current is very much safer and more effective. The shock is measured in joules and most defibrillators can deliver up to 400 joules per shock. Something less than the charge indicated actually reaches the myocardium, nevertheless the lowest possible charge that is effective should be used in order to minimize muscle damage. The timing of the shock matters if there are normal ventricular impulses. If the shock is not synchronized with the up-stroke of the R wave, it may fall on the ST segment or T wave and cause ventricular fibrillation.
[A: 155; B: 16.20; C: 161; D: 250; E: 273; F: 710; G: 1056; H: 1073]

36 Calcium ions bind with the inhibitor of the actin and myosin filaments and are an integral part of the process of contraction. Sometimes this is apparent in resuscitation when the heart monitor shows that normal electrical activity has been restored but no

pulse is felt. Provided this is not due to ventricular rupture, the pulse may return when intravenous calcium is given.

During the so-called slow phase of depolarization, calcium ions move across the muscle cell membrane. A family of drugs called calcium blockers impede this movement and are useful in the treatment of angina and arrhythmias.

Digitalized patients become more sensitive to the actions of digoxin during intravenous injections of calcium.
[B: 16.27; F: 663; G: 1057; H: 1027]

37 Digoxin. This drug appears to partially inhibit the ATP-dependent sodium–potassium exchange at the myocardial cell membrane and it competes with potassium ions for access to the site. Apart from stopping the drug, administering potassium is often necessary particularly when long-term diuretic therapy has depleted body stores.
[B: 16.27; F: 664; G: 1099; H: 1027]

38 The strength usually used is 8.4 per cent, which contains one millimole of sodium bicarbonate per ml of solution. Normal, i.e. isotonic sodium bicarbonate is a 1.4 per cent solution containing approximately 167 millimoles of sodium and bicarbonate per litre.
[A: 155; B: 16.21; C: 161; D: 250; F: 710; G: 1057; H: 185]

39 Electrical pacing. In the acute situation this is by means of a wire introduced into the right ventricle, the tip of which is lodged against the ventricular wall. If permanent pacing is required, a pacemaker can be implanted in the anterior chest wall.
[A: 156; B: 16.35; C: 166; D: 250; E: 276; F: 699; G: 1267; H: 1061]

40 No. The ECG shows right bundle branch block, but this can be a normal finding. It would have a different significance if the patient had ischaemic heart disease or chronic lung disease.
[A: 156; C: 164; D: 61; F: 696; H: 1008]

41 When the left branch of the bundle of His is blocked, depolarization occurs by spread from the right ventricle (altering the axis), and as the impulse bypasses the main Purkinje fibre bundles it takes longer to traverse the myocardium. This prolongs the QRS. The activation time (the time from initiation to the peak of the R wave) in the left precordial leads is greater than its usual 0.035 second for the same

reason. Notching or slurring is due to the abnormal pathway through the ventricle walls.
[A: 156; D: 61; F: 695; H: 1008]

42 You can't. The correct ECG interpretation depends on the clinical situation. In young adults, hemiblock would be unlikely. In a 60-year-old hypertensive cigarette smoker with ischaemic heart disease it would be unreasonable not to suspect hemiblock.
[A: 156; D: 73; F: 696–7; H: 1008]

43 In addition to his pre-existing right bundle branch block, he now has left anterior hemiblock. This combination is often termed bifascicular block. In this setting, a progression to complete heart block is an alarming possibility and most doctors would insert a temporary pacing wire.
[A: 156; D: 73; F: 696–7; H: 1008]

44 Carotid sinus sensitivity, in which the carotid sinus is abnormally sensitive due either to a localized plaque of atheroma or occasionally to the presence of a tumour. This latter should be evident on palpation. The patient should be advised to avoid tight collars and sudden neck movement.
[B: 16.4; C: 146; G: 743; H: 80]

45 Sinus bradycardia particularly and, to a lesser extent, complete heart block. Both the SA and AV nodes are influenced by the vagus which causes a slowing in the intrinsic rate of impulse formation. Atropine blocks this vagal effect. 1 mg of atropine, given intravenously, usually lasts for 2–4 hours. Accelerated idioventricular rhythm, a form of escape rhythm, can also be treated with atropine, which speeds up the sinus impulses so that they can recapture the ventricles.
[A: 153; B: 16.31; C: 166; D: 250; E: 285; F: 695; G: 1118; H: 1131]

46 Carbon dioxide retention is possible with resultant vasodilatation. Circulating volume is also probably increased with fluid retention secondary to heart failure, in this case, cor pulmonale.
[A: 117; B: 16.5; C: 147; D: 52; F: 671; H: 993–4]

47 You have made a mistake in your assessment of the pulse. A collapsing pulse is typically due to aortic incompetence and there is a wide pulse pressure and a diastolic pressure of less than 70 mmHg due to the flowback of aortic blood into the left ventricle. Patent

ductus arteriosus and a rigid atherosclerotic aorta can also produce this kind of pulse.
[A: 118; B: 16.6; C: 147; D: 53; F: 671; G: 1074; H: 1108]

48 An enlarged left ventricle, as indicated by the displacement of the apex beat, a slow forceful systolic component to the apex beat, a thrill in the aortic area and a harsh systolic ejection murmur radiating up to the neck and also to the apex. There may be a click between the first heart sound and the beginning of the murmur, and the aortic component of the second sound may be diminished in intensity.
[A: 118; B: 16.6; C: 147; D: 53; F: 671; G: 1074; H: 994]

49 Pulsus bisferiens is a pulse wave with a double impulse. It may occur in combined aortic stenosis and regurgitation. A similar impression of the pulse can be obtained by holding a normal pulse with two fingers at unequal pressure. It is an uncommon finding.
[A: 118; C: 147; D: 53; F: 671; G: 1074; H: 994]

50 Every other pulse beat is weak, yet the rate and rhythm remain normal. This is pulsus alternans. The subjective assessment of the pulse can be objectively confirmed with the sphygmomanometer. Above the systolic pressure of the weaker beats, only the stronger beats will be heard and the heart rate will appear to be halved.
[A: 118; B: 16.5; C: 147; D: 53; E: 291; G: 1090; H: 994]

51 An enlarged heart shadow, due to a pericardial effusion, or a normal-sized heart with linear calcification along the cardiac border indicating constrictive pericarditis. Pulsus paradoxus is present and the abnormal rise in JVP on inspiration is known as Kussmaul's sign. Both of these signs indicate that right ventricular filling is impeded.
[A: 118; B: 16.5; C: 147; D: 53; F: 671; G: 1273; H: 994]

52 Loss of the 'a' waves.
[A: 119; B: 16.6; C: 148; D: 54; E: 277–8; F: 671; G: 1073; H: 994]

53 The reflux of blood through the incompetent valve obliterates the 'x' descent and a single large wave remains (giant 'a' wave).
[A: 119; B: 16.6; C: 148; D: 54; F: 672; G: 1073; H: 994]

54 You should associate her hepatic pain with stretching of the capsule due to the raised venous pressure. If developing quickly it is a serious sign. A slow rise in

venous pressure may result in so-called cardiac cirrhosis.
[A: 119; B: 16.16; C: 169; D: 54; F: 670; G: 1092; H: 1039]

55 Hepatojugular reflux. Firm and sustained pressure over the liver and right hypochondrium will sweep blood in the hepatic veins and inferior vena cava up to the right atrium. If there is already some increase in circulating volume as occurs in heart failure, the extra blood will fill the neck veins.
[A: 119; D: 54; E: 278; H: 995]

56 Using too small a cuff. This problem tends to arise in the obese patient when a larger cuff is not to hand.
If inflation of the cuff is difficult there may be a blockage in the tubing and the mercury level may not indicate the actual pressure. One faulty apparatus in a consulting room can lead to many unnecessary prescriptions.
[A: 120; B: 16.7; C: 151; F: 670; G: 1200; H: 176]

57 The infarct will cause abnormal movement of the left ventricular wall which may be apparent as a diffuse and lopsided ripple or tremble.
[A: 121; B: 16.7; C: 149; D: 55; F: 672; G: 1074; H: 995]

58 Aortic stenosis or pulmonary stenosis. Typically the thrill of aortic stenosis is directed towards the right side of the neck while that of pulmonary stenosis goes to the left.
[A: 121; B: 16.7; C: 149; D: 55; F: 673; H: 995]

59 No. Normal, or physiological splitting of the second heart sound occurs during inspiration because increased right ventricular filling delays the closure of the pulmonary valve. In this patient paradoxical splitting is occurring. It could be due to mechanical prolongation of left ventricular systole resulting from myocardial ischaemia or he might in addition have left bundle branch block.
[A: 122; B: 16.7; C: 150; D: 55–6; F: 673–5; G: 1075; H: 995–6]

60 A third heart sound, or strictly speaking, a left-sided third heart sound, since it can arise in either ventricle. Occasionally there is both a left and a right S3. The sound is produced by rapid, passive ventricular filling and in the absence of evidence of heart disease is considered normal in children and young adults. Where heart pathology is present, a third heart sound

indicates increased rate or volume of ventricular filling.
[A: 123; B: 16.7; C: 150; F: 675–6; G: 1075; H: 996]

61 Fourth heart sound (S4). It occurs in the ventricle with atrial systole when ventricular compliance is reduced. This can also occur in hypertension, severe aortic stenosis and cardiomyopathies. It is a very useful sign and should always be listened for.
[A: 123; B: 16.7–9; C: 150; F: 675–6; G: 1075; H: 996]

62 It is usually best heard with the patient upright and leaning forward. It is a scratchy sound and sometimes it can be made to vary in intensity by altering the pressure with which the stethoscope is applied to the chest wall.
[A: 124; B: 16.11; C: 203; D: 56; G: 1272; H: 999]

63 Aortic stenosis. The murmur is getting louder because the improving myocardium is able to pump a larger flow of blood through the valve.
[A: 124; B: 16.9; D: 56; F: 676; G: 1177; H: 997]

64 Mitral regurgitation, tricuspid regurgitation, ventricular septal defect and occasionally shunts between aorta and pulmonary vasculature.
[A: 125; B: 16.10; D: 56; F: 676; G: 1177; H: 997–8]

65 Standing decreases heart size so the murmur gets louder.
[D: 271; F: 677; G: 1278; H: 1145]

66 Anaemia and pregnancy. Innocent flow murmurs are very common in pregnancy but the only way to be certain of their innocent nature is to re-examine some weeks after delivery when the cardiovascular changes of pregnancy have subsided.
[A: 125; F: 676]

67 The patient should be on his left side and propped up on his left elbow. The bell of the stethoscope should be placed over the apex beat. In mitral stenosis there is an opening snap following the second heart sound (at an interval determined by the severity of the stenosis: short = bad, long = milder). The opening snap is followed by a low-pitched rumbling murmur which may fade and then reappear or get louder just before the first heart sound, if the atria are contracting normally, so-called presystolic accentuation.
[A: 126; D: 56; F: 677; G: 1177; H: 998–9]

68 Austin Flint murmur. It may be confused with mitral stenosis. Echocardiography can distinguish between the two.
[A: 126; B: 16.11; D: 260; F: 678; G: 1196; H: 999]

69 A soft aortic second heart sound and an early diastolic high-pitched decrescendo murmur, loudest in the third intercostal space at the left sternal border and best heard with the patient upright and leaning forward in expiration. The murmur is usually short. Because of the increased blood flow through the valve in systole, a systolic ejection murmur is likely to be present even if there is no anatomical obstruction.
[A: 126; B: 16.10–11; D: 56; F: 678; G: 1177; H: 999]

70 +60°, +90° and −30° respectively.
[A: 127; B: 16.23; C: 152; F: 679; H: 1001]

71 Atrial rate, ventricular rate, rhythm. Axis, PR interval, QRS duration and QT interval. Character of the P waves, QRS complexes, ST segments and T waves.
[A: 128; D: 60–73; E: 311–14; F: 679]

72 Echocardiography.
[A: 128; C: 154; E: 315; F: 680–1; G: 1076; H: 1015]

73 Neither contributes to the normal PA cardiac silhouette. The left atrial appendage may lie at the edge of the upper left border, above the bulge of the left ventricle but below the pulmonary artery. Enlargement of the left atrium may produce a round double density in the centre of the shadow, while an enlarged right ventricle is best assessed on a right anterior oblique or lateral view, showing the retrosternal space.
[A: 129; B: 16.27; C: 152; F: 681; G: 1075; H: 1011]

74 Left atrium. Barium swallow with oblique views is a necessary investigation if the size of the left atrium is to be assessed.
[A: 129; C: 153; H: 1011]

75 Hypovalaemic circulatory failure, most probably due to a Gram-negative septicaemia in which the hypovolaemia is partly explained by pooling of blood in dilated splanchnic vessels.
[A: 131; G: 1109; H: 177]

76 Pump failure. The resulting drop in perfusion of the body and especially of the kidneys results in the hormonal and renal compensatory mechanisms that lead to an increased circulating blood volume,

increased interstitial fluid volume and increased body sodium.
[A: 131; B: 16.11–13; C: 168; D: 249; F: 665–6; G: 1083; H: 1132]

77 Dyspnoea at lessening grades of activity, orthopnoea, paroxysmal nocturnal dyspnoea, fatigue and weakness. On examination, elevation of the JVP, pulsus alternans, added third and fourth heart sounds, basal râles in the lungs, peripheral oedema, pleural effusion and hepatic enlargement are all common.
[A: 136; B: 16.15; C: 167; E: 278; F: 683; G: 1081; H: 1038]

78 Aggravation of pulmonary congestion by reabsorption of oedema from dependent parts of the body, relative hypoventilation during sleep causing a fall in arterial oxygen tension, reduce adrenergic stimulation of the myocardium during sleep. The paroxysm is due to acute pulmonary oedema and bronchospasm.
[A: 135; B: 16.2; C: 145; E: 267; F: 687; G: 1090; H: 1038]

79 Myocardial infarction or ischaemic heart disease, hypertension or aortic valve disease. Another cause of pulmonary oedema is mitral stenosis.
[A: 135; B: 16.15; C: 169; F: 687; G: 1089; H: 165]

80 Dyspnoea on exertion. Examples of purely right-sided lesions are pulmonary hypertension due to recurrent pulmonary embolism and pulmonary stenosis. These are uncommon compared to conditions affecting the left side of the heart and/or the lungs in which the right heart is secondarily affected.
[A: 136; B: 16.16; C: 169; F: 684; G: 1091; H: 1037]

81 Its chronotropic effect is negative, i.e. the heart rate slows. The inotropic effect is positive, i.e. the force of contraction is greater. Conduction is slowed in the nodes, and in heart failure (but not in the normal heart) digoxin is a vasodilator.
[A: 139; B: 16.18; C: 171; E: 279; F: 664; G: 1095; H: 1066]

82 All. Digoxin arrhythmias can be serious and sometimes fatal. The commonest are probably coupled ectopic beats and bradycardia. A feature of digoxin arrhythmias is that there may be evidence of simultaneous disturbance at more than one site in the conduction system, e.g. atrial tachycardia with AV block.
[A: 140; B: 16.18; C: 171; D: 250; E: 279; F: 689; G: 1098; H: 1066]

83 Shortening of the QT interval, sagging depression of the ST segments and flattening or inversion of the T waves.
[A: 139; G: 1098]

84 In the treatment of heart failure when the hypokalaemia caused by diuretics may precipitate toxicity by another drug, namely digoxin. Thiazides also have side-effects, including a slight impairment of glucose tolerance, an elevation of serum uric acid levels and a photosensitive dermatitis.
[A: 141; B: 16.18; C: 170; E: 279; F: 690; G: 1104; H: 1041]

85 A slight vasodilator effect, as evidenced by the relief that occurs in acute pulmonary oedema before a diuresis has begun, and a slight anti-arrhythmic effect.
[A: 141; B: 16.19; C: 170; E: 279; F: 690; G: 1104; H: 1042]

86 When given together with other drugs that promote potassium excretion, such as corticosteroids or carbenoxolone, hypokalaemia is likely. The combination of frusemide with the antibiotics gentamicin or cephaloridine is nephrotoxic. Frusemide, in common with the thiazides, slightly antagonizes the action of insulin and the oral hypoglycaemic drugs.

87 The development of hypokalaemia appears to be especially likely in the presence of secondary hyperaldosteronism, as in heart failure. The one condition in which this is not usually present but in which thiazides are widely used is hypertension.
[A: 142; B: 16.19; C: 170–1; F: 690; G: 1106; H: 1042]

88 Relief or prevention of angina, which is achieved by reducing left ventricular end diastolic pressure. Absorption through the oral mucosa avoids immediate hepatic metabolism and ensures a rapid action which lasts, however, only 20–30 minutes.
[A: 142; C: 171; G: 1100; H: 1043]

89 Decreased sensitivity of the respiratory centre in the medulla. During the apnoeic phase, arterial Po_2 falls and Pco_2 rises. The insensitive respiratory centre requires an abnormally large stimulus to start breathing. Deep respiration then commences. This continues until hypocapnia leading to a further period of apnoea develops. Prolonged heart–brain circulation time in heart failure may be a further factor.
[A: 244; B: 16.2; C: 145; G: 1090; H: 1276]

90 The pleural veins drain into both the pulmonary and systemic veins and effusion due to transudation occurs particularly when venous pressures in both pulmonary and systemic systems are high. The effusion collects according to gravity. Patients in heart failure apparently spend more time lying on their right side.
[A: 134; C: 169; E: 279; F: 687; G: 1092; H: 1039]

91 In tricuspid incompetence there will be V waves in the jugular veins, the murmur may get louder during inspiration and the liver may be pulsatile. The apex beat is usually palpable. In constrictive pericarditis, there may be pulsus paradoxus, Kussmaul's sign (elevation of JVP on inspiration) and pericardial calcification on chest X-ray. The ECG may show low voltages. Murmurs and cardiomegaly are not usual.
[A: 134; C: 169; E; 279; G: 1093; H: 1039]

92 There are three groups: renal, adrenal and other. The renal group consists of renal artery stenosis (renovascular hypertension) and almost any disease of the renal parenchyma. Adrenal causes comprise primary hyperaldosteronism (Conn's syndrome), Cushing's syndrome and phaeochromocytoma. Other causes include coarctation of the aorta and the contraceptive pill.

Blood pressure tends to be elevated when intracranial pressure is raised.
[A: 158; B: 16.76; C: 193; D: 252; E: 290–1; F: 809–12; G: 1209; H: 1167–9]

93 Left ventricular hypertrophy with or without strain. The criteria for LV hypertrophy include prolongation of the activation time (the upstroke of the R wave) in left precordial leads, i.e. longer than 0.035 second, increased voltages such that R in I plus S in III $\geqslant$ 26 mm or S in V1 plus R in V5 $\geqslant$ 35 mm, and a leftward axis, i.e. 0 to $-30°$. If left axis deviation is present ($> -40°$) this indicates left anterior hemiblock.
[A: 158–60; B: 16.78; C: 194; D: 252; E: 291; F: 817; G: 1203; H: 1170]

94 Apart from changes in the retinal arterioles, the presence of all the peripheral pulses must be checked, and auscultation of the large arteries (carotids, abdominal aorta, iliac and femorals) as well as of the renal arteries may reveal bruits. It is essential to check a sample of urine, by ward urinalysis, for protein and blood in all hypertensive cases.
[A: 160; B: 16.79; F: 816; G: 1203; H: 180]

95 Grade I: arteriolar narrowing; arteriolar walls appear broader but red blood column still visible;

II: greater degree of narrowing, blood column not visible; AV nipping;

III: grade II changes accompanied by flame-shaped haemorrhages and exudates; veins 'disappear' under arterioles;

IV: papilloedema accompanying marked grade III changes.

[A: 160; B: 16.79; C: 194; D: 252; E: 291; F: 817; G: 1203–5; H: 1171]

96 Occipital headaches, worse in the morning, do occur in severe hypertension although they are more commonly due to other causes. Dizziness, vertigo, tinnitus and loss of visual acuity may all accompany marked elevation of blood pressure.
[A: 160; B: 16.79; C: 195; E: 292; F: 817; G: 1205; H: 180–1]

97 Afferent glomerular arteriolar spasm and arteriosclerotic lesions of the afferent and efferent arterioles, and the glomerular tufts. These lead to a reduction in glomerular filtration with microscopic haematuria, and proteinuria.

In malignant hypertension, necrosis occurs in the vessel walls and the resulting collagen deposition occludes or obliterates the lumen of the smaller arteries and arterioles.
[A: 160; B: 16.78; C: 196; E: 292; H: 181]

98 If overweight, weight reduction should be the first step and no other treatment may be necessary. If it is, the choice at present is between a thiazide diuretic and a beta-blocker. A very large selection of preparations is available on the market. Some combine a thiazide with an aldosterone antagonist, thereby minimizing any tendency to hypokalaemia. Other preparations provide 24 hour effect from a single daily dose, thereby improving patient compliance.
[A: 162; C: 197; D: 254; E: 293; F: 819; G: 1217; H: 1172–6]

99 Hydralazine is a powerful vasodilator but it shares a disadvantage with minoxidil, another potent and recently introduced vasodilator, of eliciting a tachycardia in response to the fall in peripheral resistance. The use of a beta-blocker at the same time, however, prevents this and the separate hypotensive effect of the beta-blocker is additive.
[A: 163; C: 197; D: 254; E: 293; F: 819–20; G: 1212–17; H: 1172–6]

100 Thiazides impair glucose tolerance, elevate plasma uric acid level but most importantly may induce hypokalaemia. Beta-blockers, even the cardioselective drugs, may precipitate asthma and heart failure and they inhibit the usual sympathetic responses to hypoglycaemia. Alpha-methyldopa may cause sleepiness, depression, jaundice and a positive Coombs test. Haemolytic anaemia is uncommon. Hydralazine can cause a reversible syndrome resembling systemic lupus erythematosus. This occurs with large doses (200 mg daily) and may be provoked by interruptions in treatment.
[A: 162–4; C: 197–8; E: 293; F: 821–4; H: 1174–5]

101 The typical steptococcal infection is an acute exudative pharyngitis, i.e. a streptococcal sore throat. There is some connection between the severity of the infection and the time to onset of rheumatic fever in that carditis and arthritis may occur two weeks later. With the other manifestations, and with milder infections, the latent period may be longer. Chorea and erythema marginatum may take as much as 6 months to develop, long enough for the antecedent infection to have been forgotten.
[A: 165; B: 16.51; C: 172; D: 254; E: 294–5; F: 69; G: 377; H: 1090]

102 By convention, two major, or one major and two minor, provided there is evidence of streptococcal infection.

The major manifestations are also five in number, namely carditis, arthritis, erythema marginatum, subcutaneous nodules and chorea.
[A: 166; C: 173; D: 254–5; F: 70–2; G: 380; H: 1092]

103 The commonest presentation is painful enlargement of one large joint in the presence of fever. The migration of the arthritic signs from one joint to another is traditionally described, but several joints may hurt at the same time or only one joint may be affected. Knees and ankles are most frequently affected followed by elbows and wrists. There is no lasting deformity.
[A: 166; B: 16.53; C: 172; D: 255; F: 71; G: 380; H: 1092]

104 Cardiac enlargement, pericardial rub, abnormal murmurs and congestive heart failure, either singly or in combination. First degree heart block (prolongation of the PR interval) is common but not specific. The commonest murmur is a pansystolic murmur of mitral regurgitation. The Carey Coombs murmur is a mid-diastolic mitral murmur due to thickening of the valve leaflets.
[A: 166; C: 172; D: 255; E: 295; F: 71; G: 380; H: 999]

105 A course of penicillin to eliminate any remaining streptococci, bed rest, and soluble aspirin in large doses. The dose that relieves the symptoms can be given, subject to the development of tinnitus or other signs of toxicity. Steroids are indicated in cases of carditis showing no response to aspirin. Treatment should continue for 4–6 weeks after all signs of inflammation have subsided.
[A: 167; B: 16.55; C: 173; D: 255; F: 72–3; G: 383; H: 1094–5]

106 Choreiform movements are involuntary, purposeless and non-repetitive. They occur while the patient is awake and any voluntary muscle may be involved.
Huntington's chorea is usually familial, begins in adult life and gets steadily worse with accompanying intellectual deterioration.
[A: 169; B: 16.54; C: 720; D: 106; E: 295; F: 1365; G: 758; H: 1993]

107 The pattern corresponds to the size of the pressure gradient across which the valves have to operate. The largest gradient is between left ventricle and left atrium, the next largest between left ventricle and aorta, and so on.
[A: 170; C: 174]

108 An important auscultatory sign is the opening snap. This follows the second heart sound. Its closeness to the second heart sound gives an indication of left atrial pressure, since the valve will be forced open sooner the higher the pressure, i.e. the tighter the stenosis. The diastolic, low-pitched, rumbling murmur gives some indication of stenotic severity by its duration rather than its intensity. As stenosis increases, the murmur may get quieter.
[A: 172; B: 16.57; D: 256; E: 296; F: 749; G: 1181; H: 1098]

109 Backward transmission of raised left atrial pressure, reactive arteriolar constriction, embolic obstruction to the pulmonary vasculature and, when congestive heart failure has developed, hypoxic vasoconstriction.
[A: 171; B: 16.57; C: 176; D: 256–7; E: 296; F: 749; G: 1180; H: 1096]

110 Yes. Mitral stenosis is a cause of haemoptysis due to rupture of pulmonary–bronchial venous connections.
[A: 171; B: 16.57; C: 176; D: 256; F: 749; G: 1180; H: 1097]

111 No. Deep venous thrombosis and pulmonary embolization also occur more frequently in mitral stenosis.
[A: 172; B: 16.57; C: 176; E: 296; F: 749; G: 1181; H: 1097]

112 Echocardiography. The positions of the anterior and posterior leaflets can be observed during the events of the cardiac cycle and any adhesion detected by valve leaflet movements in relation to each other. The size of the left atrium can also be assessed.
[A: 128; D: 257; E: 296; F: 750; G: 1182; H: 1098]

113 It is common for the mitral valve damage to cause regurgitation as well and this may cause a pansystolic murmur heard over the apex and radiating to the left axilla. (Absence of the first heart sound and opening snap support the diagnosis of significant regurgitation.) When pulmonary hypertension is severe the Graham Steell murmur of pulmonary regurgitation may be present. It is high-pitched, diastolic, decrescendo and best heard down the left sternal border. Rheumatic aortic valve disease may coexist with mitral disease and give rise to aortic murmurs.
[A: 173; C: 181; E: 296; G: 1182; H: 1098]

114 The P wave changes indicate left atrial hypertrophy and this is in keeping with mitral stenosis. The voltage and ST changes are those of left ventricular hypertrophy. This does not occur in pure mitral stenosis. One of the following is likely to be present: mitral regurgitation or aortic valve disease.
[B: 16.59; C: 176; D: 257; F: 750; G: 1182; H: 1098]

115 The straight left border indicates enlargement of the left atrium and atrial appendage; prominent pulmonary vessels at the hila suggest pulmonary hypertension. Upper lobe vessel prominence indicates upper lobe diversion of blood flow. The oesophageal displacement confirms left atrial enlargement. Mitral stenosis is the most likely cause. Kerley B lines, horizontal line shadows due to distended lymphatics, may be present also.
[A: 173; B: 16.58; C: 176; D: 257; F: 750; G: 1182; H: 1099]

116 An adolescent with valve disease should be on long-term prophylaxis against streptococcal throat infections to prevent a recurrence of rheumatic fever.
An adult should receive bactericidal doses of antibiotics immediately before tooth extractions and any other minor surgery likely to cause a bacteraemia, such as a D and C.

Infective endocarditis (or SBE, subacute bacterial endocarditis) occurs on damaged valves and several weeks' antibiotic therapy is indicated for this serious condition.
[A: 175; C: 182; F: 772; G: 395; H: 1099]

117 If asymptomatic, surgery is not indicated. In patients with moderately severe and progressive dyspnoea on exertion, closed mitral valvotomy is a very effective procedure with a low mortality, and even though there is a tendency for the valve leaflets to readhere with a return of symptoms, the beneficial effects may last several years. Mitral valve replacement carries a mortality of about 10 per cent and should therefore be reserved for patients in whom ordinary daily activity is significantly limited despite medical treatment.
[A: 175; B: 16.58; C: 176; D: 257; E: 296–7; F: 752; G: 1184; H: 1100]

118 A pansystolic murmur usually easily heard over the apex and radiating to the axilla, a soft or absent first heart sound, a third heart sound and a fourth heart sound if sinus rhythm is present.
In severe cases with pulmonary hypertension, P2 will be accentuated and signs of right ventricular failure may be present.
[A: 176; B: 16.59; C: 177; D: 258; E: 297; F: 754; G: 1185; H: 1101]

119 First, the papillary muscles, which control the tension in the chordae tendinae attached to the valve cusps, can be affected by ischaemia like any other part of the myocardium and can be damaged by infarction or dragged out of normal alignment by ventricular aneurysm.
Secondly, the ischaemic left ventricle may become dilated and this can cause widening of the mitral ring with resultant failure of cusp apposition. Cardiac dilatation is an important cause of regurgitant murmurs at normal valves.
[A: 177; C: 177; D: 258; E: 298; F: 755; G: 1185; H: 1101]

120 The left ventricle tends to enlarge and the left atrium also. In severe, long-standing cases the left atrium may become enormous (bigger than can occur with mitral stenosis), and may extend and enlarge the right border of the cardiac silhouette on the PA X-ray. (The normal left atrium does not form any part of the cardiac silhouette on a PA chest X-ray.)
[A: 177; B: 16.59; D: 258; F: 755; G: 1187; H: 1102]

121 T wave inversion in inferior leads, i.e. II, III and aVF, and in left precordial leads, i.e. V5 and 6. There is also an association with ventricular arrhythmias, particularly ventricular tachycardia. The syndrome is sometimes called the floppy valve syndrome.
[A: 178; D: 258; F: 756; G: 1188; H: 1103]

122 Distended neck veins; prominent V waves in the JVP; a pulsatile enlarged liver with pain from the stretched liver capsule; a pansystolic murmur at the lower left sternal border which may become louder on inspiration. Atrial fibrillation is common.
[A: 178; B: 16.62; C: 180; D: 261; F: 764; G: 1198; H: 1111]

123 A diastolic rumbling murmur heard close to the left sternal border and at the base of the sternum, louder on inspiration; a normal P2 as opposed to the accentuation found in pulmonary hypertension. Other features of tricuspid stenosis include ECG changes of right atrial hypertrophy (tall P waves in leads II and V1) in the absence of evidence of right ventricular hypertrophy.
[A: 179; B: 16.61; C: 180; F: 763; G: 1197; H: 1110]

124 Congenital stenosis or congenitally bicuspid valve which more easily becomes stenosed; rheumatic heart disease; idiopathic calcific aortic stenosis of the elderly (a 'wear and tear' phenomenon usually of little haemodynamic significance).

The three main symptoms are dyspnoea on exertion, angina and syncope.
[A: 180; B: 16.60; C: 177; D: 259; E: 298; F: 757; G: 1191; H: 1104–6]

125 The apex beat is usually prominent, displaced downwards and laterally and may have a double impulse, the first component being the forceful contraction of the left atrium. The second component, due to ventricular contraction, may be prolonged if stenosis is marked. There is commonly a thrill, and the murmur is typically low-pitched and rasping in character, loudest in the second intercostal space at the right sternal border and radiating up to the neck.
[A: 180; B: 16.60; C: 178; D: 259; E: 298; F: 758; G: 1191; H: 1105]

126 Left atrial contraction maintains the end diastolic pressure of the left ventricle. In atrial fibrillation, a serious reduction in cardiac output may result.
[B: 16.60; F: 757; G: 1190; H: 1105]

127 Aortic valve replacement. Symptomatic relief may be striking, provided that operation is performed before the left ventricular myocardium is too damaged.
[A: 182; B: 16.71; C: 178–9; D: 259; F: 759; G: 1193; H: 1107]

128 Aortic dilatation above the valve can prevent the edges of the valve cusps meeting during diastole. Severe hypertension can cause this, and the inflammatory processes of syphilis and ankylosing spondylitis in the walls of the thoracic aorta also lead to aortic dilatation. Another famous but uncommon cause of aortic wall disease is Marfan's syndrome.
[A: 182; B: 16.61; C: 179; D: 260; F: 760; G: 1194; H: 1108]

129 A systolic ejection murmur, the presence of which may be explained by the increased flow of blood through the aortic valve (although there may be a stenosis as well) and the Austin Flint murmur, a low-pitched diastolic rumble caused by the regurgitant aortic jet hitting the anterior leaflet of the open mitral valve.
[A: 183; B: 16.61; C: 179; D: 260; E: 298; F: 760; G: 1195; H: 1108-9]

130 Yes. These are the ECG changes of left ventricular hypertrophy which occur in moderate to severe aortic regurgitation.
[A: 183; C: 195; D: 260; F: 761; G: 1196; H: 1109]

131 Blood flow through the coronary arteries to the subendocardial and deeper layers of the myocardium occurs during diastole and is therefore dependent on diastolic blood presure. This tends to be low in aortic regurgitation. Furthermore, at slower heart rates the amount of time for which there is an adequate coronary perfusion pressure is less than at faster rates (even though diastole gets shorter at faster rates). Heart rate slows at rest, during sleep and with beta-blockade. Nitroglycerin is unlikely to help the situation as it reduces ventricular end diastolic pressure.
[G: 1197; H: 1110]

132 Atherosclerosis.
[A: 185–7; B: 17.22; C: 213; D: 271; E: 299; F: 832; G: 1292; H: 1178–9]

133 Aneurysm of the arch of the aorta. Aneurysms of other parts of the aorta may produce more in the way of signs than symptoms. An ascending aortic aneurysm can compress the superior vena cava and right main bronchus while abdominal aneurysms may present as

a pulsatile mass with back pain due to erosion of the adjacent vertebrae.
[A: 185; B: 17.23; D: 271; E: 299; F: 832; G: 1293; H: 1179]

134 Experience has shown that what might appear to be a leaky graft in fact provides the best template for the patient's endothelial cells which gradually colonize the inner surface of the graft.
[A: 186–7; B: 17.23; F: 832; G: 1293; H: 1179]

135 A combination of ischaemia and 'wear and tear'. The ischaemia relates to the fact that part of the media receives its oxygen supply by diffusion across the aortic intima while the outer part is supplied by the vasa vasorum. The border between these two zones is a layer of potential weakness. The commonest site of origin for a dissection is the ascending aorta and it is this part of the aorta that is particularly subjected to repetitive expansile pulsation.
[A: 186; B: 17.22; C: 213; E: 289; F: 832; G: 1295; H: 1179–80]

136 A tearing pain is sometimes described. Hypertension tends to occur in the early stages, in contrast to myocardial infarction. Coronary, carotid, spinal, renal or mesenteric arteries may be occluded. The presence of neurological signs with a history of sudden onset of severe chest pain should arouse particular suspicion.
[A: 186; B: 17.22–3; C: 213; E: 289; F: 832; G: 1296; H: 1179–80]

137 Commonly widening of the mediastinum does not occur until a few days after the event, and the ECG is likely to remain normal with the exception of the uncommon situation where a dissecting aneurysm tracks proximally and occludes a coronary artery, causing a myocardial infarction. The X-ray and ECG findings do not therefore influence management, which consists of pain relief, reduction of systolic blood pressure to about 100 mmHg and obtaining a surgical opinion as soon as possible. In addition the patient should be monitored for complications such as mesenteric infarction or acute renal failure.
[A: 187; E: 289; F: 832; G: 1297; H: 1180]

138 Infective, namely viral (most importantly coxsackie B), bacterial (diphtheria, leptospirosis), and protozoal (South American trypanosomiasis); hypertrophic obstructive cardiomyopathy (HOCM); endomyocardial fibrosis (occurs in the tropics); fibroelastosis (usually in first few months of life).
[A: 187; B: 16.47; C: 202; D: 271; E: 310; F: 765; G: 1276–80; H: 1144]

139 Yes. The commonest involvement is a pericardial effusion in rheumatoid disease and systemic lupus erythematosus (SLE). Rheumatoid disease, SLE, polyarteritis nodosa and scleroderma can all cause myocardial fibrosis. SLE can cause Libman–Sacks endocarditis, a verrucous non-embolizing variety of valvular damage. Polyarteritis nodosa can involve the coronary arteries causing myocardial infarction. [E: 310; F: 766; G: 1283–7; H: 1142]

140 Yes. In contrast to digoxin, propranolol (like other beta-blockers) has a negative inotropic effect, i.e. it reduces the force of muscle contraction, and this helps to minimize the outflow tract obstruction. [A: 188; B: 16.48; C: 202; D: 271; E: 310; F: 767; G: 1278; H: 1145]

141 Left atrial myxoma, with systemic emboli and constitutional symptoms. [A: 188; B: 16.72; E: 296; F: 780; G: 1288; H: 1147]

142 Recurrent episodes of congestive cardiac failure, initially related to episodes of heavy drinking but later becoming permanent. Atrial fibrillation is a common arrhythmia in these cases. [A: 188; F: 765; G: 1284; H: 1142]

143 Cardiac enlargement, mainly due to pericardial effusion (with low voltage complexes on the ECG), heart failure especially when there is underlying ischaemic heart disease, prolongation of PR interval and T wave abnormalities. Long-standing hypothyroidism augments the development of atherosclerosis. Atrial fibrillation may also occur. [A: 189; B: 23.23–4; C: 468; E: 172–4; F: 779–80; G: 2122; H: 1039]

144 (a) It will be safe to conceive and go through pregnancy.
(b) Pregnancy is contraindicated.
(c) Pregnancy may be safe but careful and regular monitoring of the heart condition will be necessary. It will be important to ensure adequate rest and prompt treatment of respiratory infections.

[A: 189; B: 42.51–4. C: 210; D: 257; F: 778]

145 Hypertension; delayed or reduced pulses and reduced blood pressure in the legs; a systolic murmur; palpable, pulsatile intercostal collateral vessels in the adult. Also in the older patient the lower limbs may be relatively underdeveloped. ECG usually shows left ventricular hypertrophy (and associated cardiac

lesions may cause some right ventricular hypertrophy). X-rays may show indentation of the aorta at the site of coarctation and rib-notching (but not before the age of 6) from dilated collaterals.
[A: 191; B: 16.63; C: 206; D: 265; E: 302; F: 746; G: 1157; H: 1084]

146 Polycythaemia with attendant increase in blood viscosity; clubbing; a tendency to squatting which reduces the right-to-left shunt and increases pulmonary flow; anoxic episodes including convulsions; paradoxical embolization with venous emboli reaching the systemic circulation via the right-to-left shunt; brain abscesses, probably as a result of the loss of the filtering action of the pulmonary circulation; impaired growth.
[A: 191; D: 261; E: 302; G: 1149–54; H: 1078]

147 Kartagener's syndrome.
[G: 147; H: 1076]

148 The abnormality renders the cusps more susceptible to the stresses caused by blood flow through the valve. This damages the collagen which then becomes calcified, leading to rigidity and stenosis.
[A: 192; B: 16.63; C: 177; E: 302; F: 746; G: 1155; H: 1085]

149 A pulmonary ejection systolic murmur accompanied by an ejection click, wide splitting of the second heart sound of which the pulmonary component is of reduced intensity, and, in severe cases, signs of right heart failure. The loudness of the murmur is not an absolute guide to the severity of the lesion.
[A: 193; B: 16.63; C: 208; D: 265; E: 301; F: 745; G: 1158; H: 1082]

150 When pulmonary artery pressure is normal, as is commonly the case, there is a continuous murmur throughout systole and diastole, a 'machinery' murmur. Because of the increased pulmonary venous return to the left heart, there may be left atrial and left ventricular hypertrophy with mitral and aortic flow murmurs.

When pulmonary hypertension with reversal of the shunt occurs, unoxygenated blood is shunted to the descending aorta, resulting in cyanosis and clubbing of the toes, so-called differential cyanosis.
[A: 193; B: 16.66; C: 205; D: 263; E: 300; F: 744; G: 1162; H: 1081]

151 A diastolic murmur in the tricuspid area and/or a systolic ejection murmur in the pulmonary area, due to increased blood flow through these valves, and fixed

splitting of the second heart sound due to the inability of the right ventricle to accept the usual volume increases of inspiration, i.e. splitting is already maximal in expiration. The ECG shows right bundle branch block. In secundum defects there is right axis deviation but in primum defects left axis deviation occurs and tricuspid and mitral incompetence are commonly associated lesions.
[A: 194; B: 16.64; C: 207; D: 262; E: 301; F: 728; G: 1160; H: 1079]

152 The ECG changes depend on the haemodynamic consequences of the shunt and not on the anatomical abnormality itself. With small shunts, the ECG will remain normal but with larger shunts the left ventricle will hypertrophy and if pulmonary hypertension follows, the right ventricle will also enlarge. The ECG may show left, right or combined ventricular hypertrophy.
[A: 195; B: 16.65; C: 207; D: 263; E: 300; F: 731; G: 1170; H: 1080]

153 Small defects usually close spontaneously. Operation is indicated if the pulmonary flow rate is large or if there is a high right ventricular systolic pressure.
There is a very important situation in which surgery is definitely contraindicated and this is Eisenmenger's syndrome. In this situation irreversible pulmonary hypertension develops (with hypertrophy of the pulmonary arterial walls) causing the direction of the shunt to change to right-to-left. This can also happen in patent ductus arteriosus. The result is cyanosis and clubbing.
[A: 196; B: 16.67; D: 266; F: 728; G: 1170; H: 1077]

154 Cyanosis (developing before the age of 1 year), dyspnoea, retarded growth, clubbing and polycythaemia. Episodes of severe hypoxia and cyanosis are typical. Endocarditis, anaemia and cerebral abscess are possible complications.
[A: 196; B: 16.67; C: 209; D: 264; E: 303; F: 735; G: 1164; H: 1083]

155 The outlook is poor and nearly all cases warrant surgery. Because the operative risk of total correction can be high, time can be gained by means of a smaller preliminary operation to increase pulmonary blood flow.
Treatment of hypoxic episodes includes oxygen, placing the child in the knee–chest position and sodium bicarbonate to correct metabolic acidosis if present.
[A: 196; B: 16.67; C: 209; D: 264; E: 303; F: 736; G: 1166; H: 1083–4]

156 No. Even very minor lesions can be complicated by endocarditis. Also it may not be the lesion itself that becomes infected. For example, in a VSD, endocarditis can develop on the roughened lining of the right ventricle where it is hit by the jet of blood coming through the defect.
[A: 215; B: 16.70; C: 182; D: 268; E: 304; F: 772; G: 395; H: 1115]

157 Left ventricular hypertrophy, coronary artery spasm, aortic incompetence and polyarteritis nodosa. There are many other causes.
[A: 197; C: 184; D: 247; E: 280; F: 791; G: 1223; H: 1117]

158 Scotland, Finland, Northern Ireland, New Zealand, Australia and the United States. The epidemiological picture, however, appears to be constantly changing.
[B: 17.6; D: 247; E: 280; G: 1218; H: 1161]

159 The monoclonal hypothesis, which states that atheromatous plaques are degenerating smooth muscle cell tumours; the incrimination of dietary sucrose rather than fats; rheological theories which point out that atheroma occurs at sites where laminar flow is interrupted leading to formation of thrombi adherent to the vessel wall which then degenerate into plaques of atheroma. Genetic factors are important.
[B: 17.11; F: 787; G: 1221; H: 1159]

160 Elevated levels of systolic blood pressure, diastolic blood pressure, serum cholesterol, cigarette smoking, hyperglycaemia and obesity in approximately that order.
[A: 198; B: 17.12; C: 183; D: 247; E: 280–1; F: 788; G: 1219; H: 1161]

161 Massachusetts, USA. The Framingham Heart Disease and Epidemiology Study was a prospective study of cardiovascular disease risk factors and mortality spanning two decades with virtually complete follow-up.
[B: 17.12; G: 1202; H: 1160]

162 As regards primary prevention, an important example was the study that looked for any protective effect from lowering serum cholesterol in adult men in their 20s and 30s. As regards secondary prevention, much attention has focused on beta-blocker therapy. Benefits have not been conclusively demonstrated by either approach.
[B: 17.14; C: 185–6; D: 251–2; F: 796; G: 1236; H: 1166]

163 The commonest changes are depression or sagging of the ST segments and inversion of T waves. Less common but no less significant are ST elevation (although this is more often indicative of infarction) and 'correction' of previously inverted T waves to upright. ST and T wave changes are not exclusively caused by ischaemia. The diagnosis depends on the clinical picture. Ischaemia is the commonest cause, but left ventricular hypertrophy,drug effects, electrolyte abnormality, pericarditis and myocarditis should not be forgotten.
[A: 199; C: 184; D: 64; E: 282; F: 793; G: 1225; H: 1119–20]

164 Treadmill testing and coronary angiography. In the former, the patient goes through a preset sequence of walking speeds and gradients under continuous ECG observation. Blood pressure is checked at frequent intervals and the patient's overall tolerance of the exercise is noted. The ECG is recorded at intervals during the subsequent period of rest, and any ST changes interpreted according to criteria established for the procedure.
[B: 16.29; C: 184; D: 248; E: 282; F: 793; G: 1225–6; H: 1120–1]

165 Initially, as if an infarction had already occurred, i.e. bed rest, sedation, nitroglycerin; then propranolol and/or other antianginal drugs. Coronary angiography is necessary to determine whether bypasss surgery is indicated.
[A: 201; C: 186; D: 248; E: 282; F: 791; G: 1228; H: 1118–24]

166 Nitrites; beta-blockers: calcium blockers.
[A: 200; B: 16.38; C: 185; D: 248; E: 282–3, F: 793–4; G: 1228; H: 1122–3]

167 Major surgery with heart–lung bypass, with postoperative pain from the median sternotomy and numerous sites of blood vessel cannulation, i.e. drips, pressure lines both arterial and venous. Confusion and disorientation is a common temporary postoperative sequel. Figures vary but there is approximately a 50 per cent chance of obtaining complete relief from angina, 30 per cent chance of partial relief and 5–15 per cent chance of no relief at all. An improvement in life expectancy has not yet been unequivocally demonstrated. Dressler's syndrome may be a postoperative sequel.
[A: 210–11; B: 16.70–2; C: 185; D: 248; E: 282–3; F: 795; G: 1238; H: 1124]

168 Prinzmetal or variant angina. On coronary angiography spasm of coronary arteries may be seen without evidence of atherosclerotic obstruction of the vessels.
[A: 202; C: 184; D: 248; E: 281; F: 796; G: 1229; H: 1119]

169 Severe, crushing, central chest pain, sometimes radiating to the jaw or down the left arm but less commonly to the back; breathlessness; sweating; faint or dizzy feelings. There may be vomiting. Depending on the presence of complications, physical examination may be entirely normal. The only abnormality may be a fourth heart sound or there may be acute circulatory failure with hypotension, pulmonary oedema and arrhythmias.
[A: 203; B: 16.39; C: 187; D: 249; E: 283; F: 796; G: 1229; H: 1125]

170 Elevation of cardiac enzymes. Creatine phosphokinase (CPK) starts to rise within a few hours, glutamic-oxaloacetic transaminase (SGOT) within 12–48 hours and lactate dehydrogenase (LDH) or, more specifically, hydroxybutyrate dehydrogenase (HBD) reaches a peak at 48–72 hours. Elevation of white cell count and ESR also occur but these are not specific.
[A: 204; B: 16.41; C: 187–90; D: 61–4; E: 283–4; F: 797; G: 1231–2; H: 1126]

171 Left anterior descending, right coronary, and either right coronary or left circumflex (depending on which vessel is dominant) respectively.
[A: 204; B: 16.42; C: 188; D: 61–4; E: 283–4; F: 797; G: 1232; H: 1006–7]

172 The ECG may revert to normal but it is common for Q waves to persist. T wave inversion and ST segment elevation (and reciprocal depression) usually begin to improve within a few days and although some T wave changes may be permanent it is unusual for ST elevation to be present more than 3 weeks after the event. If it is, ventricular aneurysm may be present.
[A: 211; B: 16.41; D: 251; E: 284; F: 797; G: 1237; H: 1134]

173 Death, as the well-worn phrase goes, does not come unannounced. The occurrence of ventricular extrasystoles in myocardial infarction may be a warning of imminent ventricular tachycardia or fibrillation. Treatment is particularly indicated if there is a short coupling time (R on T), if ventricular extrasystoles occur in salvos of two or more in

succession, if they are multiform or multifocal, and if they occur more frequently than five per minute.
[A: 205–7; B: 16.40; C: 190; D: 249; E: 284; F: 798–800; G: 1235–6; H: 1130–5]

174 Although often asymptomatic, persistent heart failure or arrhythmias or systemic embolism may occur. There may be a double apex beat with visible systolic expansion in the chest wall. ECGs may show persistent ST segment elevation with or without large Q waves.
[A: 211; B: 16.41; D: 250; E: 285: F: 800; G: 1237; H: 1134]

175 While this would appear to be sound policy, some studies have shown that, statistically speaking, there is little difference between home treatment and hospital treatment in terms of survival. There is little doubt that a knowledgeable general practitioner with enough time to visit his patient two or three times daily and using antiarrhythmic drugs prophylactically has a headstart on a hectic, understaffed general medical ward or coronary care unit where the prevailing tension may be a source of anxiety, adrenaline and arrhythmias.
[A: 207; B: 16.42–3; C: 191; E: 285; F: 801; G: 1234]

176 Although serial ECGs are part of the routine follow-up of myocardial infarction, they are unlikely to detect the short salvos of ventricular ectopics which can occur during sleep or straining at stool. Telemetry is one way to continuously monitor ambulatory patients, the chest leads being attached to a small battery-operated radio transmitter, often carried in the pocket of pyjamas or dressing gown, which transmits the ECG signal to a monitoring station. Alternatively the signal can be recorded on a 24 hour tape in a portable recorder and analysed subsequently (Holter monitoring).
[A: 208; C: 190; E: 285–6; F: 799; G: 1235; H: 1130]

177 Chemical, mechanical (in a small number of centres in this country, but many more in the United States), and, in the few designated centres, heart transplant.

Chemical includes the adrenoreceptor agonists noradrenaline, isoprenaline and dopamine. This last is enjoying a vogue which may be justified on the theoretical grounds that it does not reduce renal blood flow.

Mechanical refers to aortic balloon counterpulsation, in which balloon inflation is timed to occur during diastole, obstructing aortic runoff and

increasing coronary blood flow. The technique has its advocates and critics.
[A: 210; C: 190; D: 249; E: 286; F: 798; G: 1236; H: 1133]

178 Don't smoke, lose excess weight (or don't put on weight), don't hurry and don't worry—enjoy life.
[A: 210–11; B: 17.15; C: 191–2; D: 251; E: 286; F: 802; G: 1236–7]

179 Dressler's (postmyocardial infarction) syndrome. The physical signs are due to a pericarditis with effusion, pleural effusion and pneumonitis. The two most commonly used therapeutic agents are indomethacin and prednisone. The condition usually subsides within one to two weeks.
[A: 211; B: 16.41; C: 190; D: 269; F: 801; G: 1237; H: 1135]

180 Infective (also known as subacute) endocarditis. Cerebral emboli. Microscopic haematuria. Both emboli of infected vegetations and deposition of antigen–antibody complexes contribute to the damage to the brain, kidney and other organs.
[A: 212–13; B: 16.49–50; C: 181; D: 266; E: 303; F: 770–1; G: 386; H: 1113]

181 Infective (subacute) endocarditis, although they may occur in other septicaemias. Blood culture is the diagnostic test. Treatment is with the appropriate antibiotic(s) given for up to six weeks to eradicate organisms from the avascular valve cusps and chordae tendinae (which may rupture). Valve replacement is sometimes indicated if organisms are resistant or if heart failure is intractable.
[A: 213; B: 16.50–1; C: 182; D: 267; E: 303–4; F: 771; G: 387–95; H: 1113–16]

182 In a woman of this age, the differential diagnosis is mainly between an infective cause, viral being the commonest, and an autoimmune disorder such as SLE. A recent upper respiratory tract infection would point to the former, while polyarthritis, abnormal urinary sediment, thrombocytopenia or other evidence of multisystem disease would indicate the latter. Uraemia and myxoedema should both be easily detected. Malignant invasion of the pericardium is rare.
[A: 215; B: 16.45; C: 202; D: 269; E:307; F: 782; G: 1269–72; H: 1150]

183 Pericarditis due to a myocardial infarction. Two other cardiac conditions in which pericarditis occurs are Dressler's syndrome and acute rheumatic carditis. [A: 216; C: 203; D: 269–70; E: 308; F: 783; G: 1272; H: 1150]

184 This man has a pericardial effusion, probably uraemic in origin. The chest X-ray may show an enlarged cardiac silhouette with clear edges and the ECG low voltage complexes. Variation in the size of the complexes, electrical alternans, can occur. [A: 216–17; B: 16.46; C: 203; D: 269; E: 308; F: 783–4; G: 1273–4; H: 1150–2]

185 Surgical removal of the pericardium. Conventional treatment for heart failure may give some relief. [A: 218; B: 16.46; C: 204; D: 270; E: 309; F: 785; G: 1275; H: 1154]

186 Congestive cardiac failure of any cause; chronic lung disease especially when polycythaemia is present (causing increased blood viscosity); malignancy; administration of oestrogens (synthetic ones are regarded as more dangerous than natural hormones). [A: 219; B: 18.98; C: 199; D: 242; E: 305; F: 803; G: 1129–30; H: 1249]

187 With large pulmonary emboli hypotension and cyanosis invariably occur. In the acute, critical case, the patient may prefer to lie flat (in contrast to the dyspnoea of cardiac failure). The sudden increase in pulmonary vascular resistance causes pulmonary hypertension which may be felt as a parasternal heave, and the resultant right ventricular failure may give a gallop rhythm with third and fourth heart sounds. In cases diagnosed hours or days after the event, a spike of fever is a very valuable piece of evidence. [A: 219; B: 18.99; C: 200; D: 242; E: 305–6; F: 804; G: 1131–2; H: 1250]

188 Chest X-ray—either an area of lost vessel markings, or a shadow in continuity with a pulmonary artery. Small, transient pleural effusions are common.

ECG—the S1 Q3, T3 pattern of right ventricular strain due to acute pulmonary hypertension, as well as a tachycardia.

Blood gases—low Po_2 due to the perfusion defect and low Pco_2 due to the resulting hyperventilation.

Normal chest X-ray, ECG and blood gases do not exclude the diagnosis. [A: 219; C: 200; D: 243; E: 306; F: 804; G: 1132–3; H: 1251–2]

189 It blocks the hepatic synthesis of vitamin-K-dependent coagulation factors, causing prolongation of the prothrombin time. Reversal of its effects with vitamin K takes at least 6 hours. When treatment with warfarin is first started, it may take a week to suppress all clotting factors although the prothrombin time will be prolonged before this.
[A: 220; B: 18.102; C: 201; D: 243; E: 306–7; F: 804; G: 1133; H: 1252]

190 Induction of liver enzymes reduces warfarin effect during concurrent administration but causes a rebound on withdrawal (phenobarbitone, chloral hydrate, glutethimide, meprobamate, haloperidol, griseofulvin).

Competition and displacement from plasma protein binding sites causes increased warfarin effect (aspirin, phenytoin, phenylbutazone). In turn, warfarin increases the action of phenytoin and oral hypoglycaemics. Antibiotics can augment warfarin effect by killing gut bacteria that synthesize vitamin K.
[A: 220; B: 62.18; E: 218; G: 2340; H: 379–81]

191 Streptokinase. This is a fibrinolytic agent with the property of dissolving freshly formed thrombus. It is best administered via a line introduced into the pulmonary trunk to deliver the maximum concentration to the required site. Hydrocortisone is also given to suppress any allergic reaction.
[A: 220; B: 18.103; D: 243; E: 307; F: 804; G: 1133; H: 1252]

192 Pulmonary hypertension due to recurrent, small pulmonary emboli. If tachypnoea is present at rest it will persist during sleep. Chest pains may occur but ECG changes may not develop until an advanced stage is reached, if at all.
[A: 221; B: 16.74; C: 199; F: 806; G: 1138; H: 1247–9]

193 At the stage of intermittent claudication, absent peripheral pulses and/or bruits over the larger arteries. A drop in blood presure at the ankle will occur with exercise.

At the stage of rest pain, there will be loss of hair, trophic nail changes and ulcers and gangrene may develop.
[A: 223; B: 17.16; C: 212; D: 272; E: 287; F: 829; G: 1300; H: 1183]

194 Giving up smoking. Weight reduction. Daily, systematic exercise to encourage the development of collaterals. Proper care of the feet, especially in the

presence of diabetic neuropathy, is essential. Surgery offers lumbar sympathectomy, which relieves some cases of rest pain, and vessel grafts for lesions that are localized. Very good relief of symptoms may result.
[A: 224; B: 17.18; C: 212; D: 273; E: 287–8; F: 830; G: 1301; H: 1184]

195 Buerger's disease or thrombangiitis obliterans. He must stop smoking.
[A: 225; B: 17.17; C: 214; E: 288; F: 831; G: 1302; H: 1184]

196 Acute brachial artery occlusion, due to an embolus from the heart or large vessel atheromatous plaque. Surgical embolectomy is indicated as an emergency, since irreversible tissue necrosis begins after about 6 hours. Postoperative anticoagulation should also be given, and attention given to the possibility of correcting the source of emboli.
[A: 225; B: 17.29; C: 213; D: 273; F: 830; G: 1303–4; H: 1182]

197 There are several, but the following should be particularly borne in mind: collagen vascular diseases, especially scleroderma; blood disorders including cryoglobulinaemia and dysproteinaemias; drugs, in particular ergotamine preparations used in migraine, and propranolol. Prolonged use of hand-held vibrating machinery, e.g. road drills, is another cause.
[A: 226; B: 17.24; C: 215; D: 274; E: 288; F: 829; G: 1306; H: 1185]

198 Takayasu's disease, otherwise described as pulseless disease. The disease process consists of a progressive inflammation in the walls of the aortic arch, leading to occlusion of the openings of the main branches.
[B: 25.31; C: 215; F: 831; C: 1297–8; H: 1181]

199 Ultrasound venous flow detection, radioactive fibrinogen uptake, plethysmography and venography.

The first of these is a bedside test, suitable for detecting the presence of a femoral vein thrombosis. The second test gives variable results since ideally the radioactive fibrinogen should be in the body at the time of thrombus formation and not after the bulk of thrombus has already formed. Combining radioactive fibrinogen with impedance plethysmography, however, is as effective as venography and considerably less invasive.
[A: 227; B: 17.33; C: 216–17; D: 242; E: 305; F: 834; G: 1125; H: 1187]

200 Features of the postphlebitic syndrome, namely swelling, pigmentation of the skin below the medial malleolus and slow healing of minor injuries, or chronic ulceration.
[A: 228; B: 17.33; C: 216; D: 242; F: 834; G: 1313; H: 1187]

Respiratory System

201 The oblique fissure, which separates the lower lobe from the upper and middle lobes, runs from the anterior end of the sixth rib (as it does on the left also) upwards and backwards following the line of the fifth or sixth rib to reach the vertebral column. The horizontal fissure, separating the upper from the middle lobe runs horizontally at the level of the fourth costal cartilage to join the oblique fissure in the midaxillary line.

There is no horizontal fissure on the left side because the lingula, the equivalent of the right middle lobe, is part of the left upper lobe.
[A: 231; B: 18.7–8; C: 220; F: 851]

202 Apical, anterior and posterior segments in the upper lobe and superior and inferior segments of the lingula (the lingular bronchus is the first branch of the left upper lobe bronchus), and apical, lateral, anterior and posterior in the lower lobe.
[A: 231; C: 220; F: 851]

203 Whether or not the (PA) film has been taken straight. The easiest way to confirm this is to see that the medial ends of the clavicles are equidistant from the spinous processes of the vertebrae.
[A: 232; B: 18.7–8; E: 324–5; G: 941–2]

204 In normal lungs, the markings are due to the pulmonary vasculature. The bronchi may show if they become thickened and distorted by disease but in chronic bronchitis, the commonest bronchial disease, the chest X-ray is commonly normal.
[A: 232; B: 18.7–8; E: 324–5; G: 941–2]

205 This simple device, which the patient blows into as hard as possible and then keeps blowing into until the lungs are 'empty', measures the forced expiratory volume in one second (FEV_1) and the forced vital capacity (FVC), i.e. the maximum expired volume. The values obtained are compared to the expected values for age, sex and size as given in tables. A reduction in FVC (and proportionate reduction in FEV) indicates restrictive lung disease, while a reduction in FEV_1

relative to FVC (below 75 per cent) indicates obstructive lung disease.
[A: 235; B: 18.10; C: 232; D: 51; E: 320–1; F: 854; G: 934; H: 1197]

206 Vital capacity is the volume of air which can be expired following a single maximal inspiration. The value increases with body size and decreases with age. The value obtained in a young adult male is approximately 4½ litres.
[A: 235; B: 18.10–11; C: 233; E: 320; F: 854; G: 932–3; H: 1197]

207 Obstructive—reduction in FVC with reduction in the ratio of FEV_1 to FVC to less than 75 per cent. Restrictive—reduction in FVC with normal or increased FEV_1 to FVC ratio.
In obstructive lung disease the time taken to exhale the forced vital capacity is prolonged, but not in restrictive disease.
[A: 235; B: 18.9–10; C: 232; D: 51; F: 854; G: 935–6; H: 1197]

208 Peak (expiratory) flow rate (PEFR) is measured with a peak flow meter, and minute volume (MV) with a respirometer. PEFR is used in the assessment of response to treatment either in acute asthma or in chronic obstructive airways disease, while MV (which equals the tidal volume × the respiratory rate) gives an indication of adequacy of respiratory effort in drug overdoses or following a period of mechanical ventilation (e.g. anaesthesia or fractured ribs with flail chest), and also in assessing the need for mechanical ventilation in neurological disorders (e.g. Guillain–Barré syndrome).
[A: 235; B: 18.10; C: 232; D: 51; E: 321; F: 854]

209 Hyperventilation. These blood gases show a compensated respiratory alkalosis.
[A: 236; B: 18.15–16; C: 234; D: 50; E: 322–3; F: 856; G: 939–40; H: 1198]

210 (a) Disease of the lung parenchyma in which there is either loss of lung tissue (e.g. emphysema, lobectomy) or ventilation/perfusion inequality.
(b) Thickening of the alveolar capillary membrane as occurs in sarcoidosis and other granulomatous diseases and in chronic pulmonary oedema.
[A: 237; B: 18.17; C: 225; E: 323; F: 855; G: 936–8; H: 1192]

211 Inhalation of tobacco smoke causes an immediate rise in airways resistance which perists for an hour or

longer. Studies in subjects, both men and women, who smoke 20 cigarettes daily show slight but significant reductions in all indices of lung function as compared to matched non-smokers. Smoking also enhances the decline in lung function that occurs with age.

212 Purulent sputum has pus cells in it and is a good indication of the presence of bacterial infection and probable benefit from antibiotic therapy. The commonest cause of cough is upper respiratory tract infection, but this is usually viral in origin, and the cough is seldom productive.
[A: 239; B: 18.2; C; 225; E: 318; G: 947]

213 Mitral stenosis, and acute pulmonary oedema due to left ventricular failure.
[A: 240; B: 18.4; C: 226; D: 244; E: 318; H: 160]

214 Inflammation of the pericardium may cause pain that is felt on inspiration. General practitioners and osteopaths know, however, that a very common cause of 'pleuritic' pain is musculoskeletal, arising from the shoulder girdles and cervicothoracic spine. This is diagnosed by physical examination.
[A: 241: B: 18.4; C: 226; E: 319; G: 1013; H: 30]

215 Having listened to her chest and confirmed the absence of abnormal lung signs, he checked on the full range of neck movement. He then palpated the neck and trapezius on both sides. Then he examined each intercostal space between the medial border of the scapula and the spine, on each side, firmly pressing the muscles with the balls of his thumb. At the level of T4 and T5 he felt the muscle to be like tight cords and, as he pressed, she jumped and said, 'yes, that's where the pain is'. After a few days of exercises, local heat and an anti-inflammatory preparation, her pain had settled. She continued taking the pill. Her diagnosis was musculoskeletal pain and not pulmonary embolism.
[A: 241; G: 208; H: 30]

216 It becomes prolonged. This may be evident when other auscultatory findings are not helpful.
[A: 244; H: 1207]

217 Carcinoma of the lung, pus in the chest with chronic suppuration (e.g. bronchiectasis, lung abscess, empyema) and chronic fibrosing alveolitis.

It is extremely unusual to see clubbing in patients with pulmonary TB unless severe destruction has occurred and chronic suppuration has supervened.
[A: 244; B: 18.5; C: 228; D: 48; G: 201]

218 This chest deformity may interfere with local aeration of part of the lungs. If the hypoxia is sustained, the resulting pulmonary vasoconstriction may lead to pulmonary hypertension, this, in turn, causing cor pulmonale.
[A: 245; B: 18.5; C: 306; E: 354; F: 884; G: 1020; H: 1273]

219 The position of his shoulders indicates that he has had at least moderately severe asthma for several years, probably since childhood. If one side of the chest is expanding less than the other, a pneumothorax is a possibility.
[A: 245; B: 18.5; C: 229; D: 47; E: 366; H: 1207]

220 He may of course have bilateral disease but it would have been worse on the right. The fibrosis and contracture of the lung, which is a prominent and destructive feature of TB, has pulled the trachea over. This is in contrast to the effect of a tumour which tends initially to push the trachea away from it.
[A: 245; B: 18.5; C: 229; D: 47]

221 Pneumothorax, hyperinflation as during an attack of asthma and emphysema. In the latter two instances, the area of resonance will also be greater since the upper border of the liver will be displaced downwards, sometimes making the liver edge palpable and giving the false impression of hepatomegaly.
[A: 246; B: 18.5; C: 229; D: 47]

222 It has a harsh and loud character, in contrast to the soft rustling of normal vesicular breath sounds.

Its presence indicates that there is disease in the lung parenchyma which lies between the large bronchi and the chest wall. This diseased tissue conducts bronchial sounds to the chest wall more effectively than normal lung tissue. Bronchial breathing is commonly heard over consolidation or a large cavity.
[A: 246; B: 18.5; C: 230; D: 48]

223 Inspection may reveal reduced chest wall movement on the affected side. Palpation may reveal displacement of the apex beat (if the effusion is large). Percussion will reveal the characteristically stony dullness (a more marked loss of resonance than occurs over, say, the liver). On auscultation, breath sounds will be quiet or absent. Voice conduction will be reduced over the mass of the effusion but over the upper border, aegophony is commonly heard (a nasal, bleating quality of sound). Tactile vocal fremitus will be reduced.

Physical signs can sometimes give a better idea of the position and size of an effusion than an X-ray.
[A: 243; B: 18.68; C: 230; D: 48; G: 1014; H: 1265]

224 Inspiratory rhonchi either originate in the upper respiratory tract (larynx, trachea) or indicate that a bronchus is too stiffened by pathological processes to widen as the chest and lungs expand. Expiratory rhonchi occur in the bronchial tree which reduces in diameter as the lungs empty.
[A: 247; B: 18.6; C: 229; D: 48]

225 Râles are the short, soft, crackling sounds made by air bubbling through fine bronchioles as the walls of the bronchioles snap open. In normal lungs they may be heard but should disappear following a deep breath. Persistent râles indicate the presence of abnormal amounts of fluid which may be inflammatory secretions, oedema, blood or pus. Crepitations is a synonymous term.
[A: 247; B: 18.5; C: 229; D: 48]

226 They are allergic to the protein of the house dust mite, *Dermatophagoides pteronyssinus*, and dust accumulates in houses more in winter. The first aspect of treatment of allergic rhinitis (as of extrinsic asthma and other allergic disorders) is the avoidance of the allergen. In this case, extra vacuum cleaning and removal of dusty bedding, carpets etc. is indicated.
[A: 247; B: 32.16; C: 265; E: 125; F: 839; G: 157; H: 345]

227 Rhino, adeno, ECHO, parainfluenza and respiratory syncytial viruses.
[A: 249; B: 12.17; C: 238; E: 327; F: 143; G: 230; H: 778–9]

228 Bronchogenic carcinoma, producing hoarseness by involving the recurrent laryngeal nerve (more vulnerable on the left); tuberculosis of the vocal cords in association with chronic pulmonary disease; cigarette-smoking increases the risk of laryngeal carcinoma. Damage to one or both recurrent laryngeal nerves can occur during thyroidectomy.
[A: 250, B: 32.23; C: 276; E: 495; F: 843; H: 1258]

229 Those in whom secondary bacterial infection can be anticipated, namely the frail elderly, the chronic bronchitics, patients with heart failure, severe asthmatics and others with chronic impairment of lung function and resistance to infection (e.g. bronchiectasis).
[A: 251; B: 12.17; C: 240; G: 233]

230 In the larger bronchi, hypertrophy of the submucosal mucus-producing glands occurs. In the smaller, more peripheral bronchioles, where obstruction is more serious, the normal epithelium is replaced by goblet cells.

Later stages of the disease are marked by the presence of inflammatory cells, oedema, smooth muscle hypertrophy and peribronchial fibrosis.
[A: 251; B: 18.40; C: 279; D: 224; E: 341; F: 883; G: 960; H: 1235]

231 Cough, benignly referred to as 'a smoker's cough', with sputum production is the initial symptom. Over a variable number of years, the cough changes from being a winter to a daily phenomenon and then increasing dyspnoea sets in. If this is progressive, complete disablement results, with the development of oedema and oliguria as the heart fails (cor pulmonale).

Examination in the earlier stages will reveal coarse rhonchi and râles from retained secretions. Cyanosis, barrel chest and fluid retention ('blue bloater') will be found later.

The chest X-ray is often normal but in the later stages, shadows of thickened and irregular bronchial walls may be seen. Also look for the changes of emphysema and cor pulmonale.
[A: 252; B: 18.44–5; C: 279; D: 224; E: 343; F: 883–4; G: 960–1; H: 1239]

232 Bronchodilators, such as salbutamol and aminophylline. Prednisone, in a small dose, has a valuable effect in some patients. Cough mixtures are often requested and praised by patients. Diuretics and potassium supplements are indicated once heart failure develops. Digoxin helps some patients.

Mucolytic agents are of questionable value.
[A: 252; B: 18.46; C: 279; D: 225; E: 343; F: 884; G: 962; H: 1239–40]

233 Chronic bronchitis, chronic asthma, chronic inhalation of dusts, healing of granulomatous lung diseases like tuberculosis and inherited deficiency of alpha$_1$-antitrypsin are all predisposing conditions.

The destruction of lung tissue results in a reduction in surface available for gas exchange and in ventilation/perfusion mismatching from the distorted architecture. Hypoxaemia occurs and, in pure emphysema, results in a 'pink puffer'.
[A: 253; B: 18.40; C: 281; D: 224; E: 341; F: 886; G: 960; H: 1235]

234 Some or all of the following: dyspnoea at rest; accessory respiratory muscles in action; increased PA

chest diameter (i.e. barrel chest) with poor respiratory movement; generalized increase in resonance with a reduction in cardiac and hepatic dullness; patchy or generalized reduction in breath sounds.

Rhonchi and râles may also be heard.

[A: 254; B: 18.44–5; C: 281; D: 224; E: 344; F: 887; G: 960–1; H: 1238]

235 Emphysema. Vitalograph will show an obstructive pattern with a reduced forced vital capacity. Spirometry and gas studies will show increased residual and total lung volumes with a reduced transfer factor.

[A: 255; B: 18.45; C: 281; D: 225; E: 345; F: 887; G: 961; H: 1239]

236 As with chronic bronchitis, try to prevent further deterioration—by cessation of smoking, change of climate where feasible to a warm, dry atmosphere—and by treatment of any accompanying bronchospasm and prophylaxis and treatment of infection.

Some patients make remarkable progress when general physical fitness is improved by training close to the limits of exercise tolerance.

[A: 255; B: 18.46; C: 282; D: 225; E: 345; F: 887; G: 962; H: 1239–40]

237 The first thing to check is that the film has not been rotated. If it has, the distance between the vertebral spine and the medial ends of the clavicles will not be the same on the two sides.

Unilateral emphysema can occur. If a lobe is collapsed or removed, the remainder of the lung shows compensatory emphysema. A large bulla or cyst will appear translucent. Partial obstruction of a main bronchus may trap air distally by a ball-valve mechanism, thus causing unilateral emphysema.

[A: 255; F: 888; G: 1004; H: 1241]

238 Because of the phenomenon of creeping atelectasis in which distal portions of the lungs with borderline ventilation tend to collapse.

The ventilator tubing can become disconnected and unless the possibility is kept in mind it may go unnoticed. The endotracheal tube, or the tracheostomy may block up with secretions unless these are frequently aspirated. Where oxygen is supplied by cylinder, the cylinder may run out. It has been known for a ventilator to be inadvertently unplugged to use the plug for something else.

[A: 256; B: 11.25–7; C: 236; E: 369; F: 857; G: 1039–42; H: 1282]

239 Intermittent positive pressure ventilation. This will provide adequate ventilation and enable you to give analgesia for his limb injuries and proceed with surgery if necessay.

240 Cor pulmonale.
[A: 257; B: 16.73; C: 282; F: 806; G: 960–1; H: 1139]

241 Pulmonary hypertension. Several things may contribute. Pulmonary arterioles constrict in response to hypoxia (whether this be due to the airways obstruction of chronic bronchitis or the underventilation of lungs in a grossly kyphotic chest). Distortion of lung tissue may obliterate or obstruct the blood vessels. Pulmonary oedema reduces lung compliance and increases resistance to blood flow.
[A: 257; B: 16.73; C: 282; F: 805–6; G: 1029; H: 1138]

242 Right axis deviation (axis $> +110^\circ$), P wave enlargement (P pulmonale $>$ 2.5 mm tall and $>$ 0.1 sec in duration), mainly positive deflection in V1, mainly negative deflection in V5 and left precordial leads and ST depression and T inversion in leads II, III, aVF and right precordial leads.

The PA chest X-ray will show cardiac enlargement with the dilated right atrium extending the right border of the shadow, and prominent pulmonary arteries at the hila.
[A: 257; B: 18.45; F: 807; G: 961–2; H: 1139]

243 Yes. The safety of any inspired oxygen level should be checked by arterial blood gas estimation. Some patients can be given only 24 per cent. Digoxin has often been regarded as unsafe in cor pulmonale, but many physicians find it as useful as it is in ischaemic heart disease. (Of course, its usefulness in the presence of sinus rhythm is a matter of current dispute.) Ampicillin is effective against the two most common infecting bacteria, *Haemophilus influenzae* and the pneumococcus.
[A: 257–8; B: 16.73; C: 282; E: 369; F: 807; G: 1029; H: 1139]

244 Those in whom chronic carbon dioxide retention has dulled the respiratory centre to everything except hypoxia. Giving too much oxygen then removes the respiratory drive. These patients are usually chronic bronchitics. Hypercapnia may cause restlessness and confusion, inviting sedation. Sedation will further depress the respiratory centre, however, and must be avoided.

In the absence of carbon dioxide retention as in most cases of asthma or pure emphysema, 100 per cent oxygen can be given during the acute episode with safety.
[A: 258; B: 18.23; C: 227–8; E: 368; F: 856; G: 963; H: 1274]

245 The common causes are: bronchial dilatation following pneumonias, particularly those complicating childhood whooping cough and measles; dilatation beyond a bronchial obstruction e.g. right middle lobe bronchiectasis due to compression of the bronchus by enlarged tuberculous hilar nodes in childhood—Brock's syndrome; cystic fibrosis and foreign body aspiration e.g. blood clot, peanut.

Another cause is bronchopulmonary aspergillosis.
[A: 259; B: 18.47; C: 282; D: 225; E: 352; F: 878; G: 982; H: 1230]

246 Bronchiectasis. Some patients with bronchiectasis are relatively asymptomatic, especially if their disease is confined to parts of the lung that drain spontaneously, such as the upper lobes, which may have been scarred and damaged by TB.
[A: 260; B: 18.49; C: 283; D: 226; E: 352; F: 879; G: 983; H: 1231]

247 Sputum culture for AFB and for *Aspergillus* with serology for *Aspergillus* precipitins. Cystic fibrosis is diagnosed by finding raised sodium and chloride levels in sweat.

Chest X-rays may show 1–2 cm incomplete ring shadows, representing the inflamed and thickened walls of bronchi with saccular bronchiectasis. More common are irregular line shadows representing streaky infiltration and small areas of collapse. The X-ray can also be normal.

Lung function tests and bronchography.
[A: 261; B: 18.50; E: 352; F: 879; G: 983; H: 1231]

248 Recurrent heavy haemoptysis; recurrent localized pneumonias; failure of medical management to control disabling symptoms from localized disease. Surgery is limited to the resection of localized disease, but no surgery is possible unless lung function and general condition is adequate.

Because the instillation or insufflation of the contrast medium into the airways may be irritant and provoke more secretions, patients must have had a period of physiotherapy and postural drainage to clear the lungs as much as possible. They must also be

mentally prepared and relaxed so that they can control any desire to cough during the procedure.
[A: 261; B: 18.51; C: 284; F: 881; G: 983; H: 1232]

249 At least 10 minutes twice a day, with cupped hand percussion, vibration and coughing until no more sputum comes up.

Slight elevation of the foot of the bed with the patient on his back and a pillow under the right chest is recommended for drainage of the right middle lobe.
[A: 261; B: 18.51; C: 283–4; D: 226; E: 352; F: 879; H: 1232]

250 Allergic reactions to inhaled or sometimes ingested allergens; infections; vagal stimuli, such as a heavy meal or exercise; beta-blockers; emotional states and psychological problems.
[A: 262–3; B: 18.92; C: 266; D: 226–7; E: 345; F: 889; G: 955–6; H: 1203]

251 Nothing else invariably happens, although the blood gases are likely to show a reduced carbon dioxide tension as a result of hyperventilation. Dyspnoea is due to altered reflexes and not to hypoxaemia.
[B: 18.94; E: 345; F: 890; G: 952–3; H: 1207]

252 Bronchodilators, particularly salbutamol by inhalation; intravenous hydrocortisone and oral prednisone if the case is severe; antibiotics for any infection; oxygen; bed rest and calm confidence that the attack is going to settle.

Rehydration with intravenous fluids helps the patient to cough up secretions.

Fluid and oxygen therapy must be especially carefully controlled in the presence of heart failure and carbon dioxide retention. Sedatives and tranquillizers are absolutely contraindicated.
[A: 265; B: 18.97; C: 270–1; D: 228–9; E: 349–50; F: 891; G: 959; H: 1208–9]

253 Removal or avoidance of the known allergen(s); regular or intermittent treatment with bronchodilators, and either oral prednisone in cases resistant to other forms of therapy, or beclomethasone inhaler. Occasionally, psychotherapy or a change of environment helps.
[A: 266; B: 18.96; C: 269; D: 228–9; E: 350; F: 892; G: 957–8; H: 1209]

254 If the allergen combines with IgE, the response is virtually immediate or within minutes; if with IgG, then the response takes a few hours.

An immediate hypersensitivity response usually subsides within an hour, whereas a type III reaction may take 24 hours or longer. Patterns of response have been described in which a single exposure to an allergen results in an attack of asthma at the same time each day for several days.
[A: 264; F: 889; H: 1205]

255 Incorrect use of the aerosol. Even with correctly timed triggering of the aerosol to coincide with inspiration, an appreciable part of the 'puff' is deposited on the uvula and throat because some droplets are too large to be entrained in the air-stream.
[D: 228]

256 Positive skin tests (skin-prick tests) indicate an atopic tendency but do not definitely identify the substance which is involved. RIST measures the IgE concentration of the serum, which is of interest but still not diagnostic. RAST measures the amount of IgE directed against specific antigens. This may be highly suggestive but the ultimate confirmation of an allergen lies in the patient's history and substantiation by direct allergen challenge.
[A: 263; C: 268; E: 349; F: 891; G: 159; H: 346]

257 Cigarette-smoking, both active and passive (inhaling other people's smoke); living in cities and other areas of atmospheric pollution; pulmonary asbestosis; exposure to dust from uranium, chromium and nickel ores.
[A: 267; B: 18.52; C: 288; D: 234–5; E: 360; F: 895; G: 1005; H: 1259]

258 Squamous cell—usually central, related to smoking.
Anaplastic—includes oat-cell tumours which are the tumours most commonly associated with non-metastatic endocrine disease.
Adenocarcinoma—usually peripheral, not closely related to smoking.
Alveolar cell—tumours can be single or multiple. Surgical removal of a single tumour can be curative.
[A: 267; B: 18.55; C: 288; D: 234; E: 360; F: 895; G: 1005; H: 1260]

259 Yes. Incomplete resolution or recurrence of the pneumonia is an important presentation. He should be closely followed up and bronchoscoped.
[A: 268; B: 18.57; C: 289; D: 235; F: 896; G: 1006]

260 Examine the costophrenic angle on the X-ray. If it is more dense than the lung, fluid is most probably present. X-ray the patient lying on his side (lateral

decubitus view). Fluid will move up to the apex of the lung and the appearance will change.
[A: 268; B: 18.57; C: 288–9; E: 360; F: 896; H: 1260]

261 Superior vena cava.
[A: 268; B: 18.57; C: 291; E: 360; F: 896; G: 1006; H: 1260]

262 Lymph nodes, liver, bones, brain and skin. The adrenal glands are sometimes involved.
[A: 268; B: 18.57; C: 289; D: 235; E: 361; F: 896; G: 1006; H: 1260–1]

263 Cerebral metastasis, single or multiple. Cerebellar degeneration in the absence of metastases (although metastasis to the cerebellum occurs); sensory polyneuritis; motor neuropathy; myasthenic syndrome; motor neurone disease; cerebral degeneration causing dementia.
[A: 269; B: 18.58; D: 235; F: 897; G: 1007; H: 1261]

264 Ectopic ACTH production, producing Cushing's syndrome with severe pigmentation, weakness and hypokalaemic alkalosis; hypercalcaemia due to a parathormone-like substance; inappropriate ADH secretion, causing dilutional hyponatraemia.

Carcinoid syndrome, hypoglycaemia, hyperglycaemia, thyrotoxicosis, acromegaly and gynaecomastia can also occur as can polycythaemia and red cell aplasia.
[A: 269; B: 18.58; C: 289; D: 235; E: 361; F: 896–7; G: 1006–7; H: 1261]

265 New bone is laid down at the distal ends of particularly the forearm and leg bones, leading to marked swelling at the wrists and ankles.

Other signs and syndromes which can be due to non-metastatic effects of a bronchogenic carcinoma are: clubbing; thrombophlebitis; dermatomyositis; acanthosis nigricans, urticaria and other dermatological conditions; haemolysis, bleeding tendency due to fibrinolysins and folic acid deficiency anaemia.
[A: 269; B: 18.58; C: 289; D: 235; E: 361; F: 896; G: 1007; H: 1261]

266 Lung function tests. Extensive or metastatic disease is not the only contraindication to surgery. Many patients, often by virtue of being smokers, do not have sufficient lung function to withstand lobectomy, pneumonectomy or even bronchoscopy!
[A: 270; B: 18.58; C: 231; D: 235–6; F: 898; G: 1008; H: 1262]

267 Radiotherapy is effective in relieving distressing symptoms by causing a tumour to shrink and fibrose. Superior vena caval obstruction, recurrent massive haemoptysis and pain (local or metastatic) are specific indications. Cure by radiotherapy is exceptionally rare.
[A: 270; B: 18.59; C: 289-90; D: 236; E: 361–2; F: 898; G: 1009–10; H: 1264]

268 Yes. Several drug regimens are under study and there is no doubt that tumour growth can be arrested, at least for several months. Drug side-effects, particularly nausea, vomiting, malaise and marrow suppression, often limit the amount of treatment that can be given. Methotrexate, cyclophosphamide and 5-fluorouracil are some of the main drugs used.
[A: 270; B: 18.60; C: 290; F: 898; G: 1010; H: 1264]

269 Yes. Inflammation, especially that caused by a pneumonia, can cause the appearance of cells that are indistinguishable from malignant cells. In the case of neoplastic cells seen in the presence of a pneumonia it is necessary to repeat cytology when the infection has cleared.
[A: 270; B: 18.58–9; C: 289; E: 361; F: 897–8; G: 1008; H: 1262]

270 Carcinoid syndrome, i.e. diarrhoea, flushes and asthma. The tumour would be a bronchial adenoma although most such tumours do not produce the carcinoid syndrome.
[A: 271; B: 18.60; C: 290; D: 236; E: 362; F: 900; G: 1011; H: 1261]

271 Clearly defined, rounded opacity with patchy calcification. This can be exactly the appearance of a tuberculoma or a slow-growing carcinoma. One would therefore be unlikely to diagnose a hamartoma prior to histological examination of the lesion. The presence of multiple similar shadows would favour a tuberculoma.
[A: 272; B: 18.62; E: 362; F: 900; G: 1013]

272 Lobar—*Pneumococcus, Klebsiella pneumoniae, Staphylococcus aureus* and, in some individuals and populations (e.g. East African) *Mycobacterium tuberculosis*.

Bronchopneumonia—*Streptococcus, Haemophilus influenzae*, less virulent pneumococci.
[A: 273; B: 18.27; C: 242; D: 231; E: 329; F: 864; H: 1224]

273 Bronchitis and pneumonitis due to the inhalation of gastric contents, usually during anaesthesia. It is a

constant worry in obstetrics where women may require urgent anaesthesia for Caesarean section and the stomach may not be empty.

The acidity of the inhaled material sets up a particularly severe inflammatory reaction and impairment of oxygenation may be serious. Treatment includes corticosteroids, antibiotics and oxygen.

Further causes of inhalation pneumonia include hiatus hernia and oesophageal obstruction, e.g. achalasia of the cardia.

[A: 273; B: 18.36–7; C: 245; D: 233; E: 334–5; F: 868; H: 1224]

274 *Mycoplasma pneumoniae* (remember cold agglutinins); *Chlamydia*, causing psittacosis or ornithosis (contact with budgerigars, other birds); *Coxiella burneti* causing Q fever (raw milk, contact with farm animals); *Legionella pneumophila* causing Legionnaire's disease.

[A: 279; B: 18.28; C: 244; D: 233; E: 333–4; F: 867; G: 343; H: 760]

275 Lung abscess; empyema necessitatis; pericarditis; arthritis; endocarditis and meningitis.

Sickle cell disease, multiple myeloma and splenectomy predispose to pneumococcal infection.

[A: 274; B: 18.28; C: 242; D: 231–2; E: 331; F: 866; G: 347; H: 1224]

276 During an influenza epidemic. It can occur at any age.

[A: 276; B: 18.29; C: 243; D: 232; F: 864; G: 401; H: 1224]

277 Alcoholism, diabetes mellitus and chronic bronchopulmonary disease.

Klebsiella is not usually sensitive to the penicillins and has to be treated with cephalosporins or aminoglycosides.

[A: 277; B: 18.29; C: 243; D: 232; E: 332; F: 864; G: 357; H: 1224]

278 Review the bacteriological studies and antibiotic sensitivities but making a special point of looking for acid-fast bacilli and excluding tuberculosis.

Tuberculous pneumonia varies in incidence with ethnic group and is uncommon in Europeans and Chinese. Its occurrence in the latter groups usually signifies poor resistance and serious disease.

[A: 278; B: 18.29; C: 256; F: 873; G: 482; H: 703]

279 Bilateral, multiple shadows, appearing to spread from the hila and involving the lower parts of the lungs.

Cold agglutinins are present in serum and easily detected.

Mycoplasma pneumoniae is sensitive to tetracycline and erythromycin.

[A: 280; B: 18.32; C: 244; D: 233; E: 333; F: 867; G: 344; H: 760]

280 Q fever, caused by the rickettsia *Coxiella burneti*, also causes a pneumonitis accompanied by headache and fever but the acute illness is usually shorter. The organism is also sensitive to tetracycline.

Granulomatous hepatic disease and endocarditis may result from a chronic variety of infection with this organism.

Contact with sheep, goats, cows, their milk or their ticks' faeces (handling hides) is the source of infection.

[A: 280; B: 12.98–9; C: 244; E: 333–4; F: 867; G: 337; H: 770]

281 Acute—cough, fever, dyspnoea, malaise, occurring within hours or days of drug administration.

Chronic—gradually progressive dyspnoea, developing over months or years.

[E: 363; F: 895; G: 974–5; H: 1213]

282 Lung abscess. Bacteriological study is important, because some of the possible organisms are resistant to the first-choice antibiotics e.g. *Staphylococcus aureus, Klebsiella pneumoniae, Mycobacterium tuberculosis*. Anaerobic culture should be specifically requested.

Clubbing may occur in chronic lung abscess,without there necessarily being an underlying bronchial carcinoma.

[A: 281; B: 18.38; C: 247; D: 234; E: 332; F: 868; G: 980–1; H: 1228]

283 Anaerobic organisms are commonly present as well as aerobes in abscesses and some are resistant to penicillin. The persistence of the abscess may be due to survival of these anaerobic organisms and a suitable antibiotic such as clindamycin or metronidazole (both active against *Bacteroides*) should be added.

[A: 282; B: 18.39; D: 234; E: 333; F: 869; G: 981; H: 1229]

284 The possibility of increased secretions blocking a bronchus and causing collapse of a lobe or even a whole lung. Because of her incision, peritonitis and complicating ileus, she has been unable to cough. If physiotherapy fails to clear the mucus plug, bronchoscopy and aspiration is necessary.

Her symptoms may also indicate pulmonary embolism, myocardial infarction or pneumonia. [A: 284; E: 335; F: 859]

285 *Taenia echinococcus*, the dog tapeworm, causing hydatid disease.

If a cyst ruptures then the contents may be coughed up and these consist of small off-white envelopes, about 1 cm in length, the daughter cysts. Eosinophilia may or may not be present. Serological tests show fewer false positives than the intradermal Casoni test. [A: 287; B: 18.107; E: 602; F: 857; G: 1002; H: 918]

286 Yes. There is a number of morphologically similar but culturally and clinically different mycobacteria which are collectively known as the atypical mycobacteria. Clinically they are distinguished by a liking for damaged lungs, a slow, protracted course, and relative or complete resistance to the anti-TB drugs. Fortunately their incidence is low.
[A: 287; B: 14.17; C: 251; D: 238; F: 872; G: 498–500; H: 700]

287 Africans; inhabitants of the Indian subcontinent; American Indians; Eskimos.

Because TB heals by fibrosis, the fact that someone's disease is chronic does not imply that the resulting damage will be any less. The reverse may be true. [A: 288; B: 14.2; C: 251; D: 239; F: 872; H: 700]

288 Massive haemoptysis; bronchiectasis; cor pulmonale; emphysema; recurrent pneumothorax.

Deaths also occur with treatment failure due to drug resistance or poor patient compliance, but there may be other underlying factors impairing host resistance. [B: 14.2]

289 A Ghon focus is a small pneumonic tuberculous lesion, representing the first seat of infection. The combination of this focus and the hilar lymph nodes, which enlarge and subsequently calcify on healing, is the primary complex. This happens to be the pattern of response in most people to their first encounter with the tubercle bacillus (which used to be in childhood but nowadays may not be until adult life).

The Mantoux test converts to positive during primary infection, and small calcified spots in the hilar lymph nodes in a chest X-ray are further evidence of primary tuberculous infection. Their significance is that they may harbour some dormant but living bacilli.
[A: 288; B: 14.2; C: 253; D: 238; E: 336–7; F: 872; G: 484; H: 701]

290 Miliary TB is an important cause of PUO and malaise, night sweats and weight loss which may precede the appearance of the fine mottling on the chest X-ray. The Mantoux test may remain negative until later in the illness, either because of a weak antigenic challenge or because of poor host response. Tuberculous meningitis may occur as part of miliary tuberculosis.
[A: 289; B: 14.5; C: 255; E: 339; F: 873; G: 492; H: 706]

291 Tubercle bacilli ingested in infected cow's milk or other contaminated food may infect the terminal ileum and set up a primary complex involving the mesenteric lymph nodes. This is uncommon nowadays, but it may present like acute appendicitis or Crohn's disease, or silently progress to tuberculous peritonitis with ascites. Calcified lymph nodes are often seen on abdominal films of older people, and tuberculous peritonitis or miliary spread in later life may result from breaking down of the primary disease.
[A: 289; B: 14.10; F: 873; G: 492; H: 704]

292 Systemic upset is very variable and enlargement of a group of nodes may be silent.

It is common for glands to reach 3–4 cm in diameter, be matted together but with some fluctuation. They may point and rupture, and although the pus should be cultured, it is commonly sterile. Treatment is as for other forms of TB but may need a more conventional duration of 12–18 months. An interesting feature of tuberculous lymphadenitis is that the nodes may temporarily enlarge during the course of correct and adequate treatment.
[A: 290; B: 14.9; G: 495; H: 705]

293 Not with complete certainty, but, with the proviso that the only reliable indicator of activity is the culturing of bacilli in the sputum, lesions that have a soft or fluffy appearance with indistinct margins are likely to be active, while shadows that look denser and consist of clearly defined streaks are likely to be healed and fibrotic. Cavities, formed by the discharge of the caseous and necrotic centres of tuberculous foci may be old or fresh.
[A: 291; B: 14.7; C: 257; D: 239; E: 337; F: 874; G: 486; H: 703]

294 Bronchogenic carcinoma; aspiration pneumonia as in alcoholics and oesophageal regurgitation; *Klebsiella* pneumonia shows a preference for upper lobes over the rest of the lungs; histoplasmosis; melioidosis—an infection endemic in parts of S.E. Asia due to

Pseudomonas pseudomallei. All of these conditions can show cavitation at different stages of the illness. [G: 486–7; H: 704]

295 The fluid is formed in what appears to be a pleural hypersensitivity reaction for which the presence of small numbers of bacilli is sufficient.

Pleural biopsy may show tuberculous granulomata and is a routine test in the investigation of an effusion.

Blood-stained effusion (in the absence of traumatic aspiration) is nearly always a reliable sign of malignancy.
[A: 305; B: 14.9; C: 300–1; F: 922; G: 491; H: 703]

296 The routine method employs the Ziehl–Neelson technique. In cases where this stain is negative but the presence of bacilli is strongly suspected, a fluorescent dye can be used, helping to highlight sporadic bacilli.

The usual time to culture tubercle bacilli is 4–6 weeks and no culture should be considered negative before 6 weeks has elapsed.
[F: 874]

297 The Mantoux test is an intradermal test, achieved by injecting 0.1 ml of test solution with a fine needle introduced into the skin horizontally. It is important not to reach the dermis because the slight bleeding that results distorts the response. The reaction at 48 hours is noted in terms of millimetres of induration. Greater than 5 mm of induration is positive.

Old tuberculin is approximately what its name suggests and should not be used any more. PPD comes in different strengths so that response to one unit, ten units or one hundred units can be observed. Which strength is used initially depends on the expected severity of the reaction. Usually either one or ten units is used first.
[A: 292; B: 14.7; C: 254; E: 336; F: 874; G: 482; H: 706]

298 Provided that the organisms are fully sensitive to isoniazid and rifampicin, treatment is continued with these two drugs alone for a further 7 months.
[A: 293; B: 14.14–15; C: 261; E: 338–9; F: 875; G: 487–90; H: 708]

299 Only two are fully bactericidal, isoniazid and rifampicin; the remainder are bacteriostatic to a varying degree. The combination of streptomycin and pyrazinamide is the equivalent of one bactericidal drug, due to a combined spectrum of action across the pH range encountered.

Patient compliance and lack of interruption in therapy are probably the two most important factors. In the minority of patients with drug side-effects, a successful outcome may be much delayed. The presence of diabetes, chronic fibrotic lung disease (such as silicosis) or conditions requiring steroid therapy make successful treatment more difficult. [A: 293; B: 14.12–13; G: 487–8; H: 708–10]

300 BCG is a live, attenuated tubercle bacillus, named after its originators ('bacille Calmette-Guérin'). It is used in vaccination of tuberculin-negative people worldwide.

Its contribution is difficult to assess and is disputed by some. A large fall in the incidence of tuberculosis occurred due to better public health measures and standards of living in the first part of this century before either chemotherapy or vaccination was available. Nevertheless, it is officially held to be an effective weapon in preventing TB. For the individual, it confers at least partial protection, although state of health and the degree of exposure to active disease continue to be relevant factors in contracting the disease.
[A: 294; B: 14.10; C: 263; E: 339; F: 874; G: 483; H: 711]

301 In the presence of liver disease. There are very few drugs free of hepatic side-effects. Rifampicin usually causes a transient elevation of hepatic enzymes in normal people, but in liver disease this may be exaggerated and hepatitis may occur. Isoniazid does not usually cause hepatitis but it is usually severe when it does. PAS can cause severe hepatitis or cholestasis and both pyrazinamide and ethionamide are more likely to affect hepatic function than the other drugs.

Of the commonly used drugs, only streptomycin and ethambutol have no adverse effect on the liver.
[A: 293–4; B: 14.13; C: 260; D: 240; E: 338; F: 876; G: 487–8; H: 708–9]

302 Although a dry cough and vague chest discomfort may occur, the disease is commonly asymptomatic. Chest X-ray shows one or two dense and discrete infiltrates. Treatment is with flucytosine and/or amphotericin B.

The organism, in most cases, originates from old pigeon droppings, and infection tends to occur where host defences are suppressed.
[A: 295; B: 12.92; C: 885; E: 340; F: 172–3; G: 543; H: 736]

303 The two distinctive ones are mycetoma, a ball of fungus colonizing an old cavity, and

bronchopulmonary aspergillosis in which an acute hypersensitivity reaction causes inflammation of the larger bronchi. Scarred and dilated bronchi result and the condition is responsible for tram-line shadows on chest X-ray.

Other conditions are extrinsic asthma, extrinsic allergic alveolitis and acute necrotizing pneumonitis in the immunosuppressed.

[A: 295; C: 264; E: 340; F: 878; G: 546; H: 742]

304 A ball of fungal growth, often *Aspergillus*, occupying a cavity remaining from some other lung condition, often tuberculosis. The radiological appearances are usually of a crescent-shaped air space above a soft shadow in a cavity, with alteration of the position of the shadow in a decubitus view.

Most are asymptomatic which is as well because there is no effective treatment short of surgical resection. This may be considered when the disease causes gross haemoptysis or chronic, purulent expectoration.

[A: 295; B: 12.93; C: 264; E: 340; F: 878; G: 546–7; H: 743]

305 This condition comprises eosinophilia, fever, dyspnoea and recurrent pulmonary infiltration with *Aspergillus* hyphae present in the sputum. The proximal bronchi become obstructed with large plugs of mucus and the radiological appearance is of characteristically date-sized shadows proximally situated which have a tendency to affect the upper lobes. Distal atelectasis and collapse may be evident.

It can occur at any age but only in the presence of asthma. Both immediate and IgG-mediated hypersensitivity to the fungus are implicated.

The affected bronchi subsequently manifest cylindrical bronchiectasis, which may cast tram-line shadows on a plain chest X-ray.

[A: 295; C: 264; E: 340; F: 878; G: 547; H: 743]

306 *Nocardia asteroides* is a fungus-like bacterium and the hyphae can be seen on a Gram stain of infected sputum. Treatment is sulphonamide or co-trimoxazole for up to 18 months. Dapsone is also effective.

Pneumocystis carinii is a protozoan. Special stains and fluorescent antibody examination of infected sputum or biopsy specimens are needed. Co-trimoxazole is the treatment of choice, for 2–3 weeks. Pentamidine is an alternative.

Candida albicans, a yeast-like fungus, is readily identified on wet smear or on culture. Treatment is with amphotericin B and/or flucytosine, for several weeks.

[A: 281; C: 244; D: 233; E: 335; G: 362; H: 1228]

307 Chest infection; dyspnoea due to pneumothorax or cor pulmonale; symptoms of complicating tuberculosis; scleroderma.

Once the disease is detected exposure to the dust should be prevented, but the lung deterioration may proceed despite this.
[A: 296; B: 18.79; C: 296; D: 241; E: 358–9; F: 905; G: 989; H: 1220]

308 Chronic interstitial pulmonary fibrosis, affecting chiefly the lower lobes; bronchogenic carcinoma; plaques of pleural calcification; pleural mesothelioma.
[A: 297; B: 18.80; C: 297; D: 241; E: 359; F: 906; G: 990; H: 1220]

309 Simple pneumoconiosis, with three grades according to the size of the nodules; and progressive massive fibrosis.
[A: 297; B: 18.78; C: 295; E: 358; F: 905; G: 986; H: 1221]

310 Large dense masses develop in the upper parts of the lung fields, sometimes coalescing or breaking down to give cavitation. Surrounding lung is emphysematous.

Dyspnoea and productive cough are usually present but coexisting chronic bronchitis is the likely cause.
[A: 297; B: 18.76–7; C: 296; D: 241; E: 358; F: 904; G: 992–3; H: 1221]

311 Caplan's syndrome, originally described in Welsh miners.
[A: 297; B: 18.77; C: 296; E: 358; F: 902; G: 992; H: 1221]

312 The dyspnoea is due to bronchospasm which occurs not because of an atopic tendency in the sufferer but because of the presence in cotton bracts of a substance which can liberate histamine.

Repeated exposure over several years leads to chronic bronchitis and emphysema.

Chest X-ray is thus usually normal until the late stages of chronic bronchitis and emphysema.

Exposure to platinum salts in the electronics industry causes a similar kind of disease.
[A: 298; B: 18.86; C: 297; F: 911; G: 997; H: 1219]

313 It can be a complication or feature of asthma, sometimes involving *Aspergillus* spores; worm and parasite infestations in some of which there is actually a migratory phase through the lungs; polyarteritis nodosa can involve the lungs, often following a history of asthma.

Loeffler's syndrome is a particular form of pulmonary eosinophilia which shows transient, migratory infiltrates lasting less than a month with a relative absence of symptoms. It may be due to drugs such as PAS or nitrofurantoin.
[A: 298; B: 18.103; C: 273; D: 227; E: 335; F: 893; G: 969; H: 1210]

314 Intradermal injection of a suspension of sarcoid tissue. Within 4–6 weeks, a nodule develops at the site of the injection which shows non-caseating granulomatoma (epithelioid tubercles) on histology. False negatives are not uncommon and may occur during steroid therapy.
[A: 299; B: 15.1; F: 917–18; G: 210; H: 930]

315 Serum angiotensin-converting enzyme (ACE) is elevated, but it is not entirely specific for sarcoidosis. Another common 'presentation' is bilateral hilar lymphadenopathy on routine chest X-ray of an asymptomatic patient.
Whenever the diagnosis is suspected, chest X-ray is an essential investigation.
[A: 299; B: 15.2; C: 293; D: 236–7; E: 354–5; F: 916–17; G: 212; H: 929]

316 Skin lesions including lupus pernio in which purple plaques occur on the nose, ears, cheeks, hands and feet. Involvement of the scalp causes alopecia and infiltration of old scars is another feature. Bone lesions consist of dramatic, punched-out lesions in the distal phalanges of the hands and feet. Usually there are overlying skin changes with them and periarticular swelling also occurs. Chronic iritis is a cause of blindness and myocardial involvement can cause a cardiomyopathy. Also it occurs in an older age group ($>$ 40 years) than acute sarcoidosis.
[A: 300; B: 15.3–5; C: 294; D: 237; E: 355; F: 917; G: 213; H: 930]

317 Sjögren's syndrome. In this autoimmune condition, there is lymphocytic infiltration in contrast to the non-caseating granulomas of sarcoid.
Uveitis or iridocyclitis is an indication for steroid therapy.
[A: 300; B: 15.3–4; C: 294; D: 237; E: 355; F: 917; G: 213; H: 929]

318 No. If effusions occur, the diagnosis is not sarcoidosis.
The progress of parenchymal lesions is also checked with serial lung function studies, particularly vital capacity and transfer factor.
[A: 300; B: 15.2; C: 294; D: 236; E: 355; F: 916; G: 212–13; H: 929]

319 Cellulose phosphate 5 g t.d.s. This binds calcium in the gut and reduces its absorption.
[A: 300; B: 15.5; C: 293; D: 237; F: 918; G: 215; H: 930]

320 Increasing dyspnoea, dry cough, marked clubbing and coarse cracking ('firecracker') râles. The lungs are contracted on X-ray and diffuse pulmonary shadowing may give the appearance of 'honeycomb lung'.
Hamman and Rich described a particularly aggressive form of the disease with death in less than a year.
[A: 302; B: 18.90; C: 292; D: 245; E: 356–7; F: 911; G: 967; H: 1245]

321 Extrinsic allergic alveolitis. The allergic response involves alveoli and the smallest bronchioles and depends on IgG and cell-mediated responses. This is why it is possible serologically to detect precipitins.
Many causative agents have been identified and their corresponding names include farmer's lung, bird-fancier's lung, pigeon-fancier's lung, maltworker's lung, mushroom worker's lung, etc.
[A: 302; B: 18.87; C: 274; D: 241; E: 351; F: 909; G: 970; H: 1210]

322 Idiopathic pulmonary haemosiderosis.
Goodpasture's syndrome is the combination of this with glomerulonephritis and is characterized by the presence of antiglomerular basement membrane antibody.
The eventual result of idopathic pulmonary haemosiderosis is interstitial pulmonary fibrosis in which the appearance of the lungs is indistinguishable from fibrosing alveolitis.
[B: 18.105; C: 293; F: 915; G: 976; H: 1244]

323 Pneumonia; pulmonary infarction; lung abscess; Bornholm disease, also called epidemic pleurodynia, which is a coxsackie B virus infection affecting the intercostal muscles and the pleura.
[A: 303; B: 18.67; C: 298; E: 365–6; F: 921; G: 1013; H: 1265]

324 Cytology; cell count; protein; glucose; Gram stain and culture for pathogens; Z–N stain and culture for AFB.
This is almost a standard list for fluid removal from any body cavity.
[A: 304; B: 18.70–1; C: 299–300; D: 49; E: 365–6; F: 921; G: 1014; H: 1266]

325 Empyema is the name for a collection of pus in the pleural cavity. It usually results from spread of infection from the lung (pneumococcal pneumonia),

from tuberculous infection of the pleural cavity or from chest wall infection.

Empyema necessitatis is the name for an empyema that points and ruptures through the chest wall.
[A: 308; B: 18.71; C: 301; F: 923; G: 1015; H: 1267]

326 Treatment may have been instituted too late; unrecognized tuberculous origin; underlying malignancy; presence of a foreign body.
[A: 308; B: 18.71; C: 302; F: 924; G: 1015; H: 1267]

327 Emphysema; asthma; healed and fibrotic tuberculosis.

Pneumothorax is sometimes a feature of Marfan's syndrome. Pneumothorax is a possible complication of mechanical ventilation.
[A: 310; B: 18.72; C: 303; D: 243; E: 364; F: 294; G: 1016; H: 1268]

328 Reduced chest movement over the pneumothorax, increased resonance and reduced breath sounds. There may or may not be dyspnoea, cyanosis or evidence of mediastinal displacement. There may be no abnormal physical signs with a small pneumothorax.
[A: 310; B: 18.73; C: 303; D: 243–4; E: 364; F: 925; G: 1016–17; H: 1268]

329 The underwater seal is usually enough to assist the lung to re-expand. If the lung remains collapsed, suction can be applied. If a bronchopleural fistula is present (as may happen with mechanical ventilation) suction may still be ineffective. Surgery may be necessary.

Once the lung has re-expanded as confirmed by X-ray, the tube is clamped for 48 hours and a repeat X-ray taken. If the lung has remained expanded the tube is removed by a gentle but rapid movement during inspiration, and the hole in the chest wall immediately squeezed shut and covered with a plug of Vaseline and a dressing.
[A: 311; B: 18.73; C: 305; D: 244; E: 364–5; F: 925; G: 1017; H: 1268]

330 Mid-mediastinal swellings—bronchogenic carcinoma or enlarged lymph nodes (lymphoma, metastatic spread, sarcoidosis etc.)

Posterior mediastinum—neurofibroma or ganglioneuroma. These usually lie in the paravertebral gutter.

Anterior mediastinum—retrosternal goitre (upper zone) thymoma, dermoid cysts and teratomas (midzone) and (in the lower zone in the right cardiophrenic angle) pericardial cysts.
[A: 311–12; B: 18.64; C: 290–1; E: 325; F: 927; G: 1018–19; H: 1269]

Alimentary Tract, Liver & Pancreas

331 Mesenteric vascular insufficiency.
[A: 76; B: 19.1; E: 47; G: 1477; H: 35–6]

332 Urinary tract conditions, especially renal colic; aortic aneurysm.
[A: 76; B: 19.1; E: 47; G: 1476; H: 36]

333 Mallory–Weiss syndrome.
[A: 77; B: 19.3; C: 311; E: 49; F: 634; G: 1477; H: 198]

334 Hiatus hernia. The symptoms are due to gastro-oesophageal reflux. Elevation of the head end of the bed, avoidance of bending over and weight reduction will lessen the symptoms.

There is an association between hiatus hernia, cholelithiasis and diverticular disease.
[A: 77; B: 19.2; C: 311; D: 210; F: 616; G: 1479; H: 196]

335 Laxative abuse and irritable bowel syndrome are both common. Laxative abuse is sometimes carefully concealed.

Alactasia occurs in 20 per cent of Caucasians and is normal in the adults of other races, but it uncommonly gives rise to diarrhoea which the patient has not already linked to dairy products.

The Zollinger–Ellison syndrome is due to a gastrin-producing tumour, usually lying in the pancreas. Diarrhoea is prominent. Hypersecretion of other intestinal hormones such as VIP (vasoactive intestinal polypeptide) also results in diarrhoea.
[A: 77; B: 19.5; D: 44–5; E: 50; F: 636; G: 1480; H: 200–1]

336 Magnesium-containing antacids, digoxin and methyldopa can cause diarrhoea.
Aluminium-containing antacids, ferrous sulphate, tricyclic antidepressants, and phenothiazines can cause constipation.
[A: 78; B: 19.5; C: 311; E: 52; F: 635; G: 1481; H: 201]

337 Bacterial overgrowth of the small intestine can be demonstrated by breath analysis following ingestion of ^{14}C-labelled cholylglycine. Bacteria metabolize this bile acid, liberating ^{14}C-labelled carbon dioxide, some of which is exhaled. The time interval between ingestion and breath detection indicates the site of bacterial overgrowth.

Intraluminal bacterial metabolism of undigested lactose produces hydrogen. This can be detected by

breath analysis for hydrogen at an appropriate time interval after lactose ingestion.
[A: 92; E: 75; F: 639; G: 1531; H: 1399]

338 Anaemia—smooth, red and sore tongue (glossitis).

Leukaemia—petechiae, ulcers and gingival bleeding. Gingival hypertrophy is prominent in monocytic leukaemia.

Addison's disease—bluish black or brownish pigmentation of buccal mucosa.

Pemphigus—ruptured bullae and ulcerated areas, mainly of buccal mucosa.

Ulcerative colitis—some patients have recurrent aphthous ulcers.

Infectious mononucleosis—petechiae at junction of hard and soft palate, with pharyngeal or tonsillar exudates.
[A: 79; B: 19.6–10; C: 317; F: 602–10; H: 188–90]

339 Iron deficiency which causes koilonychia, a shallow spoon-shaped deformity of the nails.
[A: 595; B: 19.18; C: 319; D; 44; F: 620; G: 1483; H: 193]

340 Gradually progressing dysphagia over several years.
[A: 80; B: 19.22; C: 322; D: 44; E: 48; F: 615; G: 1487; H: 1369]

341 By no means. Apart from evidence of weight loss, physical signs do not occur until the malignancy is advanced. Urgent barium swallow and/or oesophagoscopy is indicated.
[A: 81; B: 19.25; C: 323; D: 44; E: 85; F: 620; G: 1597; H: 1369]

342 Varices change in size with respiration due to changes in intrathoracic pressure.
[A: 108; B: 20.22; F: 559; H: 1481]

343 Alcohol, aspirin and other anti-inflammatory drugs.
[A: 82; B: 19.31; C: 325; E: 56; F: 624; G: 1504; H: 202]

344 A drink. It may be deduced from this that the nausea and vomiting are symptoms of withdrawal rather than of gastric irritation.
[A: 82; C: 336; H: 971]

345 Cigarette-smoking and heredity both contribute to duodenal ulceration as do chronic renal failure and cirrhosis of the liver.

In gastric ulceration, reflux of bile acids through the pylorus is considered by many to be an important factor.
[A: 83; B: 19.33; C: 324; E: 58; F: 625; G: 1504–7; H: 1371–4]

346 Pain at night is a feature of duodenal ulcer. Vomiting can occur with both forms of ulcer, and it often indicates some obstruction of the gastric outlet.
There is considerable overlap in the symptomatology of the two forms of ulcer.
[A: 83; B: 19.35; C: 326; D: 206; E: 59; F: 625; G: 1507; H: 1374]

347 Situations in which gastric acid measurement is of diagnostic help include:
(a) when a gastrinoma is suspected or when an ulcer has recurred after surgery;
(b) to detect achlorhydria, in pernicious anaemia and in cases of gastric ulcer. The occurrence of a gastric ulcer in the presence of achlorhydria is indicative of malignancy since most cases of benign gastric ulcer have some acid secretion.
[A: 84; B: 19.36; C: 327; D: 207; E: 59; G: 1509–12; H: 1375]

348 Upper abdominal distension and a succussion splash may be present. Vomit typically contains identifiable remnants of previous days' food. Because of the repeated vomiting there is a net loss of acid resulting in a metabolic alkalosis.
[A: 85; B: 19.44–8; C: 329–34; D: 206; E: 59; F: 628–30; G: 1516–18; H: 1379]

349 Antacids relieve symptoms by neutralizing gastric acid. For a liquid antacid like mist. magnesium trisilicate, an effective dose is not less than 30 ml, at least three to four times daily.
The milk–alkali syndrome occurs when the antacid calcium carbonate and milk are both taken in large quantities for the relief of ulcer symptoms. Hypercalcaemic nephropathy and metabolic alkalosis result.
[A: 86; B: 19.38; C: 328; D: 207; E: 60; F: 626; G: 1513; H: 1376]

350 Gastric acid production returns to its pretreatment level.
[A: 86; C: 328; D: 207; E: 60; F: 626; G: 1514; H: 1376]

351 Avoid cigarettes, alcohol, aspirin and other anti-inflammatory drugs. Avoid undue stress. Take regular meals, avoiding foods that provoke symptoms.

Colloidal bismuthate has been shown to give healing rates in duodenal ulcer as high as those found with cimetidine.
[A: 86; G: 1515]

352 Gastrin release is unaffected or may be increased by vagotomy.
[A: 87; B: 19.40; C: 329; G: 207–8; F: 626; G: 1519; H: 1379–80]

353 Both these syndromes result from the rapid emptying of gastric contents into the proximal small intestine. In the early syndrome, abdominal discomfort, lightheadedness and tachycardia occur. It is thought to be due to a shift of fluid into the gut lumen, drawn in by the hyperosmolar contents.

The late syndrome, also consisting of lightheadedness, sweating and sometimes confusion is due to reactive hypoglycaemia.

Both syndromes can be avoided by taking small meals.
[A: 88; B: 19.43; C: 335; E: 61; F: 627; G: 1520; H: 1381]

354 There is a slightly increased incidence of stomach cancer in people with blood group A. Approximately 1 in 20 patients with pernicious anaemia develops carcinoma. Atrophic gastritis also predisposes to carcinoma but the risk is slight.
[A: 89; B: 19.49; C: 337; E: 85; F: 630; G: 1600–1; H: 1385]

355 In some cases, radiological features are diagnostic. Cytological examination of material obtained by gastric brushing detects the majority of cases. The highest rate of positive results is obtained by endoscopic biopsy.
[A: 90; B: 19.50; C: 338; F: 630; G: 1601; H: 1386]

356 Transperitoneal seeding. This results in peritoneal metastases, ascites or Krukenberg tumours which masquerade as ovarian or adnexial masses.
[A: 89–90; B: 19.50; C; 338; F: 630; G: 1601; H: 1386]

357 In some patients, symptoms improve after leaving the tropical environment. Folic acid should be given for at least 6 months, and a 2–4 week course of tetracycline should be given initially. This produces a rapid remission. Deficiency of B_{12}, calcium, vitamin D and other essential factors must be corrected.
[A: 90; B: 19.61; C: 797; D: 217; F: 642; G: 1545; H: 1402]

358 (a) Dermatitis herpetiformis. (b) Intestinal lymphoma.

[A: 91; B: 19.60; C: 350; D: 215; E: 76; F: 641; G: 1539; H: 1405]

359 Weakness may be due to either anaemia or hypokalaemia. A painful tongue results from anaemia which itself is due to deficiency of iron, folic acid or vitamin B_{12}. Paraesthesiae are likely to be due to B_{12} malabsorption. Bone pain may result from osteomalacia due to vitamin D depletion. Tetany is due to hypocalcaemia and bruising to malabsorption of vitamin K.
[A: 91; B: 19.58; C: 346–7; D: 216; E: 74–5; F: 637–40; G: 1530–1; H: 1397]

360 Measurement of serum gastrin levels. Fasting levels are nearly always raised. In borderline cases the secretin infusion test is the best provocative test, causing a rise in gastrin levels only when a gastrinoma is present.
[A: 93; B: 19.48; C: 334; D: 208; E: 88; F: 589; G: 1508; H: 1382]

361 On clinical grounds, intestinal lymphoma is often indistinguishable from coeliac disease. Failure to respond to a gluten-free diet and the presence of abdominal pain and fever are suspicious of lymphoma. Intestinal obstruction may occur. The condition affects men more often than women.
[A: 93; B: 19.62; C: 623; F: 642; G: 1541; H: 1403]

362 Dilatation and alteration of calibre of segments of small bowel, coarse mucosal pattern and flocculation (or clumping) of the barium.
[A: 92; B: 19.54–7; C: 549; D: 218; E: 95; F: 638–9; G: 1530–2; H: 1396–8]

363 The aetiology has yet to be established. There is conflicting evidence for an infectious agent. Impaired immune mechanisms may play a part in the pathogenesis of the disease, as may genetic factors. Relatives of patients with Crohn's disease have an increased incidence both of Crohn's disease and of ulcerative colitis. Patients who develop sacroiliitis in association with the bowel disease very often carry the tissue antigen HLA B 27.
[A: 93; B: 19.65; C: 351; D: 213; E: 79; F: 651; G: 1561; H: 1411–12]

364 The peak incidence of Crohn's disease is in young adults.

In the earlier stages of the disease, barium studies reveal a loss of the normal mucosal pattern and rigidity of segments of the bowel. There may be a cobblestone appearance to the mucosa. Later, strictures and fistulous tracts may be seen.
[A: 93–4; B: 19.67; C: 352; D: 214; E: 80; F: 651; G: 1563–4; H: 1413]

365 The disease typically follows a fluctuating course. In acute exacerbations, corticosteroids are often necessary and effective but they do not prevent relapses. Azathioprine has a steroid-sparing effect. Sulphasalazine has some effect in mild disease.

As important as drug treatment are bed rest and nasogastric suction during acute episodes, and careful attention to diet during remission to avoid morbidity from malabsorption.

Surgery may be needed for draining abscesses, removing fistulae, relieving obstruction, and bowel resection in selected cases. Postoperative recurrence is common.
[A: 94; B: 19.66; C: 352–4; D: 214; E: 80; F: 651–3; G: 1566–7; H: 1415]

366 Sacroiliitis, iritis, erythema nodosum, clubbing and cholangitis.
[A: 94; B: 19.67–8; C: 353; D: 214; E: 80; F: 651–2; G: 1563; H: 1414]

367 The highest incidence of ulcerative colitis is between the ages of 20 and 40, but it can occur at any age.

Bacillary dysentry, amoebic dysentry, viral gastroenteritis, carcinoma, diverticular disease and ischaemic colitis are all causes of bloody diarrhoea.
[A: 95; B: 19.101; C: 360; D: 211; E: 81; F: 654; G: 1570; H: 1425]

368 Loss of haustral markings, saw-tooth appearance to the mucosal surface, collar stud ulcers and pseudopolyps. Stricture and carcinoma may also be demonstrated.
[A: 95; B: 19.103; C: 361; D: 211; E: 82; F: 652–5; G: 1571; H: 1426]

369 Pyoderma gangrenosum is a skin lesion associated with active colitis which subsides as the colitis is treated. It may develop rapidly. Ulceration, erythema and gangrene of the skin occur. The lower limbs are usually affected.

The risk of carcinoma of the colon is increased by (a) a long duration of illness, e.g. disease starting before the age of 15; (b) extensive involvement of the colon; and (c) family history of colonic malignancy. How best

to achieve early detection is an unresolved problem. Annual colonoscopy is one possibility.
[A: 96; B: 19.104; C: 363; D: 212–13; E: 83–4; F: 655; G: 1572–4; H: 1428–9]

370 ESR; stool culture; stool occult bloods; sigmoidoscopy and mucosal biopsy; barium enema.
[A: 97; B: 19.99; C: 373; D: 221; E: 51; F: 634; G: 1493; H: 1422]

371 Acute diverticulitis; paracolic abscess; fistula formation to the bladder, uterus or other intra-abdominal organ; haemorrhage.
[A: 97; B: 19.108; C: 365; D: 220; F: 647; H: 1420]

372 Crohn's disease. In ulcerative colitis, macroscopic ulceration is not seen.
Fifty per cent of large bowel malignancy occurs within the distal 25 cm of the bowel, i.e. within reach of the sigmoidoscope.
[B: 19.95; C: 314; H: 1419]

373 Congestive cardiac failure; cholestasis; diabetes mellitus.
[C: 376; D: 36; G: 1639; H: 1444]

374 Gamma-glutamyl transpeptidase (GGT). It is not, however, specific for alcohol damage.
[A: 103; B: 20.1–4; C: 381–4; D: 41; E: 95; F: 557–9; G: 1646–7; H: 1447]

375 Ultrasound and computerized axial tomography (CAT) scanning.
[B: 20.4; C: 387; E: 96; F: 559; G: 1465–70; H: 1453]

376 Endoscopic retrograde choledochopancreatography (ERCP) and percutaneous trans-hepatic cholangiography.
[B: 20.5; C: 413; G: 1622; H: 1452]

377 Bed rest for a few weeks at a time; a good diet with 80–100 g protein, devised according to the patient's preferences; abstinence from alcohol; maintenance of haemoglobin level above 10 g per 100 ml with folic acid supplements and transfusion if necessary; avoidance of sedatives.
[A: 107–8; B: 20.19; C: 404; D: 200; E: 69; F: 567; G: 1645; H: 1444]

378 Removal of nitrogen from the gastrointestinal tract by (a) withdrawal of dietary protein; (b) reducing the population of colonic bacteria by oral neomycin and lactulose, and magnesium sulphate enema; avoidance

of hypokalaemia; avoidance of hypoglycaemia; prevention of gastrointestinal bleeding with cimetidine and vitamin K. Finally, sedatives and narcotics must not be used.
[A: 107; B: 20.24; C: 397; E: 69–71; F: 575; G: 1666; H: 1482–3]

379 Salt-free diet—the practical minimum is 20–30 mmol of sodium per day; gentle diuresis with a potassium-sparing diuretic such as amiloride or spironolactone to give a weight loss of not more than 0.5 kg daily. A loop diuretic such as frusemide can also be used with careful attention to potassium supplementation.

The patient should weigh himself daily at home to monitor the weight loss.
[A: 108; B: 20.22; C: 405; D: 202; E: 68–70; F: 574; G: 1640; H: 1481]

380 Dilated abdominal wall veins with blood flow away from the umbilicus; splenomegaly; the liver may be shrunken. There may be ascites. Haemorrhoids may also be present but they are not specific for portal hypertension.

Haematemesis is the commonest presenting feature.
[A: 107–8; B: 20.20; C: 404; D: 201; E: 68–9; F: 573; G: 1639; H: 1480]

381 Mild impairment of liver cell function and centrizonal hepatic necrosis due to hypoxia; cardiac cirrhosis; bilirubin released from pulmonary infarcts.
[F: 576; G: 1661; H: 1478]

382 Patients with haemolytic jaundice tend to have a lemon-yellow tinge, and they may be anaemic with a history of previous episodes of a known haemolytic tendency. In hepatic jaundice the patient usually manifests the effects of liver disease, either the fever and anorexia of acute hepatitis or the malaise and stigmata of chronic liver disease. In cholestatic jaundice, the retention of bile salts causes itching and the patient may feel normal apart from any symptoms due to the underlying cause. Stools are pale and the urine is tea-coloured.

An enlarged palpable gall bladder suggests carcinoma of the head of pancreas rather than cholelithiasis. This is known as Courvoisier's law.
[A: 100; B: 20.2; C: 388; D: 38–9; E: 63; F: 563; G: 1638; H: 208]

383 The serum of a patient with hepatitis B may show spherical and tubular particles, which are surplus viral protein (HB_sAg), and larger Dane particles. Each Dane particle is a complete virus.

The core of each virus contains core antigen and e antigen, HB_cAg and HB_eAg respectively. Persistence of the e antigen or of antibodies to core antigen implies continuing infectivity, whereas fluids containing only the surface antigen, HB_sAg, are not necessarily infectious. Blood, semen and saliva can transmit infection. The presence of antibody to the surface antigen, HB_sAg, appears to correlate with immunity.

It is of epidemiological interest that different antigenic subtypes exist for the surface antigen, and these are labelled with the letters a, d, y, w and r.
[A: 104; B: 20.9–13; C: 393; D: 196; E: 64–7; F: 565–8; G: 1650–1; H: 1459]

384 Chronic persistent hepatitis and chronic active hepatitis. Chronic active hepatitis exists in mild and severe forms. Only the severe form of chronic active hepatitis progresses to cirrhosis or carcinoma.

In chronic persistent hepatitis the total serum globulin level is not usually raised and signs of chronic liver disease are absent. The opposite is generally true of chronic active hepatitis. Full differentiation, however, rests on liver biopsy appearances.
[A: 106; B: 20.17; C: 402; D: 198; E: 71; F: 570; G: 1661; H: 1470]

385 Cirrhosis due to Hb_sAg (Australian antigen)-negative chronic active hepatitis is associated with smooth muscle antibodies. That due to primary biliary cirrhosis is associated with mitochondrial antibodies.
[A: 106–9; B: 20.14–28; C: 404; D: 199; E: 68; F: 569; G: 1663; H: 1473]

386 Zieve's syndrome is the name for the combination of acute haemolysis with acute alcoholic hepatitis and hyperlipidaemia.

Dupuytren's contracture and parotid enlargement are seen in cirrhotics and are related to an alcoholic aetiology. A macrocytic anaemia and features of Wernicke's encephalopathy, Korsakoff's psychosis, peripheral neuropathy or delirium tremens all point to alcoholism.
[B: 20.16; D: 199; E: 72; F: 573; G: 1663; H: 1473–5]

387 Liver cell function is usually minimally impaired in haemochromatosis.

Other signs of haemochromatosis include bronze or slate-grey pigmentation of skin folds, genitalia and buccal mucosa, and an arthropathy affecting the metacarpophalangeal joints and some large joints. X-ray may reveal calcification of menisci and joint cartilage. An associated cardiomyopathy may produce arrhythmias and cardiac failure.

[A: 110; B: 20.31; C: 410; D: 202; E: 72; F: 571; G: 1791; H: 489]

388 In cholestatic jaundice of pregnancy pruritis is common and jaundice is variable. There is little derangement of biochemical liver function. Vitamin K should be given to avoid any increased risk of haemorrhage at the time of delivery. The condition recurs in subsequent pregnancies or with oral contraceptive use.

Tetracyclines stain the bones and teeth of the fetus. Tetracycline administration also shows an association with the serious maternal condition of acute fatty liver.
[B: 20.30; F: 563; G: 1658; H: 1487]

389 Sclerosing cholangitis causing strictures of the bile ducts, and cholangiocarcinoma.
[B: 20.17; C: 418–19; F: 562; G: 1575; H: 1498]

390 Non-metastatic features of hepatocellular carcinoma include hypoglycaemia, raised cholesterol levels, polycythaemia and raised levels of alpha-fetoprotein.

Gynaecomastia and hypercalcaemia also occur.
[A: 113; B: 20.33; C: 412; E: 71; F: 579; G: 1668; H: 1485]

391 Oestrogens; cholestyramine, which binds bile acids and reduces enterohepatic circulation; clofibrate which increses cholesterol excretion into the bile.
[B: 20.38; C: 414; D: 222; E: 90; F: 581; G: 1619; H: 1491]

392 Chronic biliary tract disease, as a result of which infected bile may reflux into the pancreatic duct; alcohol consumption, although not necessarily alcoholism; steroid therapy; hyperparathyroidism.
[A: 114; B: 20.46; C: 340; D: 219; E: 92; F: 586; G: 1551; H: 1503]

393 The secretin stimulation test will reveal a subnormal response; malabsorption of vitamin B_{12} is present in many cases as a result of binding of B_{12} by proteins which are usually digested by pancreatic proteases.
[A: 114–15; B: 20.48; C: 342; D: 220; E: 92; F: 587; G: 1554; H: 1507–10]

394 Liver function tests will show marked elevation of bilirubin and alkaline phosphatase with only moderate elevation of transaminases. Glucose tolerance may be impaired. The stools may contain fat and occult blood and are said to be silvery in colour.

Barium meal examination may reveal deformity of the duodenal loop. Ultrasound examination is useful in demonstrating the enlarged extrahepatic bile ducts of extrahepatic cholestasis. CT scanning may confirm the presence of a pancreatic tumour.

More invasive tests include endoscopic retrograde choledochopancreatography (ERCP), trans-hepatic cholangiography and coeliac angiography. The diagnosis is confirmed at laparotomy.
[B: 20.51; C: 344; D: 219; E: 87; F: 588; G: 1557; H: 1511–12]

395 Cystic fibrosis. Morbidity and mortality are largely determined by the respiratory complications which include frequent pulmonary infections, bronchiectasis, recurrent pneumothorax, haemoptysis and cor pulmonale.
[A: 259; B: 20.49; C: 344; F: 586; G: 1559; H: 1234]

Nervous System

396 Head injuries may shear the olfactory fibres where they pierce the cribriform plate of the ethmoid under the olfactory bulb. A meningioma growing in the olfactory groove may compress the bulb and tract.
[A: 317; B: 34.55; C: 666; E; 485; F: 1304; G: 899; H: 2021]

397 Either in the periphery of the retina, as in retinitis pigmentosa or affecting the peripheral retinal fibres where they lie superficially and are vulnerable to the increased intraocular pressure of glaucoma.
[A: 318; G: 2322; H: 104]

398 The lesion is in the optic nerve of the blind eye right up against the anterior edge of the chiasma. The temporal hemianopia in the other eye is explained by the fact that fibres from the nasal side of the retina loop into the optic nerve of the opposite eye at the chiasma.
[A: 318; C: 663; D: 6; G: 899; H: 104]

399 A pituitary tumour expanding upwards and compressing the optic chiasma. Most commonly this is asymmetrical so that one eye is more affected than the other. Also, since the initial damage comes from below the chiasma, the lower retinal fibres are first affected and the early field defect is therefore an upper quadrantanopia.
[A: 318; B: 34.57; C: 663; D: 6; E: 487; F: 1304–6; G: 899; H: 104]

400 Non-congruous defects, i.e. the eyes are not affected to the same extent, arise from lesions of the optic tract

(between chiasma and lateral geniculate body of the thalamus). Pituitary tumours and aneurysms of the posterior communicating or internal carotid arteries may be responsible as may temporal lobe lesions or meningitis.
[A: 318–19; B: 34.57; C: 663; F: 1305–6; H: 104]

401 In the optic radiations, fibres serving corresponding parts of each visual field lie close together so that any lesion will affect each eye's visual field equally, causing a congruous defect. In the optic tract, this is not the case and non-congruous defects result.
[A: 318–19; B: 34.57; C: 663; F: 1305–6; H: 104]

402 A left lower homonymous quadrantanopia and a right upper homonymous quadrantanopia respectively.
[A: 318–19; C: 663–4; D: 6; F: 1305–6; H: 104]

403 Visual impairment which may be marked. There may also be pain behind the eye, and the direct light reflex may be sluggish while the consensual reflex is intact. If there is papillitis, then the disc will tend to have the appearance of papilloedema. The distinction from papilloedema due to raised intracranial pressure rests on the presence of normal visual acuity in the latter, at least in the earlier stages.
[A: 319; B: 34.56; C: 666–7; E: 488; F: 1305; G: 899; H: 2021]

404 Optic atrophy and permanent visual impairment.

Papilloedema, when bilateral, strongly indicates raised intracranial pressure, such as may be caused by a tumour or by malignant hypertension. Obstruction of the central vein of the retina such as may occur in cavernous sinus thrombosis is also a cause.
[A: 319; B: 34.55; C: 666; E: 486–7; F: 1305; G: 2327; H: 104–5]

405 By testing visual acuity.

Any significant degree of optic atrophy is invariably associated with some loss of visual acuity.
[A: 319; B: 34.57; C: 667; E: 488; F: 1305; H: 104]

406 Oculomotor (III) nerve palsy. The ptosis is due to loss of action of levator palpebrae superioris, the dilated pupil to the loss of pupillary constrictor fibres, the inferolateral deviation of the eye to the weakness of all the eye muscles except the lateral rectus and superior oblique. The more complete the palsy, the more the eye will deviate laterally rather than inferiorly.

Close to where it emerges from the midbrain, the oculomotor nerve passes between the posterior cerebral and superior cerebellar arteries. Aneurysm of either of these could have ruptured, causing compression of the nerve and headache.
[A: 321; B: 34.58; C: 668; D: 8; E: 490; F: 1306–7; G: 899; H: 106]

407 Aneurysm of the posterior cerebral artery. Inability to look downwards when the eye is adducted.
[A: 322; B: 34.58; C: 668; D: 8; E: 490; F: 1306–7; G: 899; H: 106]

408 Weakness of the lateral rectus muscle with loss of abduction of the eye and acoustic neuroma, since all these nerves emerge from the pons and lie close together in the cerebellopontine angle.
[A: 322–3; B: 34.58; C: 668; D: 8; E: 490; F: 1306–7; G: 899; H: 106]

409 Present since birth or early childhood; normal range of eye movements in each eye; absence of diplopia. Usually the angle of deviation between the visual axes is constant in all directions of gaze.
[A: 324; C: 668; D: 7; H: 105]

410 Left inferior oblique.
[A: 324; B: 34.59; C: 668; D: 7; H: 105]

411 Nothing. They are normal.
[A: 327; B: 34.60; D: 8; E: 489; F: 1307; H: 108]

412 Absent knee and ankle jerks. The combination of a myotonic pupil with these absent jerks is called Adie's syndrome. It is benign, and not the cause of the headaches.
[A: 327; B: 34.60; D: 9; E: 489; F: 1307; G: 900; H: 108]

413 All that can be confidently diagnosed is that the lesion is on the same side as the signs. The sympathetic fibres originate in the hypothalamus, run down in the brain stem to the cervical cord, emerge at the level of T1 to join the cervical sympathetic ganglion from where they run up the carotid artery, re-entering the skull to reach the eye. Horner's syndrome may be due to a lesion anywhere along this course. The most important causes of damage include vascular lesions in the medulla, syringobulbia, syringomyelia, carcinoma of the lung and enlarged cervical lymph nodes. A carotid artery lesion can produce an ipsilateral Horner's syndrome and a contralateral hemiplegia.

[A: 327; B: 34.60; C: 675; D: 9; E: 489; F: 1307; G: 787; H: 108]

414 Argyll Robertson pupils. They are very suggestive of syphilis, but syphilis is rare now and other causes include diabetes, hypertrophic polyneuritis and vascular or neoplastic lesions of the midbrain. The exact site of the lesion in syphilis is contested.
[A: 327–8; B: 34.60; C: 704; D: 8; E: 489; F: 1307; G: 900; H: 108]

415 Two of his children are seen to have the same bilateral ptosis indicating that this is familial.
[B: 34.58; C: 668; D: 4; H: 108]

416 Lesions of the upper cervical cord can cause loss of pain and temperature sensation over the face.
Another important fact about the trigeminal nerve is that it forms the afferent limb of the corneal reflex. Loss of the corneal reflex can be an early sign of a tumour in the cerebellopontine angle.
[A: 328; B: 34.60–1; C: 670–1; E: 491; F: 1307; G: 900]

417 After passing through the geniculate ganglion it first gives off the greater superficial petrosal nerve which supplies secretomotor fibres to the lachrymal gland, then the nerve to the stapedius muscle after which there is the junction with the chorda tympani.
Lesions of these nerves will cause loss of lachrymation, hyperacusis and loss of taste from the anterior two-thirds of the tongue respectively.
[A: 330; B: 34.62; F: 1308; G: 900; H: 2023]

418 In upper motor neurone lesions, facial weakness is confined to the lower part of the face while movement of the muscles around the eye and of the forehead will be intact. Bell's palsy is a lower motor neurone lesion, causing complete paralysis of the affected side of the face. In a cerebellopontine angle lesion, one would expect to find evidence of damage to the fifth, sixth and eighth cranial nerves as well as loss of taste in the anterior two-thirds of the tongue and facial palsy.
[A: 331; B: 34.63; C: 672; D: 11; E: 492; F: 1308; G: 900; H: 2023]

419 That eventual complete recovery can be expected. Even without this early evidence of recovery, an optimistic attitude should be adopted. If the patient is seen early on, some physicians give ACTH or prednisone for a few days.
[A: 331; B: 34.63; C: 672; D: 11; E: 492; F: 1308; G: 900; H: 2023]

420 Sarcoidosis.
[A: 332; B: 12.32; D: 11; F: 1309; G: 900; H: 2024]

421 Weber's and Rinne's tests.
In Weber's test, the vibrating tuning fork is applied to the forehead in the midline. It is normal to hear the sound in the midline. In conductive deafness, it seems louder in the affected ear whereas in nerve deafness it seems louder in the normal ear.

In Rinne's test, the vibrating tuning fork is applied to the mastoid process until the patient ceases to hear it. It is then held at the ear. In middle-ear deafness, the sound cannot be heard by air conduction after bone conduction has ceased to transmit it. In nerve deafness, as in normal individuals, it can.
[A: 332; D: 9; G: 734; H: 109]

422 The presence of long tract signs would point to the lesion being in the brain stem. Impairment of fifth, sixth and seventh cranial nerves would point to the cerebellopontine angle, while a facial nerve palsy (with loss of taste from the anterior two-thirds of the tongue) would suggest the petrous temporal bone as a possible site. The commonest causes of acquired nerve deafness are fractured skull, acoustic neuroma and Paget's disease.

In audiometric tests, cochlear deafness is distinguished by the presence of loudness recruitment.
[F: 1310; G: 734–5; H: 109]

423 Check the patient's medications; check the blood pressure; examine the ears; check the blood sugar; X-ray the cervical spine.
[B: 34.13; C: 673; D: 10; E: 494; F: 1309; G: 737; H: 83]

424 (a) Ocular—defective vision is the cause.
(b) Vestibular—the slow phase points to the side of the lesion.
(c) Central (cerebellar or brain stem).
[A: 325; B: 34.59; C: 669; D: 10; F: 1303; G: 738; H: 107]

425 Ménière's disease. The abnormality is in the semicircular canals.
[A: 333; B: 34.65; C: 674; D: 10; E: 495; F: 1310; G: 739; H: 2024]

426 Caloric testing.
[A: 333; B: 34.65; C: 674; F: 1310; G: 738; H: 84]

427 Its name is helpful. Its sensory fibres supply the posterior third of the tongue with taste and ordinary sensation. Motor fibres supply the pharyngeal constrictor muscles. As well as the posterior third of

the tongue, the nerve supplies sensation to the adjacent soft palate and pharynx. The tonsillar fossa is a reliable place in which to test for anaesthesia. Secretomotor fibres to the parotid gland are also in the glossopharyngeal nerve.
[A: 333; B: 34.66; C: 674; E: 495; F: 1311; G: 727]

428 After emerging from the skull it lies in the carotid sheath and enters the thorax behind the great veins. Both right and left vagi come to lie on the posterior surfaces of the lungs, but the left first runs over the aortic arch. The left recurrent laryngeal has a longer course than the right and is more vulnerable to compression by upper thoracic tumours.
[A:333; B: 34.66; C: 674; E: 495; F: 1311]

429 The fibres arise from nuclei in the cervical cord between C1 and C5. They emerge from the cord as separate rootlets which merge to form a trunk which travels up the spinal canal, through the foramen magnum into the posterior cranial fossa where they join the nerve emerging from the XI nucleus in the medulla to pass through the internal jugular foramen.
[A: 334; B: 34.67; C: 674; E: 495; F: 1311]

430 Lower motor neurone lesions cause wasting. In the tongue this occurs within days, and results in the tongue being pulled over to the normal side as it lies in the mouth but pushed to the weak side on protrusion.

With an upper motor neurone lesion, e.g. pseudobulbar palsy, wasting is not prominent but stiffness (or spasticity) causes difficulty in putting out the tongue and articulating the letters 'd, j, l, n.' etc.
[A: 334; B: 34.67; C: 675; E: 496; F: 1311; G: 900]

431 The muscles of articulation are innervated from both cerebral cortices, so unilateral upper motor neurone damage will not cause dysarthria. In progressive cerebrovascular disease, for example, there can be bilateral internal capsule damage, causing a pseudobulbar palsy, of which dysarthria is a striking feature. Lower motor neurone lesions of the seventh, ninth, tenth or twelfth cranial nerves may cause dysarthria. Disseminated sclerosis causing cerebellar damage typically causes a dysarthria described as 'scanning speech'. Myasthenia gravis can cause weakness of the muscles of articulation.
[A: 334; B: 34.9; C: 661; D: 12; F: 1303; G: 656; H: 144]

432 Receptive dysphasia means that the patient cannot properly process words that he hears or reads. This will be clear from inability to give appropriate responses to questions and commands, and also from

the inappropriateness of what he says since he cannot judge whether his own speech is correct.

In expressive dysphasia, comprehension is intact and the patient clearly knows what he wants to say but cannot select the right words. Since he can correctly 'hear' himself speaking, he is aware of the problem and tries to correct himself.
[A: 316; B: 34.8; C: 661; D: 12; F: 1296–9; G: 656; H: 141]

433 The CSF is abnormal, organic disease is present and there is probably a space-occupying lesion (tumour or abscess) compressing the dominant frontal lobe in the anterior cerebral fossa.
[A: 316; C: 661; F: 1299; G: 656–7; H: 141]

434 They arise from the motor cortex (on the precentral gyrus) on which somatic representation is a striking feature. The fibres converge on the internal capsule and pass down in the cerebral peduncle to the midbrain from where they pass to the pons. Some fibres decussate in the midbrain and pons to supply cranial nerve nuclei. The main bundle lies anteriorly in the brain stem, forming the pyramids (hence the name pyramidal tracts). The main tracts decussate in the lower medulla to acquire a lateral position in the white matter of the cord. The small number of fibres that do not decussate lie anteriorly and close to the midline.
[A: 335; C: 650; D: 22; F: 1293; H: 86]

435 Muscle weakness, increased tone, loss of skin reflexes, increase in tendon reflexes and extensor plantar reflexes. Any one of these may predominate. There are many other signs more specific to upper motor neurone lesions at particular sites.

In a lesion of sudden onset, as in a cerebrovascular accident, there is likely to be diminished tone, i.e. flaccidity for the first few days before spasticity develops.

An extensor plantar reflex indicates an UMN lesion but a flexor response does not exclude one.
[A: 336; C: 650; F: 1293; H: 86]

436 Pin-prick and temperature decussate two to three segments above entry to the spinal cord and travel up in the lateral spinothalamic tract. Light touch (cotton-wool) decussates several segments above entry to the cord and travels up in the anterior spinothalamic tract. Proprioception (position sense), vibration, deep pain and some light touch travel up in

the posterior columns and do not decussate until they have formed the medial lemniscus in the medulla.
[A: 343; B: 34.6; C: 655; F: 1294; H: 111–12]

437 Symmetrical, peripheral muscular weakness and wasting, loss of tendon reflexes, pain (of a persistent burning quality) and tenderness of muscles, and sensory impairment.

In the early stages all of these features may not be present. It is common also for damage to be selective (e.g. in diabetes, vibration sense and reflexes are usually lost first, whereas in lead poisoning and porphyria, motor changes predominate).
[A: 353; B: 34.37; C: 657; D: 21; F: 1312; H: 112]

438 Pain, lancinating or burning in nature, and exacerbated by coughing or sneezing, with hyperaesthesia over the corresponding dermatome. If adjacent roots are affected, there will be sensory loss. The important aspect of these symptoms and signs is that they are segmental.
[A: 350; C: 657; F: 1321; G: 889; H: 113]

439 Metastatic bronchogenic carcinoma with extradural cord compression. The spine is longer than the spinal cord, hence the discrepancy between the radiological and neurological levels (and hence also the safety of lumbar punctures, provided the needle is inserted below L2).
[A: 347; B: 34.50; C: 727–8; D: 116; E: 507–8; G: 890; H: 2019]

440 Interference with conduction in the roots and the cord itself by direct pressure. Oedema of the cord below the site of compression from pressure on the ascending longitudinal spinal veins. Ischaemia from compression of spinal arteries, either longitudinal or radicular or both.
[C: 727; F: 1325; G: 896–7; H: 2019]

441 Evidence of compression on one half of the cord, unilateral root pains and a high CSF protein suggest extramedullary compression, whereas bilateral motor symptoms and a dissociated sensory loss with a less elevated CSF protein favour an intramedullary lesion.
[C: 728; F: 1304; G: 892; H: 2019]

442 Spinal cord compression on the left side at the level of L3 and L4. Brown-Séquard syndrome.
[A: 348; C: 728; D: 21; F: 1323; G: 890; H: 113]

443 Contralateral impairment of pain and temperature sensation; ipsilateral impairment of facial pain and

temperature sensation (descending tract of trigeminal nerve); vertigo and nystagmus (ipsilateral vestibular nucleus); ipsilateral Horner's syndrome (descending sympathetic tract); dysphagia and hoarseness (tenth nerve) and loss of taste (nucleus and tractus solitarius). Ataxia also occurs, with a tendency to fall to the side of the lesion, but UMN signs are absent.
[B: 34.68–9; C: 658; F: 1302; H: 114]

444 Severe pain over the contralateral side of the body. The threshold to pain on the affected side is usually increased but when stimuli are felt, the sensation is usually exaggerated and unpleasant.
[B: 34.78; C: 658; F: 1295; H: 114]

445 One test of parietal function is the ability to hold the arms outstretched (palms upward) with eyes closed. If one arm slowly drifts downwards, this is a good sign of abnormality.

Touching identical parts of the body on left and right at the same time elicits sensory inattention. Faulty recognition of objects placed in the hand (with eyes closed) is called astereognosis. Another test of this is 'writing' numerals on the patient's palm with the examiner's finger. Two-point discrimination is another parietal function which is tested with a pair of dividers.
[A: 317; B: 34.7; C: 658; D: 13–14; F: 1295–6; H: 114]

446 Loss of muscle tone; alteration of tendon reflexes, best demonstrated by tapping the knee with the patient sitting on the edge of the bed—the leg goes on swinging backwards and forwards—a 'pendular' knee-jerk; ataxia which may affect a limb or the trunk, i.e. positive Romberg's sign; dysdiadochokinesis which is difficulty or inability to perform a repetitive movement rapidly; dysarthria, in which the voice may be too loud and the syllables produced jerkily and separated from each other—this is sometimes called scanning speech.
[A: 346; B: 34.73–5; C: 653–4; D: 24; F: 1303; H: 97]

447 Putamen—athetosis; caudate nucleus—chorea; subthalamic nucleus—hemiballismus; globus pallidus and substantia nigra—Parkinsonian tremor and rigidity.

In the inherited disease of copper metabolism (Wilson's disease), the lentiform nuclei are most affected although damage occurs to other nuclei as well. The liver shows cirrhosis, hence the other name for the disease, hepatolenticular degeneration. It typically affects young adults.
[A: 343; B: 34.146; C: 653; F: 1363; G: 750; H: 92]

448 Application of pressure to the jugular veins during lumbar puncture should cause a rapid rise in the fluid pressure measured in the graduated tube attached to the needle. The pressure should drop quickly to its original value when the jugular veins are released. This is Queckenstedt's test, and it indicates free communication of fluid between the intracranial sinuses and the lumbar puncture needle.

Failure of the fluid pressure to rise occurs with spinal cord compression or with a venous sinus thrombosis, i.e. a block in the CSF system between the jugular veins and the LP needle.
[B: 34.16; C: 665; F: 1303; G: 2351; H: 1905]

449 Exhaustion, stress, watching television, stroboscopes and flickering lights of any type, e.g. a single fluorescent light tube or driving under sunlit trees, hypoglycaemia, alcohol, hypocalcaemia, cerebral ischaemia, fever.
[A: 365; B: 34.160; C: 676; D: 97; E: 517; F: 1373–5; G: 852–3; H: 133]

450 History or evidence of injury during an attack; an aura before the loss of consciousness; incontinence; tongue-biting; abnormal movements during the attack.
[D: 96; E: 518; F: 1378; G: 740–5; H: 81]

451 The attacks are the same but there is no recovery of consciousness between attacks. Fever, deepening coma and death occur unless the fits can be stopped.
[A: 366; B: 34.161; C: 676; D: 97; E: 518; F: 1373; G: 853; H: 131–6]

452 The patient may become confused, anxious or aggressive and display automatism, i.e. complex actions performed in an automatic way. There may be hallucinations of smell, taste or vision, powerful feelings of fear and a sense of altered reality. Déjà vu, an intense feeling of familiarity with the environment, also occurs.
[B: 34.161–3; C: 677; D: 97–8; E: 518; F: 1373; G: 854–5; H: 131]

453 Phenytoin, 150 mg daily in one or two doses, increasing as necessary up to 600 mg daily, subject to the development of toxicity.

Carbamazepine, starting at 100 mg twice daily and slowly increasing up to 400 mg twice daily or occasionally larger doses.
[A: 367–8; B: 34.165; C: 679; D: 97–8; E: 519; F: 1376; G: 859; H: 137]

454 Carbamazepine may cause dizziness, drowsiness and gastrointestinal upset. These usually subside but are the reason for starting treatment with a low dose. Inappropriate secretion of ADH can occur with prolonged use.
[A: 367–8; B: 34.165–6; C: 679; E: 519; F: 1376; G: 859; H: 137]

455 It may affect the ophthalmic division of the trigeminal nerve, the geniculate ganglion or the spinal cord, with serious consequences.

It occurs in patients in whom cellular immunity may be depressed, e.g. lymphoma, malignancy, tuberculosis.

Post-herpetic neuralgia is common and can be extremely severe.

People not immune to the varicella-zoster virus can catch chickenpox from a person with shingles.
[A: 351; B: 12.31; C: 711; E: 550; F: 135; G: 825; H: 802]

456 Yes. Ramsay Hunt syndrome.
[A: 332; E: 550; F: 135; G: 826; H: 802]

457 Acupuncture, neuroelectric therapy, for both of which Wall's gate theory provides a physiological basis.
[A: 351; B: 34.61; C: 711; D: 92; E: 524; F: 135; G: 725; H: 803]

458 There may be an aura, commonly some form of visual disturbance. At this stage there is vasoconstriction of some of the vessels of the extracranial or intracranial systems. Subsequent relaxation of these vessels causes the headache which is often severe, prostrating and accompanied by vomiting.

There may be a family history.
[A: 370; C: 688; D: 91; E: 520–1; F: 1379; G: 731; H: 21]

459 Coffee, chocolate, cheese, citrus fruits and bananas. Alcohol is a potent cause of migraine.
[B: 34.157; F: 1380; H: 21]

460 Methysergide, a serotonin antagonist, which can cause retroperitoneal fibrosis.

Propranolol is effective in some cases.

Clonidine in small but frquent doses is also sometimes effective.

Some doctors stress the anxious nature of migraine sufferers and prescribe a regular dose of tranquillizer e.g. diazepam 2 mg t.d.s.
[A: 370–1; B: 34.158; C: 668; D: 91; E: 522; F: 1380; G: 731–2; H: 25]

461 Migrainous neuralgia or cluster headaches. The treatment is ergotamine, but because oral tablets are too slowly absorbed to abort the headache, the drug is best taken as either a subcutaneous injection or as a suppository on retiring to bed.
[A: 371; B: 34.158; C: 687; D: 91; E: 524; F: 1381; G: 731; H: 22]

462 There may be a lucid period of 20–30 minutes after injury to the side of the head followed in quick succession by headache and ipsilateral pupil contraction, then drowsiness, loss of consciousness and a fixed dilated pupil as the expanding haematoma forces the brain to herniate through the tentorium.

If there is no recovery of consciousness after the injury, the presence of an extradural haemorrhage can be diagnosed from deepening of the level of unconsciousness and development of asymmetrical neurological signs. Careful and frequent examination is therefore essential.
[A: 371; C: 695; D: 94; E: 516; F: 1344; G: 883; H: 1939]

463 At the time of injury oozing occurs from the subdural veins, leading to the slow formation of a flat haematoma. As this haematoma organizes it develops a skin and the centre liquefies. Fluid is drawn into the centre by osmosis and the haematoma expands, compressing the brain. Subdural haematomas are often bilateral.

The patient may have a slight fever. A fluctuating level of consciousness, changing neurological signs, restlessness and irritability are all common features. Surgical drainage of the haematoma frequently produces a dramatic cure.
[A: 372; C: 696; D: 95; F: 1345; G: 884; H: 1939]

464 Aneurysms can seldom be removed but the chance of further bleeding can be lessened by applying a clip to the neck of the aneurysm, or wrapping it. In other words, neurosurgery can do nothing for the bleed that has already occurred. Only patients who have a normal level of consciousness are candidates for surgery.
[A: 372; B: 34.97; C: 694–5; D: 95–6; E: 527; F: 1335–6; G: 796; H: 1936–8]

465 The most important clue is the duration of onset of the symptoms and signs. Thrombosis usually takes at least a few minutes and the symptoms may evolve over hours. Embolism and haemorrhage, however, are usually sudden. Haemorrhage usually presents with more severe damage which may progress. The presence of neck stiffness or a preceding history of

hypertension are suggestive of a haemorrhagic cause. Several days or weeks of symptoms preceding the stroke is evidence of a space-occupying lesion. An embolic cause for a stroke should be considered when a source of emboli is present, e.g. mitral stenosis, atrial fibrillation or recent myocardial infarction.
[A: 373–4; B: 34.93–6; C: 691–3; D: 92; E: 530–6; F: 1331–5; G: 784–6; H: 1923]

466 Cerebral angioma. There may be a bruit over the malformation. It is usually best heard over the eyeball on the side of the lesion.
[A: 373; B: 34.72; F: 1336; G: 863; H: 1938]

467 Vertigo, ataxia, drop attacks, diplopia, dysarthria and even blindness, hemiparesis or quadriparesis.
[A: 374; B: 34.71; C: 692; D: 93; E: 531–2; F: 1331–2; G: 784; H: 1926–7]

468 Progressive cerebral atherosclerosis.
[C: 693]

469 Cavernous sinus thrombosis secondary to the facial boil.

Middle ear infection can cause lateral sinus thrombosis. Papilloedema may occur.
[A: 375; B: 34.104; C: 700; E: 546; F: 1337; G: 789; H: 1965]

470 Headache, fever, nausea, vomiting and drowsiness. Neck stiffness and a positive Kernig's sign are two important signs of meningeal irritation.

Meningococcus, pneumococcus and haemophilus are the three most common causative organisms.
[A: 357; B: 34.123; C: 702; D: 99–102; E: 542; F: 58–61; G: 412; H: 1961]

471 The CSF pressure is usually raised. The cell count is raised to 100 or more per ml with a predominance of lymphocytes. Protein is increased and glucose is reduced although not as markedly as in acute pyogenic meningitis.

Evidence of TB elsewhere in the body e.g. on chest X-ray, makes a tuberculous aetiology of meningitis more likely.
[A: 358; B: 34.124; C: 703; D: 99; E: 544; F: 90; G: 493; H: 706]

472 Fever, asymmetrical lower motor neurone paralysis and neck stiffness. Pain and hyperalgesia over the affected muscles may occur but there is no sensory loss. Bladder and bowel may be affected.

Rest until 3–4 days after defervescence of the fever should be followed by an active programme of physiotherapy.
[A: 361; B: 34.130; C: 710; D: 113; E: 548; F: 146; G: 829–32; H: 813]

473 Loss of position and vibration sense in the legs, loss of deep pain sensation in the calves and Achilles tendons and loss of knee and ankle jerks. There may also be loss of pain sensation below the knees and over the upper chest and down the medial side of the arms.
These deficits cause ataxia. In addition Argyll Robertson pupils occur and ptosis, Charcot joints, trophic ulcers and optic atrophy may develop.
[A: 363; B: 34.133; C: 705; D: 111; E: 551; F: 1330; G: 814; H: 720]

474 Pain, usually paroxysmal, severe 'lightning pains' affecting one spot at a time; paraesthesiae, especially numb or cold feelings in the feet with a 'walking on wool' sensation; tabetic crises, which are episodes of pain arising in any hollow viscus, most commonly the stomach, causing vomiting; impotence; urinary retention with overflow; loss of sensation of micturition or defaecation; failing vision or diplopia.
[A: 363; B: 34.133; C: 705–6; D: 111; E: 551; F: 1330; G: 814–15; H: 113]

475 Optic atrophy. A syphilitic gumma can behave like a space-occupying lesion.
[A: 364; B: 34.134; C: 705; D: 111; E: 551; F: 1329; G: 814; H: 720]

476 Focal epilepsy; gradual personality change (this is often a sign of frontal lobe tumours); gradual development of weakness, or impaired intellectual function (e.g. speech, memory); vertigo.
[A: 376; B: 34.114; C: 681–2; D: 107; E: 538; F: 1337–8; G: 864–6; H: 1952]

477 The lesion may be calcified. The pineal may be displaced from the midline. Erosion of the posterior clinoid process is a sign of raised intracranial pressure. A pituary tumour may cause expansion or destruction of the sella turcica. Sometimes hyperostosis of the skull vault occurs adjacent to a meningioma. A malignant tumour may cause local erosion of the bone.
[A: 376; B: 34.15; C: 683; E: 539; F: 1341; G: 866]

478 Benign intracranial hypertension (pseudo-tumour cerebri). The condition is misnamed since blindness

can result from associated long-standing papilloedema.
[B: 34.119; C: 678; D: 108; F: 1342; G: 870; H: 1955]

479 Electroencephalography may show abnormal, slow activity either localized to the site of a cerebral lesion or diffusely when intracranial pressure is raised.

Isotope brain scanning will show lesions if the lesion takes up more or less isotope than the surrounding brain tissue. Meningiomas commonly show up clearly, abscesses may be silent areas. Uptake by gliomas and metastatic deposits is less reliable.

Cerebral angiography shows abnormal vessel patterns, which may be of diagnostic value and also shows lesions by the displacement of adjacent vessels.
[A: 377–8; B: 34.20–23; C: 684; D: 107; E: 539; F: 1341; G: 746–50]

480 Surgery offers the best chance of cure because it may be possible to completely excise a benign tumour. In most cases, however, all treatment is palliative, and although removal or shrinking of tumour mass may relieve symptoms and reduce intracranial pressure, the neurological deficit often remains. Sometimes tumour removal increases the deficit, regardless of intraoperative or postoperative complications.
[A: 378; B: 34.118; C: 684–5; F: 1341; G: 869]

481 (a) Disease of the vertebral column, e.g. metastatic neoplastic disease, tuberculosis, crush fracture of vertebrae or prolapsed intervertebral disc.
(b) Disease of the meninges, e.g. epidural abscess, meningioma, lymphoma.
(c) Tumours of the cord itself, e.g. glioma, angioma.
[A: 347; C: 728; D: 117; E: 507; F: 1323–6; G: 891; H: 2019]

482 Anteroposterior and lateral views of the spine at the level involved. Oblique views are necessary also to show the intervertebral foramina. Posteroanterior and lateral chest X-rays should also be taken. The commonest source of malignant metastasis to the nervous system and bones is bronchogenic carcinoma.
[D: 117; E: 507; F: 1324–6; G: 892; H: 2020]

483 The finding of a very high CSF protein level (more than 500 mg/dl) without an increase in cells.

This occurs when there is a partial or complete block in the subarachnoid space. Queckenstedt's test may also be abnormal.
[C: 728; D: 117; G: 892–3; H: 2019]

484 Progressive muscular atrophy, in which the lower motor neurone lesions predominate, often starting with wasting and weakness of the hands.

Lateral sclerosis in which the predominant lesion is in the upper motor neurones, resulting in spastic weakness. The clinical picture depends on the combination of upper and lower motor neurone signs.

Progressive bulbar palsy due to involvement of the medullary nuclei. Dysphagia and dysarthria result. [A: 337; B: 34.52; C: 721–2; D: 108; E: 511; F: 1353; G: 765; H: 2002]

485 Peroneal muscular atrophy or Charcot–Marie–Tooth disease. It is a familial condition with little effect on life expectancy. All modalities of sensation are impaired over the affected muscles. [A: 381; B: 34.40; D: 116; F: 1320; G: 913; H: 2035]

486 Cutaneous pigmentation and neurofibromas. Pigmentation is nearly always present and consists of café au lait spots, brownish as their name is meant to suggest, and varying in size from a small dot to large patches. The trunk is typically affected.

Neurofibromas are most often felt on the extremities or the sides of the neck. Tumours on specific nerves cause characteristic symptoms, acoustic neuroma being one of the most serious conditions. [A: 382; B: 34.43; C: 725; E: 512; F: 1351; G: 769; H: 2006–7]

487 Dissociated sensory loss, by which is meant impairment of pain, heat and cold sensation (the modalities carried in the spinothalamic tracts) with preservation of posterior column modalities; loss of reflexes at the level of the sensory loss but spastic weakness of the lower limbs.

Trophic changes and Charcot joints are common in later stages.

The cerebrospinal fluid usually shows no abnormality. [A: 349; B: 34.48; C: 724; D: 114; E: 509; F: 1326; G: 768; H: 2018]

488 Festinant gait, monotonous speech, excessive salivation, restlessness and tolerance of cold. Sensory and reflex changes are not present unless there is another disease process (e.g. diffuse cerebrovascular disease) and intellect and emotions may be unaffected. [A: 343; B: 34.149; C: 716; D: 104; E: 553; F: 1361; G: 752; H: 1997]

489 With drugs. Chlorpromazine, haloperidol and the other phenothiazines and butyrophenones all may

cause extrapyramidal side-effects, notably tardive dyskinesia and oculogyric crises. Metoclopramide, a widely used antiemetic, is chemically related to the phenothiazines and Parkinsonian features may appear when the drug is used in frequent dosage.
[A: 344; B: 34.147; C: 715; D: 104; E: 553; F: 1361; G: 753–4; H: 1997–8]

490 The decarboxylase inhibitor, which is either carbidopa or benserazide, prevents destruction of L-dopa outside the brain, enabling more L-dopa to enter the brain. This in turn makes it possible to use a smaller dose of L-dopa, reducing side-effects.

In patients who do not respond, bromocriptine or amantadine are alternatives.
[A: 344; B: 34.152; C: 717–18; D: 105; E: 554; F: 1362; G: 754–6; H: 1998]

491 Progressive dementia.
[A: 345; C: 720; D: 106; E: 555; F: 1365; G: 758; H: 1993–4]

492 Subacute combined degeneration of the cord due to vitamin B_{12} deficiency.
[A: 381; B: 34.76; C: 723; D: 110; E: 511; F: 1349; G: 767; H: 2017]

493 Antibodies to the muscle cell acetylcholine receptors are present, and the disease is therefore an autoimmune disorder. Other autoimmune disorders may coexist.
[A: 338; B: 34.31; C: 737; D: 119; E: 556–9; F: 1396; G: 925; H: 2066]

494 Thymectomy, especially if a thymoma is present; steroids; azathioprine; plasmapheresis with removal of circulating antibodies.
[A: 339; B: 34.32; C: 738; D: 119; E: 559; F: 1397; G: 928; H: 2067]

495 Young adults in their 20s and 30s are mainly affected. Before puberty and over the age of 60 the disease is virtually unknown.

Weakness of one or both lower limbs, or visual disturbance in the form of blindness in one eye or diplopia, together account for the presenting symptom in about two-thirds of all cases. Upper limb weakness and paraesthesia (often numbness and formication) each account for a further 10 per cent.
[A: 379; B: 34.141; C: 712; D: 102; E: 540; F: 1356; G: 846; H: 1974]

496 Visual evoked potentials, tested by electroencephalography.

These are common symptoms in multiple sclerosis but physical signs of organic disease are usually present, namely pallor of the optic discs, particularly the temporal halves, absent abdominal reflexes and extensor plantar reflexes.
[A: 380; B: 34.140; C: 713; D: 103; E: 541; F: 1358; G: 846–7; H: 1975]

497 Latitude. The disease is commoner in higher latitudes. Studies of migrating populations suggest that one's risk of developing the disease is determined or acquired before the age of 15. A change of latitude therafter does not alter the incidence.
[A: 380; B: 34.143; C: 714; D: 103; E: 541; F: 1359; G: 847–8; H: 1976]

498 Bilateral retrobulbar neuritis occurs either simultaneously or consecutively, followed by a transverse myelitis. Blindness, spastic paraplegia, sphincter disturbance and sensory changes result.

Many cases recover completely. Others show rapid deterioration. Corticosteroids have a more important role than in multiple sclerosis.
[A: 380; B: 34.144; C: 715; F: 1360; G: 849; H: 1975]

499 Two types; first, symptoms of root compression i.e. pain in the motor, sensory or visceral distribution, or paraesthesiae in the dermatome of the root involved; secondly, spinal cord compression with the anterior tracts predominantly affected, i.e. spastic paraparesis and sensory loss at the level of the compression. This form of spinal cord compression develops slowly, a feature shared by subacute combined degeneration of the cord and the spinal form of late onset multiple sclerosis.
[A: 348; C: 730; D: 117; E: 497; F: 1322; G: 894–5; H: 2016]

500 In the leg: loss of the ankle jerk, weakness of eversion and plantar flexion, sensory loss over the outer border and sole of the foot.

In the lumbosacral spine; loss of normal lordosis, spasm of the erector spinae muscles, scoliosis and tenderness over the level of the affected disc.

Lasègue's sign is pain in the hamstrings on flexion of the hip with the leg straight. This movement stretches the sciatic nerve and aggravates any root or nerve compression. The test is described according to the angle the patient's leg makes with the bed in active and passive straight leg raising. Normal should be 90° or more.

[A: 350; B: 25.56–8; C: 732; E: 502; F: 1322; G: 894–5; H: 42]

501 The disc between L4 and L5. Because there are only seven cervical vertebrae the answer to this question for the C4 root is the disc between C3 and C4. The C4/C5 disc compresses C5, the C5/C6 disc compresses C6, the C6/C7 disc compresses C7, the C7/T1 disc compresses C8, the T1/T2 disc compresses T1, and so forth.
[A: 350; B: 25.57; C: 732; F: 1322; G: 891; H: 42]

502 The lower roots of the brachial plexus, namely C8 and T1. Weakness and wasting of the muscles of the hand and hyper- or analgesia can occur in the corresponding dermatomes.
The same syndrome can result from a fibrous band which will not be visible radiologically.
[A: 352; C: 733; E: 497; F: 1313; G: 902]

503 Radial nerve damage, depending on its site, may cause paralysis of triceps (elbow extension) brachioradialis, supinator (supination) and the extensors of the wrist and fingers. Sensory loss is usually confined to the dorsum of the hand between thumb and index finger.
Ulnar nerve damage causes weakness of the ulnar half of flexor digitorum profundus, the hypothenar muscles (little finger abduction), the interossei (abduction, adduction of the fingers) and adductor pollicis (adduction of the thumb). Sensory loss is usually over the little finger and the ulnar border of the ring finger and of the palm.
[A: 354; B: 34.35; C: 733; D: 23; F: 1314–15; G: 901–2; H: 2037]

504 The patient rests the hand palm upwards on a flat surface and tries to point the thumb at the ceiling against resistance.
[A: 353; C: 733; D: 22; E: 501; F: 1315; G: 901; H: 2037]

505 Numbness and pain over the lateral aspect of the thigh, brought on typically by exercise. Rest brings relief over a few minutes so that the history may resemble that of intermittent claudication. Weight gain may precipitate the condition.
[A: 355; C: 733; D: 23; E: 502; F: 1317; G: 902; H: 2038]

506 Pains in the back and limbs, headache, ascending or mainly proximal paralysis, loss of tendon reflexes and variable sensory loss following a febrile illness, usually a viral infection. The condition often goes by the name of Guillain–Barré syndrome. The sphincters are rarely affected. The cerebrospinal fluid shows a

great excess of protein with a normal or minimally raised cell count.
[A: 356; B: 34.39; C: 733–4; D: 109–10; E: 504–5; F: 1312–21; G: 903–10; H: 2029]

507 Non-metastatic effects of malignant disease can account for a large number of neurological features, viz.: peripheral neuropathy, proximal myopathy, a motor neurone disease picture, cerebellar degeneration, and dementia due to leucoencephalopathy. The neurological disturbance may occur before the malignancy is clinically detected and may persist despite satisfactory treatment of the underlying condition. Carcinoma of the bronchus is most commonly implicated.
[A: 383; B: 34.122; C: 741; D: 24; E: 504; F: 1320, 1368; G: 867–9; H: 2029–36]

508 Isoniazid therapy in slow-acetylators causes a peripheral neuropathy which responds to pyridoxine. Some cases of oral contraceptive-associated depression respond to pyridoxine as do some cases of premenstrual tension, but pyridoxine deficiency in these two situations has not been definitely demonstrated.
[A: 382; C: 725–6; D: 109; F: 1371; G: 773; H: 426]

509 Subacute combined degeneration of the cord, peripheral neuropathy, optic atrophy, dementia and megaloblastic anaemia.
[A: 383; C: 725–6; D: 109; E: 510; F: 1327; G: 776; H: 1988–9]

510 None, unless surgical attempts at treatment have been made, i.e. injection of the gasserian ganglion. Trigeminal neuralgia can accompany multiple sclerosis but the presence of abnormal neurological signs suggests the presence of a tumour or other underlying pathology and further investigation is indicated.
[A: 329; B: 34.61; C: 671; D: 91; E: 523; F: 1307; G: 727; H: 2023]

Kidney Function & Disorders; Water, Electrolyte & Acid–Base Balance

511 Approximately three and a half vertebrae in length, or roughly 13 cm long.
Overlying of the psoas shadow indicates loss of renal mass.
[B: 22.15; C: 429; D: 181; E: 219; G: 1341]

512 The mesangial cells (also called axial cells) are supporting cells, lying in a matrix between adjacent capillary loops. They are of endothelial origin and the matrix in which they lie resembles the basement membrane.
[A: 448; B: 22.19; C: 421; E: 220; F: 991; G: 1317; H: 216]

513 The juxtaglomular apparatus (JGA) is a collection of granular cells, situated in the wall of the afferent arteriole at the point where it lies next to the distal convoluted tubule.
It produces renin.
[A: 453: B: 22.8; C: 424; E: 220; F: 992; G: 1321; H: 1715]

514 Creatinine clearance is 20 ml per minute. This is derived from the formula UV/P, where U = urine concentration of creatinine in μmol/l, V = volume of urine per minute and P = plasma concentration of creatinine in μmol/l.
Inulin is neither reabsorbed nor secreted by the tubular cells. This is ideal. Creatinine may be reabsorbed in heart failure, but secreted in some normal people. For convenience, however, these shortcomings are usually ignored.
[A: 458; B: 22.2; C: 428; E: 226; F: 996; G: 1339]

515 Tubular maximum rate of reabsorption, abbreviated to *Tm*.
Glucose does not normally appear in the urine because the enzyme systems inside the renal tubular cells (especially in the proximal tubule), in conjunction with the huge surface area of the brush border, succeed in reabsorbing all the glucose present in the glomerular filtrate. The *Tm* indicates the maximum capacity of this process.
Similar considerations apply to amino acids.
[A: 517; C: 22.64; F: 993]

516 The Fick principle applied to the kidney to calculate renal plasma flow (not blood flow since the red cell mass is not involved), gives the amount of PAH extracted from the blood divided by the arteriovenous difference in PAH concentration. For practical purposes (hence the 'estimated' in the name), this is equal to UV/P. In the normal it is about 600 ml/min.
Filtration fraction is the fraction of total renal plasma flow which is being filtered by the glomeruli. For example, if inulin clearance is 120 ml/min and ERPF is 600 ml/min, the filtration fraction is 0.2.
[F: 996; G: 1340]

517 In the collecting tubules as they run through the hyperosmotic medulla.

The presence of antidiuretic hormone (ADH), which renders the walls of the collecting ducts permeable to water, controls the process.
[A: 459; B: 22.4; C: 421–2; F: 993; G: 1321; H: 1686]

518 Concentrating ability depends on the medulla being hypertonic, since this is what pulls water out of the collecting tubules. It has been demonstrated that a redistribution of renal blood flow can occur in renal impairment, especially acute renal failure, with increased flow going to the medulla. This 'washes out' the hypertonicity and destroys the concentrating ability.

Urine in renal failure has a specific gravity of 1010, which is equivalent to 285 mosmol per litre, the osmolality of plasma.
[A: 450; B: 22.3; C: 422; E: 222; F: 993; G: 1318–20; H: 1289]

519 Virtually all the potassium in the glomerular filtrate is reabsorbed before the filtrate reaches the distal convoluted tubule. Potassium is secreted in the distal convoluted tubule in exchange for sodium ions. The activity of this exchange is influenced by aldosterone and corticosteroids.
[A: 451–3; B: 22.5; C: 422; E: 221; F: 993; G: 1321–3; H: 1288–93]

520 ADH increases their permeability to water, allowing water to pass out of the urine thus making it concentrated. In addition, ADH increases permeability to urea, allowing more urea to diffuse into the hypertonic medulla. This increases the hypertonicity and generates more concentrating power.
[A: 450; B: 22.3; F: 993; H: 1289]

521 Bence Jones proteins are light chains of gammaglobulins, produced in excess in myelomatosis and appearing in the urine in about 50 per cent of cases.

On heating urine they precipitate between 45 and 55°C and redissolve at 95°C. Electrophoresis of urine protein shows a peak between beta- and gammaglobulins or close to the gamma band.
[A: 454; B: 22.6; C: 426; D: 180; F: 1000; G: 1331; H: 215]

522 Postural proteinuria is the name for proteinuria that occurs when a person is upright but disappears when he lies down. In most cases, it appears to be due to

lordosis in the erect position and there is no renal lesion. Slight proteinuria can occur in a fever, and also after heat stroke or heavy exercise.
[A: 455; B: 22.14; C: 427; D: 180; F: 1001; G: 1331–2; H: 1319]

523 There is little or no albumin. Alpha$_2$-globulin, beta$_2$-microglobulin and gammaglobulin predominate. This kind of proteinuria occurs, for example, in the Fanconi syndrome.
[B: 22.6–7; C: 426–7; D: 180; G: 1337; H: 215]

524 During upper gastrointestinal haemorrhage; dehydration especially if there is coincident catabolism as in infections; treatment with corticosteroids (sometimes).
[A: 457; B: 22.2; C: 428; E: 225–6; F: 997; G: 1340; H: 1306]

525 Reduces concentrating ability since less urea is formed and hence the hypertonicity achieved by the medulla is less.

526 A dose of vasopressin (Pitressin) is given by either intramuscular or subcutaneous injection. Urine is collected hourly for 4 hours and tested for a rise in osmolality.

When dilute polyuria is long-standing, normal kidneys may take a few days to regain full sensitivity to ADH and the test may need to be extended over a few days to check for this. The vasopressin may precipitate angina or infarction in patients with coronary artery disease.
[B: 22.67; F: 999; G: 1341; H: 1690]

527 A normal person should be able to acidify his urine to below a pH of 5.3, the lowest the kidneys can achieve being between 4 and 5.

The ammonium chloride acidification test consists of administering 0.1 g/kg body weight of ammonium chloride orally in capsules and measuring urine pH over the following 6 hours. Measurements of blood pH are made just before and 3 hours after giving ammonium chloride. Urinary pH should fall below 5.3.
[A: 460; B: 22.5; C: 426; F: 1000; G: 1357; H: 1346]

528 Renography consists of intravenous injection of a radioactive isotope (usually PAH labelled with ^{131}I). Counters are positioned over each kidney, bladder, and the heart (for a background level). A normal renal blood flow is indicated by a rapid increase in activity after injection. Uptake and secretion of the labelled PAH by the tubules is signalled by a further but

slower rise in activity, after which the absence of lower urinary tract obstruction is inferred from a steady decline in activity over each kidney and the appearance of activity in the bladder.

The test takes about 20 minutes and can be done at the bedside.

[B: 22.69; C: 430; G: 1345; H: 1339]

529 After noting the naked-eye appearance, spin 10 ml at 1000 r/min for 5 minutes. Observe the naked-eye appearance of the sediment then decant the supernatant and resuspend the sediment in the residual drop of urine. Put a drop of this on a microscope slide and cover with a cover-slip.

[A: 456; B: 22.14–15; D: 182; E: 225; G: 1338]

530 Hyaline casts, composed of Tamm–Horsfall protein (coming from the tubules) occur in normal urine. They may be cylindrical and are more or less homogeneous.

Renal failure casts are formed in the wider tubules of the collecting system when there is little urine flow. They are consequently broader.

Red cell casts indicate glomerular disease. White cell casts occur when glomeruli and tubules are invaded by polymorphs, as in glomerulonephritis or SLE. Granular casts, considered to be degenerated cellular casts, are a reliable sign of abnormality.

Waxy or fatty casts also occur but their origin is uncertain.

[A: 456; B: 22.15; C: 428; D: 182–3; E: 225; F: 1000; G: 1338–9; H: 217]

531 Tell the patient; dehydration for 6–8 hours before the test, or overnight; bowel preparation with laxatives to expel as much gas as possible.

Any history of allergic reaction to contrast media should be elicited and alternative investigations (renography, ultrasound) pursued if there is a prospect of anaphylaxis. Patients with multiple myeloma and diabetes are at risk of acute renal failure. This risk can be largely avoided by omitting the dehydration and maintaining a good urine output before the test.

Uraemia and renal failure are not contraindications to an IVP, but larger doses of contrast medium will be necessary.

[A: 460; B: 22.15; D: 181; F: 1001; G: 1342]

532 In urinary tract obstruction, all calyces are equally involved and the cortical thinning that occurs later in the condition is diffuse. In chronic pyelonephritis, on the other hand, calyceal involvement and associated cortical scarring is patchy.

[A: 489; E: 226; G: 1342]

533 Polycystic kidneys.

The normal size is $3\frac{1}{2}$ vertebrae in length. A localized abnormality indicates a space-occupying lesion which could be a cyst, abscess or solid tumour.
[B: 22.74; C: 429; D: 192; E: 226; F: 1093; H: 1344]

534 Retrograde pyelograms are resorted to when an IVP or other investigations have failed to provide clear or sufficient information. The main situations are: suspected obstruction of ureters or renal pelvis; renal or ureteric stones; renal tumours; investigation of a non-functioning kidney; investigation of anuria.

The hazards of the procedure are those of cystoscopy and ureteric catheterization.
[B: 22.16; C: 429; D: 184; E: 226; F: 1001; G: 1343]

535 Demonstration of abnormal or multiple renal arteries which may be obstructing urine drainage; demonstration of renal artery stenosis—usually fibromuscular hyperplasia in the young, atheromatous in the elderly; demonstration of renal artery occlusion, which may result from emboli; diagnosis of a silent area on IVP. Tumours nearly always show an abnormal vessel pattern, while cysts and abscesses are avascular.

Ultrasound and CAT scanning have been shown to be as good as renal arteriography in this last situation.
[B: 22.15–16; C: 429; E: 227; F: 1002; G: 1343; H: 1339]

536 In anuric acute renal failure not due to obstruction—to distinguish between acute tubular necrosis and cortical necrosis of infarction; in the nephrotic syndrome, to determine the cause; in asymptomatic proteinuria, to determine the cause.
[A: 455; B: 22.17; C: 430; E: 227; F: 1002; G: 1346]

537 About 8–10 days. Patients at greatest risk of developing nephritis are those who have microscopic haematuria at the height of the streptococcal infection, and those who develop high antistreptococcal antibody titres.
[A: 465; B: 22.18–24; C: 430–4; D: 189; E: 235; F: 1025; G: 1394; H: 1312]

538 Immune complex disease. The antigen is thought to be a streptococcal protein and the antigen–antibody complex binds complement on the epithelial side of the glomerular basement membrane. The resulting aggregates of immune complexes are seen as humps on electron microscopy. By light microscopy, fluorescent anti-IgG staining shows a granular appearance.
[A: 468; B: 22.18; C: 431; E: 235–6; F: 1022–4; G: 1325–7; H: 1312]

539 In malignant hypertension, complement levels are not reduced as they are in acute glomerulonephritis. Pyelonephritis is usually marked by fever and dysuria. Henoch–Schönlein purpura is distinguished by the purpura, arthritis and abdominal pain. Focal nephritis is usually distinguished by the presence of red cells alone in the urine and by a short course. Hypertension is the rule in acute glomerulonephritis but early or mild cases of nephrotic syndrome are usually normotensive.
[C: 433; G: 1396; H: 1312]

540 Bed rest—traditional but of uncertain value. Fluid intake restricted to urine output + insensible losses. A 2000 calorie, low protein diet is advisable. Penicillin should be given to eliminate any residual streptococci.
If fluid overload is present, peritoneal dialysis with 4.5 per cent dextrose in the PD fluid may be necessary. A low sodium diet should then also be given.
[B: 22.32; C: 433; E: 237–41; F: 1025–6; G: 1396; H: 1313]

541 Development of hypertension and renal failure after apparent recovery from acute glomerulonephritis. The latent period may be long (up to 20 years). There may have been some persistence of proteinuria after the acute illness.
[C: 437; E: 238; F: 1027–9; H: 1319]

542 Membranous and proliferative types may respond. Membranoproliferative or mesangiocapillary types usually do not.
[A: 475; B: 22.31; C: 437; E: 238; F: 1027–9; G: 1399; H: 1319]

543 Membranoproliferative, 'minimal change' and membranous glomerulonephritis, amyloidosis, diabetes, systemic lupus erythematosus, renal vein thrombosis, renal artery stenosis, focal glomerulonephritis, congestive cardiac failure, penicillamine and other drugs.
In Nigeria, quartan malaria is the commonest cause. Syphilis can cause it also.
[A: 470; B: 22.29; C: 434–6; D: 181; E: 239; F: 1031; G: 1387; H: 1315]

544 Increased incidence of atheroma, coronary artery disease, myocardial infarction and cerebrovascular disease.
Renal artery stenosis may occur due to aortic atheroma occluding the opening of the renal artery.
[A: 470; B: 22.30; C: 435; D: 181; E: 240; F: 1033; G: 1388; H: 1315]

545 Aldosterone levels are raised as a result of which the urine contains very little sodium. Thyroxine-binding globulin levels are lowered, so that thyroxine appears to be low also. In some cases it may really be low due to excessive urinary loss. Glycosuria is common, as is a diabetic glucose tolerance curve in uraemia (although diabetes is, of course, one cause of the nephrotic syndrome).

Glycosuria can result from the damage caused to the proximal tubules by chronic proteinuria, and it may be accompanied by aminoaciduria.
[A: 470; B: 22.29; C: 435; E: 239–40; F: 1033; G: 1388; H: 1315]

546 The 'minimal change' lesion responds well to steroids. Membranous glomerulonephritis has a 25 per cent chance of spontaneous remission with symptomatic treatment alone, steroids not so far conferring any advantage. Immunosuppressives are slightly better in that approximately one in three will remit. Proliferative glomerulonephritis treated with both steroids and immunosuppressives will respond in approximately half the cases.

There are two other histopathological types which respond badly to treatment; membranoproliferative (mesangiocapillary) and focal sclerosing glomerulonephritis. This latter may initially masquerade as 'minimal change', but then fails to improve.
[A: 474; B: 22.29; C: 435; D: 188–90; E: 241; F: 1025–9; G: 1392; H: 1316]

547 Malignant tumours, tumour antigens taking part in the immune complex deposition on the glomerular basement membrane. Hepatitis B surface antigen (Australia antigen) has also been isolated from membranous deposits. In some patients with SLE, DNA-anti DNA complexes are implicated in a membranous lesion.
[B: 22.26–8; D: 188–90; E: 237; F: 1026; G: 1393; H: 1317]

548 Reduced levels of both C3 and C4 indicate complement activation by the normal pathway. A low C3 but normal C4 indicates alternate pathway activation. Immune complexes, as in SLE, activate complement by the normal pathway whereas endotoxin is a cause of alternate pathway activation.
[C: 28; E: 126–7; F: 381–2; G: 135; H: 323]

549 Multiple myeloma, although only 3 per cent of cases are complicated by renal amyloidosis; chronic suppurative or chronic inflammatory disease, such as

rheumatoid disease; malignancies including Hodgkin's disease; familiar Mediterranean fever.
[A: 475; B: 22.33; C: 436; E: 246; F: 1085; G: 1405; H: 1324]

550 Loin pain on one or both sides with deterioration in renal function. Proteinuria increases as renal function decreases. Sometimes rapidly progressive renal failure occurs with haematuria as evidence of infarction.
[A: 475; B: 22.71; C: 436; E: 249; F: 1036; G: 1408; H: 1315]

551 First, the relief of the oedema. This is with diuretics, low sodium diet and occasionally albumin infusions or even dialysis. Diuretic therapy must be guarded by attention to electrolyte balance.

Secondly, the suppression of the underlying disease process. This means corticosteroids and/or immunosuppressive drugs such as azathioprine, cyclophosphamide or chlorambucil. Steroids are contraindicated in amyloidosis and are not helpful in nephrotic syndrome secondary to diabetes.
[A: 474; B: 22.30; C: 436; D: 182; E: 240–1; F: 1034–6; G: 1389; H: 1315]

552 The few cases of 'minimal change' that do not improve progress to membranous or focal sclerosing glomerulonephritis, meaning death or dialysis within a few years.

Membranous glomerulonephritis progresses to renal failure but may take 20 years to do so.

Prognosis in proliferative glomerulonephritis ranges from 18 months where more than 80 per cent of the glomeruli are involved to a few years in more chronic disease.
[A: 474; B: 22.32; C: 436; D: 182; E: 241; F: 1034–6; H: 1316–17]

553 Urinary tract obstruction by stone, prostatic enlargement, neoplasm or periureteric fibrosis (retroperitoneal fibrosis); urinary stasis in pregnancy and the puerperium; diabetes mellitus; hypokalaemia; hypercalcaemia; analgesic nephropathy.
[A: 484; B: 22.35; C: 441; D: 190; E: 242–3; F: 1040; G: 1409–10; H: 1328]

554 100 000 bacteria per ml and 1000 yeasts per ml.

Another guide to the significance of a positive culture is the presence of white cells in the urine. It is unusual to have significant infection without white cells.
[A: 483; B: 22.34–5; C: 442; D: 190; E: 243; F: 1043; G: 1411; H: 1327]

555 Mild proteinuria is usual. Urine cultures may be positive, especially when protoplast forms and anaerobes are looked for. White cells may be increased in the urine. The IVP may show typical changes of patchy calyceal distortion with overlying cortical thinning and scarring.
[A: 488; B: 22.37; C: 443; D: 191; E: 244; F: 1042; G: 1411; H: 1332]

556 The first biochemical changes are in the urine. The urine/plasma ratio of urea and creatinine falls. A urine sodium of less than 20 mmol/l indicates major sodium retention and commonly accompanies minor degrees of renal impairment.

It may take 24–48 hours for blood biochemistry to begin to indicate abnormality.

Oliguria is usual but not invariable.
[A: 461–2; C: 447; D: 184; E: 229; F: 1018; G: 1373–4; H: 1294]

557 There may be urinary tract obstruction (which may be causing the renal failure). Complete anuria must lead to a search for causes of obstruction, starting with cystoscopy and retrograde pyelography.
[B: 22.44; C: 449; D: 183; E: 230; F: 1018; G: 1374; H: 1295]

558 Fluid overload: avoid giving the patient more than his fluid losses i.e. urine, gastrointestinal losses, insensible loss; daily weighing is essential.

Hyperkalaemia: dialysis to remove potassium, but intravenous dextrose and insulin in an emergency, or ion-exchange resins as a temporary measure.

Maintain accurate sodium balance; feed the patient well with at least a 2000 calorie 60 g protein diet; dialyse early, before severe metabolic derangement has occurred. Infection remains a major cause of mortality in acute renal failure—good aseptic technique and correct antibiotic therapy are mandatory.
[A: 463; B: 22.52; C: 447–8; D: 185; E: 231–2; F: 1018; G: 1372; H: 1296]

559 Pain. pneumonia due to elevation of the diaphragms and collapse of the basal segments. Peritonitis, which may be treated successfully by adding the appropriate antibiotic to the PD fluid. Loss of the cannula into the peritoneal cavity. Perforation of the bowel during cannula insertion. There is also loss of protein in the PD fluid, resulting in hypoalbuminaemia in chronic dialysis.
[B: 22.49; C: 449; F: 1008; G: 1377–8; H: 1306]

560 The hypotheses says that with the majcrity of nephrons damaged by disease, the few remaining healthy ('intact') nephrons have to cope with the uraemic filtrate on their own. They are thus subjected to an osmotic diuresis and it is this that impairs their function.

A patient's sodium loss has to be measured (24 hour urine sodium for a few days on a 20 mmol sodium diet) and the observed loss added to his diet so that the patient balances between deficit (causing hypovolaemia) and excess (causing overload).
[A: 476; B: 22.10; C: 437; E: 233; F: 1003; G: 1348–9; H: 1287–8]

561 Lack of erythropoietin due to renal damage; marrow-depressant effect of uraemia; bleeding tendency in uraemia, as a result of impaired platelet function and circulating inhibitors to clotting factors; reduced red cell survival time.
[A: 477; B: 22.9; C: 437; D: 186; E: 233; F: 1003; G: 1363–4; H: 1304]

562 Phosphate retention occurs in chronic renal failure and this initially causes serum calcium levels to fall. Osteomalacia may develop, but hypocalcaemia stimulates the parathyroid glands and increased parathormone may bring calcium back to normal or even above normal levels, thus causing the solubility product of calcium and phosphate to be exceeded. Common sites for calcification are the conjunctivae and periarticular soft tissues.

Oral aluminium hydroxide binds phosphate in the gut and decreases phosphate levels in the blood.
[A: 478–9; B: 22.9; C: 438; E: 233; F: 1005; G: 1359; H: 1303]

563 Twitching; flapping tremor; peripheral neuropathy with decreased nerve conduction times.
[A: 478; B: 22.11–12; C: 437–9; E: 233; F: 1005; G: 1364–5; H: 1305]

564 Yes. The Giovannetti diet was specially designed to provide the daily requirement of essential amino acids, thereby minimizing endogenous protein turnover, but at the same time restricting total protein intake to about 20 g. Considerable biochemical and symptomatic improvement results from this.
[A: 480; B: 22.53; C: 439; D: 187; E: 235; F: 1006; G: 1360–1; H: 1305–6]

565 A shunt is a loop of silicone-rubber tubing with one side inserted into an artery and the other into a vein. It is put in via cutdowns under local anaesthesia and is

the means of access for urgent haemodialysis and for the first few weeks or months. For continued dialysis, a fistula is used. This is a subcutaneous anastomosis between artery and vein, near the elbow or wrist, which has the effect of arterializing the adjacent veins, making them readily accessible for needle insertion when putting the patient on the dialysis machine. [A: 481; B: 22.53–4; C: 440; D: 188; E: 235; F: 1008–10; G: 1378; H: 1306]

566 Systemic lupus erythematosus; polyarteritis nodosa; rheumatoid disease; scleroderma; thrombotic thrombocytopenic purpura.
[B: 22.32; E: 236–40; F: 1029–30; G: 1400; H: 1320]

567 Collagen vascular disease, especially SLE or polyarteritis nodosa. The renal pathologies of these two conditions include immune complex glomerulonephritis, which can be both proliferative and membranous, the nephrotic syndrome (hypercholesterolaemia may be absent) or asymptomatic proteinuria.
[B: 22.32; C: 629; E: 246; F: 1029; G: 1400]

568 There may be a focal glomerulonephritis; amyloidosis may be present; chronic pyelonephritis and papillary necrosis occur as a result of reduced resistance to infection and analgesic consumption; specific forms of therapy e.g. gold, penicillamine, can cause nephritis.
[C: 632; E: 247; F: 1090; G: 1401; H: 1324]

569 Transfusion, dialysis, corticosteroids and very carefully controlled heparin.
[C: 446; D: 192; E: 246; F: 1030; G: 1401; H: 1341]

570 Diffuse glomerulosclerosis with, in some cases, nodular glomerulonephritis which is the Kimmelstiel–Wilson lesion; pyelonephritis; necrotizing papillitis; atherosclerosis of the renal vessels (in company with the vascular damage elsewhere in the body).
[A: 494; B: 23.79; C: 523; D: 159; E: 245; F: 1086–7; G: 1403; H: 1325]

571 (a) Oliguria may occur in renal failure which, in diabetes, is usually due to development of the nephrotic syndrome. An important complication of the nephrotic syndrome is renal vein thrombosis and this results in a sudden deterioration of renal function.

(b) Anuria, which as a rule indicates complete urinary tract obstruction, may occur when one kidney is already non-functioning and a necrotic papilla sloughs off and blocks the drainage of the other kidney.
[H: 1328]

572 Either chlorothiazide or chlorpropamide. The diuretic works by increasing sodium excretion which reduces glomerular filtration and the water load on the tubules. Chlorpropamide appears to have a vasopressin-like effect on the tubules.
[B: 22.67; C: 466; E: 165; F: 1067; G: 1435; H: 1346]

573 Appropriate sodium retention may be impaired with sodium 'leaking' into the urine; there may be inability to acidify the urine causing a reduction in the titratable acidity.
[B: 20.60–3; C: 450; F: 1049; G: 1448; H: 1353]

574 40–50 per cent increase in glomerular filtration rate (creatinine clearance); increased renal plasma flow; plasma urea reduced to 2.5–3.5 mmol/l; increased uric acid clearance; decreased renal threshold for glucose. The calyces, pelvis and ureter on each side undergo marked dilation due to the effect of progesterone.
[A: 486; B: 42.47; F: 1053; G: 1414–16; H: 1328]

575 These are all features of pre-eclampsia. Renal biopsy in pre-eclampsia has shown hypertrophy of the glomeruli and hyperplasia of the endothelial cells, with thickening of the basement membrane. This lesion accounts for the albuminuria, while hypertension and oedema are explained by greater sodium retention due to higher aldosterone and progesterone levels.
[F: 826; G: 1414–16; H: 1342]

576 There are three signs: the affected kidney is smaller than its partner; in the first 5 minutes after contrast injection, the pelvicalyceal system of the affected kidney fills more slowly (films will be needed every minute to catch this); subsequently the concentration of contrast in the affected kidney will be greater than on the normal side.
[A: 493; B: 22.69; F: 1045–6; H: 1339]

577 Renin converts angiotensinogen to angiotensin I, a decapeptide. Angiotensin-converting enzyme cleaves this molecule to an octapeptide, angiotensin II, which is one of the most potent vasoconstrictors known. In

addition, angiotensin II stimulates the adrenal cortex to produce more aldosterone.
[B: 22.8; C: 424; E; 222; F: 997; G: 1321; H: 1714]

578 In essential hypertension there is hyaline thickening of the arterioles with only a very slow reduction in renal function.

In malignant hypertension there is endothelial proliferation of the arterioles, fibrinoid necrosis of the arteriolar walls and damage and necrosis of the glomeruli with rapid progression of renal failure if the hypertension is not controlled.
[B: 22.71; H: 1339–40]

579 Cystine stones are radio-opaque, although less so than calcium oxalate.

Alkalinization of the urine and maintenance of 3 litres per 24 hours fluid input dissolves the stones.
[A: 490–1; B: 22.64; C: 451; E: 628; F: 1065; G: 2023; H: 1347]

580 Yes, very. These are the findings of the Fanconi syndrome with multiple defects of proximal tubular function. The osteomalacia is due to the phosphate loss in the urine.
[A: 490; B: 22.68; C: 423; E: 628; F: 1056; G: 2023; H: 1348]

581 The basic defect is failure to excrete hydrogen ions into the urine. This results in systemic acidosis but alkaline urine. There is an inability to produce a urine pH below 5.4, even after an administered load of ammonium chloride. The accompanying biochemical features are low serum bicarbonate, phosphate and potassium but high chloride.

Treatment is with a mixture of sodium and potassium citrate in increasing amounts until plasma pH and potassium are within the normal range.
[A: 490; B: 22.66–7; C: 423; F: 1058; G: 1441; H: 1346]

582 Alkalinization of the urine and high fluid intake—3 litres every 24 hours equally divided between day and night. The stones will dissolve. Allopurinol should be given if 24 hour uric acid excretion exceeds 45 mmol/l.
[A: 438; B: 22.57; C: 451; E: 249; F: 1072; G: 1443–5; H: 1351]

583 Loin pain; haematuria; ureteric colic due to stone formation; pyelonephritis.

Hypertension, usually mild, occurs in half the cases.
[B: 22.73–5; C: 453; D: 192; E: 247; F: 1092–3; G: 1453; H: 1343]

584 Recurrent pyelonephritis, due to urinary stasis in redundant urinary pathways; hypertension; renal calculus formation.

Surgery may be indicated to remove the seat of recurrent infection.
[B: 22.76; F: 1099–1100; G: 1457]

585 Acute glomerulonephritis, with proliferative changes as in post-streptococcal nephritis, except that the antibody deposition on the basement membrane is linear rather than granular.
[A: 469; B: 22.33; C: 431; D: 188; E: 241; F: 1025; G: 1324; H: 1322]

586 Because both hypernephroma and renal tuberculosis may present with otherwise symptomless haematuria.

Other signs are calyceal distortion by a silent area on the IVP or calcification in the case of tumour. TB causes cavitation along the edges of the calcyces in the early stages and distortion of calyceal pattern with calcified scarring later.
[A: 456; B: 22.42–3. 22.81; C: 445; E: 245; F: 1095–6; G: 1458–9; H: 1355]

587 One of the drugs used for migraine prophylaxis, methysergide, can cause retroperitoneal fibrosis. In this condition the ureters become encased in fibrous tissue from which it is possible to free them by surgery if there is no response to steroid therapy. Back and loin pain, a raised ESR and hydronephrosis are the main features of the condition.
[A: 482; E: 248; F: 1055; G: 223; H: 1353]

588 Cessation of analgesic consumption, at least of analgesics that are excreted by the kidneys.
[A: 496; B: 22.50–1; C: 454; D: 186; E: 248; F: 1041–2; G: 1419; H: 1334]

589 250 mg every 8 hours.
[A: 496; B: 22.44; C: 454; D: 188; F: 1076; G: 1425; H: 1335]

590 Graft rejection; vascular complications in the form of graft artery or vein thrombosis; 'plumbing' problems in the insertion of graft ureter into recipient bladder, mainly due to ischaemia of the graft ureter; opportunistic infection in the immunosuppressed recipient.

One year kidney survival rates are 90 per cent for live donor transplants and 60 per cent for cadaveric grafts.
[A: 481; B: 22.54; C: 440; F: 1011–15; G: 1382–6; H: 368]

591 The main symptoms of water intoxication are nausea, headache and drowsiness. These may be followed by vomiting, seizures and coma. Peripheral oedema is not found when water excess occurs alone, i.e. without coexisting sodium retention.
[A: 503; B: 49.8; C: 134–5; D: 193; E: 256; F: 390; G: 2110; H: 1691]

592 Causes of severe deficiency of water include cranial and nephrogenic diabetes insipidus, non-ketotic hyperosmolar diabetic coma, and hyperparathyroidism.
[A: 502; B: 23.14; C: 465; D: 148–9; E: 254–5; F: 396; G: 2110; H: 1686]

593 Findings include reduced plasma osmolality with a urine osmolality greater than that of the plasma. There is hyponatraemia maintained by continued urinary sodium excretion. All of these features occur in the absence of any dehydration.
[A: 503; B: 49.8; D: 193; F: 390; G: 1953; H: 1691]

594 Acute and chronic renal failure, the injudicious use of potassium supplements or potassium sparing diuretics (e.g. spironolactone), Addison's disease and systemic acidosis may all cause hyperkalaemia.
[A: 507; B: 49.29; C: 133; D: 195; F: 400; G: 1959; H: 443]

595 First, potassium supplements or potassium containing diuretics must be stopped. Intravenous calcium gluconate may prevent cardiac arrest in severe hyperkalaemia, and a dextrose and insulin infusion should be started. This drives potassium back into the cells. Bicarbonate may have a similar effect and should be used, but only in the absence of sodium excess. An ion-exchange resin should be given and severe cases or those with renal failure may require dialysis.
[A: 506; B: 49.30; C: 133; D: 195; E: 258; F: 401; G: 1959; H: 1010]

596 Diarrhoeal states, Zollinger–Ellison syndrome and ureterosigmoidostomy may cause hypokalaemia and acidosis.
[A: 505; B: 49.23; C: 131; D: 194; E: 257; F: 398–9; G: 1957; H: 441]

597 Four major conditions: renal failure, diabetic ketoacidosis, lactic acidosis and ingestion of drugs

such as salicylates, paraldehyde or poisons such as methanol or ethylene glycol.
[A: 511; C: 141; D: 194; E: 262; F: 403; G: 1961–5; H: 446]

598 Biguanide ingestion, ethanol and methanol ingestion and severe liver disease may all give rise to lactic acidosis despite the fact that circulation and tissue perfusion may be normal.
[B: 49.40; C: 141; D: 164; E: 262; F: 403; G: 1962; H: 446]

599 Excessive ingestion of alkali as in the milk–alkali syndrome may cause metabolic alkalosis. Potassium deficiency may produce a similar effect due to renal tubular hydrogen ion loss.

In metabolic alkalosis, plasma bicarbonate and pH are elevated and respiratory compensation for alkalosis produces a rise in $P\text{CO}_2$.
[A: 512; B: 49.47; C: 142; E: 263; F: 403; G: 1965–6; H: 448]

600 The commonest cause of overventilation is hysteria, but it may also be due to excessive artificial ventilation, meningitis, encephalitis, salicylate intoxication and hepatic failure.
[A: 511; B: 49.53; C: 144; D: 50; E: 263; F: 403; G: 1969; H: 449]

Endocrine & Metabolic Disorders

601 A pituitary tumour will frequently extend above the sella turcica to compress the optic chiasma which is situated above the fossa. This compression frequently causes bitemporal hemianopia and, if not treated, may progress to produce optic atrophy and blindness.
[A: 578; B: 23.7; C: 462; D: 147; E: 161; G: 2095; H: 1673]

602 A plain lateral skull X-ray should be done in all suspected pituitary tumour cases. The earliest evidence of tumour is erosion of the posterior clinoid process. With large tumours this may be completely destroyed.
[A: 578; B: 23.7; C: 462; F: 483; G: 2095; H: 1672]

603 Optic atrophy is always associated with significant visual impairment. Therefore the patient should be asked whether he can see clearly with the eye in question and if necessary visual assessment should be carried out.
[A: 578; C: 462; D: 147; G: 2095; H: 1673]

604 A significant number of acromegalics have impaired glucose tolerance and a smaller number have overt diabetes mellitus. About one-third of cases develop hypertension and a few appear to develop a specific cardiomyopathy. About 5 per cent of cases have hypercalcaemia. A myopathy with muscular weakness is common.
[A: 576; B: 23.7; C: 462; D: 147; E: 162; F: 482; G: 2105; H: 1681]

605 Drugs are an important cause of hyperprolactinaemia. These include dopamine antagonists such as phenothiazines and metoclopramide and cathecholamine depletants such as methyldopa and *Rauwolfia* alkaloids.
[A: 577; B: 23.9; C: 463; E: 163; F: 483; G: 2092; H: 1680]

606 A life-threatening coma may occur in cases on inadequate hormonal replacement therapy. This is due to a combination of hypoglycaemia, hypothyroidism and hypothermia.
[A: 578–80; B: 23.4–5; C: 464–5; D: 146; E: 163–4; F: 484; G: 2100; H: 1676]

607 First, the TRH test may be done. Intravenous administration of thyrotrophin-releasing hormone (TRH) stimulates output of thyrotrophin-stimulating hormone (TSH) and prolactin. Secondly, administration of luteinizing hormone-releasing hormone (LHRH) stimulates output of follicle-stimulating hormone (FSH) and luteinizing hormone (LH). Thirdly, the insulin tolerance test may be done. Intravenous administration of soluble insulin causes hypoglycaemia which in turn stimulates the anterior pituitary to secrete growth hormone and ACTH. Plasma cortisol will rise as a result of ACTH release, and is easier to measure than plasma ACTH.
[A: 579; B: 23.1–4; C: 460–1; D: 154–5; F: 480–1; G: 2091–4; H: 1676]

608 Cranial diabetes insipidus is due to deficiency of the posterior pituitary hormone, antidiuretic hormone (ADH) or vasopressin. Many cases are idiopathic. Head injury or cranial surgery may damage the pituitary stalk and cause transient cranial diabetes insipidus. Other causes include pituitary tumours, craniopharyngiomas and conditions such as meningitis or encephalitis.
[A: 532; B: 23.14; C: 465; D: 148–9; E: 165; F: 487; G: 2110; H: 1686]

609 The diagnosis is confirmed by carrying out the water deprivation test. Urine which continues to be hypotonic following fluid deprivation but which is concentrated following administration of exogenous vasopressin, indicates cranial diabetes insipidus.
[A: 532; B: 23.15; C: 466; D: 149; F: 488; G: 2110–11; H: 1688]

610 An increase in plasma oestrogen such as occurs in women on anovulant therapy or pregnant women produces an elevation of plasma thyroxine-binding globulin. This raises the total serum T_4 but the small 'free' fraction of serum T_4 remains normal. This free fraction of serum T_4 is the metabolically available form and hence in this situation the patient remains euthyroid.

The true situation may be elucidated by estimating the free thyroxine index or directly assaying the circulating free T_4, both of which will remain within normal limits in cases where elevated total T_4 is due to increased thyroxine-binding globulin levels.
[A: 550–1; B: 23.17–19; C: 468–9; D: 155–6; F: 490–1; G: 2117–19; H: 1703]

611 Agranulocytosis is an uncommon but dangerous side-effect of antithyroid drugs. This presents with a sore throat and patients must be warned to stop taking the drugs immediately should a sore throat develop, and to report for a white cell count.
[A: 552; B: 23.27–8; C: 470; D: 142; E: 173; F: 496; G: 2123–4; H: 1706]

612 Bowel motions may be increased in frequency in thyrotoxicosis—occurring several times per day. The stools are formed, so that true diarrhoea is not in fact a feature of thyrotoxicosis.
[A: 546; B: 23.23–4; C: 467; D: 141; E: 172; F: 494; G: 2122; H: 1704]

613 In thyrotoxicosis the hands are usually both warm and sweaty, and there is frequently a fine tremor. Examination of the radial pulse may reveal sinus tachycardia, atrial fibrillation or ectopic beats. The pulse is usually of large volume and in these circumstances it is associated with capillary pulsation of the nail beds. Rare additional findings in the hand include thyroid acropachy which resembles clubbing, and onycholysis in which nails may be partly lifted from their beds.
[A: 549; B: 23.26; D: 141; E: 172; F: 494; G: 2122; H: 1704]

614 The most serious complication of exophthalmos is exposure keratitis which may lead to blindness. It is important to avoid medically induced hypothyroidism as this may aggravate exophthalmos.

Lateral tarsorrhaphy may prevent exposure keratitis in moderately severe cases. In more severe cases high dose steroid therapy may be necessary. If this fails surgical orbital decompression should be considered.

[A: 548; B: 23.24; C: 474; D: 142; E: 172; F: 495; G: 2126; H: 1704]

615 Features of thyroid crisis include a delirious state with delusions, tachycardia and cardiac failure, dehydration and hyperthermia. Mortality is high.

Management includes rehydration with intravenous dextrose, intravenous hydrocortisone because of possible adrenal exhaustion, and sedation with chlorpromazine.

Beta-blockers should be used to reduce sympathetic overactivity provided cardiac failure is not too severe. However, the most rapidly effective antithyroid drug is potassium iodide which should be given intravenously.

[A: 553; B: 23.27; C: 468; D: 143; F: 495–7; G: 2127; H: 1709]

616 The only complication of radioactive iodine therapy is hypothyroidism in the years following treatment. The incidence of hypothyroidism rises with each succeeding year and is about 50 per cent 20 years following therapy. Accordingly all patients treated with this substance should have annual thyroid function tests done and thyroxine supplements introduced if necessary.

[A: 552; B: 23.29; C: 472; D: 142; E: 173; F: 496; G: 2124; H: 1706–7]

617 Complications of subtotal thyroidectomy include the following: postoperative hypothyroidism which is more frequent in those with high titres of circulating antithyroid antibodies preoperatively; damage to a recurrent laryngeal nerve produces transient hoarseness; transient or permanent hypoparathyroidism with hypocalcaemia occasionally occurs.

In a few cases thyrotoxicosis will relapse postoperatively and is then best treated with radioactive iodine.

[A: 552; B: 23.28; C: 471; D: 142; E: 173; F: 496; G: 2125; H: 1707]

618 Transplacental passage of antithyroid drugs may occasionally cause neonatal hypothyroidism or goitre.

To avoid this, overtreatment of the mother must be avoided and if possible the drugs should be reduced in dosage or stopped during the last 3 weeks of pregnancy. The baby of a mother on antithyroid drugs should not be breast fed. Finally, an index of thyroid function that is not altered by the high circulating oestrogen levels of pregnancy should be used—for example the free thyroxine index.
[A: 552; B: 23.31; C: 473; F: 496; G: 2125; H: 1706]

619 Menorrhagia is a common feature of hypothyroidism. Deafness or hoarseness may cause ENT referral. Rheumatological features include generalized joint and limb pains. Psychiatric manifestations of hypothyroidism include mental slowing and psychosis (myxoedematous madness).
[A: 554; B: 23.31; C: 475; D: 143; E: 174; F: 500; G: 2132; H: 1701]

620 Although some controversy surrounds the optimum dose of thyroid hormone, many authorities would give $400\mu g$ of L-thyroxine intravenously or via nasogastric tube, following drawing of blood for biochemical confirmation of diagnosis. Hypothermia is treated by exposure to normal room temperature. Intravenous dextrose is normally given, plus oxygen to overcome respiratory acidosis. Cardiac arrhythmias may occur during resuscitation.
[A: 556; B: 23.36; C: 475; F: 502; G: 2134; H: 1702]

621 Primary hypothyroidism is usually confirmed by finding a low serum T_4 but estimation of serum TSH is probably the most useful single test. In primary hypothyroidism serum TSH is elevated due to loss of feedback inhibition by T_4 on the anterior pituitary TSH secreting cells.
[A: 555; B: 23.35; C: 476; D: 143; E: 175; F: 501–3; G: 2133; H: 1702]

622 Rapid increase in size, fixation to surrounding tissues, obstructive symptoms, vocal cord palsy causing hoarseness and lymphadenopathy all suggest malignancy. Benign lesions are usually soft, mobile and have a long history with no recent increase in size.
[A: 556; B: 23.47; C: 478; D: 145; E: 176; F: 499; G: 2142; H: 1709]

623 The most notable biochemical finding is an elevated plasma calcitonin level. This is a useful marker for the presence of this tumour. It may also be used to monitor for recurrence of the tumour following thyroidectomy,

and also to screen first degree relatives who are at increased risk of developing the tumour.
[A: 557; B: 23.48; C: 478; D: 145; F: 500; G: 2143]

624 Following bilateral adrenalectomy for pituitary dependent Cushing's disease, Nelson's syndrome may develop. In this condition a locally invasive pituitary tumour is associated with progressively rising ACTH levels and deepening pigmentation. Chiasmal compression may cause optic atrophy and blindness, and other cranial nerves such as the third may be damaged. Because of this complication, partial pituitary excision preferably by the trans-sphenoidal route may be the treatment of choice in pituitary dependent Cushing's disease.
[A: 558; B: 23.65; C: 485; E: 168; F: 483; G: 2098; H: 1682–3]

625 Plasma ACTH assay, although difficult to carry out, is extremely useful in this situation.

In pituitary dependent Cushing's disease plasma ACTH is usually somewhat elevated at midnight, although the 9 a.m. value may be in the higher part of the normal range.

Undetectably low plasma ACTH levels are found in adrenal adenoma or carcinoma.

Very high plasma ACTH values are found in the ectopic ACTH syndrome.
[A: 558; B: 23.66; C: 486; F: 517; G: 2155; H: 1722]

626 Obesity is a feature of all three conditions but only in Cushing's syndrome is the obesity confined to the truncal area. Thinning of the skin and pigmentation are conspicuous in Cushing's syndrome but not in the other two conditions. In Cushing's syndrome a characteristic proximal myopathy may be demonstrated by showing that the patient is unable to rise from a squatting position without assistance. This feature does not occur in cases of simple obesity or polycystic ovarian syndrome.
[A: 565; B: 28.7; C: 486]

627 The overnight dexamethasone suppression test is useful in this regard. A 9 a.m. plasma cortisol value of less than 170 nmol/l following 2 mg of dexamethasone taken orally at midnight excludes Cushing's syndrome. Also urinary cortisol levels are elevated in most cases of Cushing's syndrome and normal in conditions such as simple obesity.

On rare occasions excess steroid output in Cushing's syndrome may be intermittent, and if suspicion persists, these tests could be repeated after some weeks.

[A: 559; B: 23.66–7; C: 486; D: 154; F: 511–13; G: 2154–5; H: 1720]

628 Cushing's syndrome due to production of ACTH from an ectopic site is usually due to a bronchogenic neoplasm. It is more frequent in males, is of rapid onset and is associated with weight loss and marked skin pigmentation. Truncal obesity and moon face are characteristically absent.
[A: 558–9; B: 23.67; C: 485–6; E: 167; F: 517; G: 2155; H: 1722]

629 Hyperpigmentation is most obvious first in areas which are normally exposed to light—face, neck, backs of hands; secondly, areas subject to pressure and friction—palmar creases, elbows, knees, knuckles, the belt area and beneath brassière straps; thirdly, areas which are normally pigmented such as nipples and scrotum; fourthly, mucosae such as buccal mucosa, conjunctiva and vagina. Finally scars acquired after the onset of adrenal failure become pigmented whereas those acquired beforehand do not.
[A: 562; B: 23.61; C: 489; D: 152; E: 169; F: 514; G: 2148; H: 1730]

630 Findings suggestive of a tuberculous aetiology include a positive tuberculin test, adrenal calcification on X-ray, evidence of pulmonary tuberculosis on chest X-ray and the absence of serum antibodies to the adrenal cortex.
[A: 562; B: 23.60; C: 488; D: 152; E: 169; F: 514; G: 2147; H: 1729]

631 A low plasma sodium concentration with elevated plasma potassium and urea levels support this diagnosis. Reactive hypoglycaemia may also occur unless of course there is an associated diabetes mellitus.
[A: 563; B: 23.62; C: 490; D: 152; E: 169; F: 515; G: 2147–8; H: 1730]

632 In cases of acute adrenal crisis one litre of normal saline with 5 per cent dextrose should be given over one hour intravenously, followed by 2–4 litres of normal saline over the next 24 hours. Hydrocortisone 100 mg 6 hourly should be given intravenously over the first 24 hours and gradually tapered as the patient improves. Precipitating causes such as infection must be treated simultaneously.
[A: 562; B: 23.64; C: 494; D: 152; F: 513; G: 2149; H: 1730]

633 The main biochemical features of Conn's syndrome are due to the effect of excess aldosterone secretion which produces sodium retention and hypernatraemia. There is also severe hypokalaemia with secondary metabolic alkalosis (increased plasma pH and plasma bicarbonate). Plasma aldosterone is of course elevated with secondary depression of plasma renin. A considerable number of cases have glucose intolerance.

Surprisingly, despite sodium retention, oedema is unusual.

[A: 561; B: 23.68; C: 487; D: 151; E: 168; F: 520; G: 2157; H: 1724]

634 Diagnosis is confirmed by finding excess normetanephrine, metanephrine and vanillylmandelic acid (VMA) in the urine. These estimations may be interfered with by drugs such as methyldopa, hydralazine, phenothiazine, tetracycline, monoamine oxidase inhibitors and some vitamin preparations.

[B: 23.56; F: 523–4; G: 2204; H: 1739]

635 Attacks may be associated with paroxysmal hypertension. Sustained hypertension may occur between attacks. Postural hypotension may also occur. Tachyarrhythmias and fever may also occur during attacks.

[A: 567; B: 23.56; C: 496; D: 153; E: 170; F: 523; G: 2202–3; H: 1737]

636 Deep pressure over the tumour when examining the abdomen may precipitate a hypertensive attack and should therefore be avoided in suspected cases.

[F: 523]

637 Diabetes mellitus, multiple sclerosis and tabes dorsalis may all be associated with impotence.

Some cases of impotence are associated with hyperprolactinaemia and may respond to bromocriptine therapy.

[B: 35.34; C: 498; E: 178; F: 545; G: 2174; H: 230]

638 The comatose hypoglycaemic patient is usually well hydrated with a moist pink tongue, bounding pulse, normal or raised blood pressure, normal breathing, brisk tendon reflexes and extensor plantar reflexes. In contrast, the hyperglycaemic ketoacidotic patient usually shows marked dehydration with dry skin and a dry furred tongue, weak pulse, low blood pressure, hyperventilation (Kussmaul breathing), diminished

tendon jerks and a flexor plantar reflex. In addition the breath may smell of acetone.
[B: 23.91–2; C: 522; D: 161; F: 443; G: 1983–4; H: 1747]

639 Acromegaly is due to excess circulatory growth hormone and about 30 per cent of cases are diabetic. Excess adrenocorticoid hormone in Cushing's syndrome also produces a state of impaired glucose tolerance.

Some cases of hyperthyroidism show impaired glucose tolerance. Cases of phaeochromocytoma with excess circulating adrenaline are frequently diabetic.

Pregnancy is associated with increased levels of hormonal insulin antagonists and genetically predisposed individuals may develop gestational diabetes.
[A: 519; C: 501–2; D: 158; E: 184; F: 435; G: 1982; H: 1753]

640 Latent diabetics are individuals with a normal glucose tolerance test who are known to have had an abnormal test in conditions associated with certain forms of beta-cell stress, for example during pregnancy or infection, when obese, or during treatment with drugs such as corticosteroids.
[B: 23.81; C: 504–5; E: 183; F: 437; G: 1974–5; H: 1742]

641 Maturity onset diabetes usually presents insidiously after the age of 40 and is frequently associated with obesity. Ketosis is rare. Cell mediated immunity to beta-cells, and circulating islet cell antibodies are quite unusual. Concordance in identical twins is 100 per cent and there is no HLA association. There is no increased association with other autoimmune disorders. Circulating insulin levels are frequently high and the majority of cases should be controlled with diet alone.
[A: 519; B: 23.81; C: 500–1; D: 158; E: 184; F: 436; G: 1975; H: 1743]

642 Clinical features of cardiovascular dysfunction due to diabetic autonomic neuropathy include persistent tachycardia, disappearance of normal respiratory arrhythmia and development of postural hypotension. The usual heart rate changes in response to the Valsalva manoeuvre disappear. Of more importance than any of these features is the fact that myocardial infarction may be painless.
[A: 521; B: 23.98; C: 735; D: 160; F: 446; G: 1980; H: 1752]

643 Features of proliferative retinopathy include preretinal haemorrhage, new vessel formation and

fibrous proliferation. A further possible complication is retinal detachment. Prognosis for vision is bad and approximately 50 per cent of cases with proliferative retinopathy will be blind in 5 years.
[A: 520; B: 23.96; C: 523–4; D: 159; F: 445; G: 1976–8; H: 1750]

644 In the later stages of diabetic nephropathy, oedema, hypertension and progressive renal failure develop. Serial estimations of serum creatinine, creatinine clearance or 24 hour urinary protein are useful. Renal biopsy may be indicated to distinguish the lesion from other causes of the nephrotic syndrome.
[A: 494; B: 23.96; C: 523; D: 159; F: 446; G: 1977; H: 1751]

645 Sulphonylureas promote the synthesis and secretion of insulin from pancreatic beta-cells and are therefore not effective in situations where these cells have lost the capacity to produce insulin (i.e. juvenile onset diabetes). In addition they are not the drug of first choice in obese maturity onset diabetics who usually have high levels of circulating insulin, associated with a degree of insulin resistance.
[A: 523; B: 23.87; C: 512; E: 186; F: 438–9; G: 1986; H: 1746]

646 Lactic acidosis is the most serious side-effect of this group of drugs. This is less likely with metformin than with phenformin, which should no longer be used. Patients with increased risk of hypoxia such as those with cor pulmonale, ischaemic heart disease and alcoholics should not be treated with biguanides. In addition, these drugs should not be used in those with renal or hepatic dysfunction.
[A: 523–5; B: 23.88; C: 513; E: 186; F: 438–9; G: 1986; H: 1746]

647 After the first trimester of pregnancy, diabetic control should be monitored by weekly blood glucose profiles. If possible a four point profile should be obtained i.e. blood glucose should be estimated in the fasting state and 2 hours after each of the three main meals.
[A: 531; B: 23.100; C: 527; D: 85; F: 447; G: 1988]

648 The criteria for good diabetic control in pregnancy which should now be aimed for are fasting blood glucose levels of 5 mmol/l or less and postprandial levels of 6.5 mmol/l or less whilst endeavouring to avoid hypoglycaemia. Fortunately the fetus appears to tolerate maternal hypoglycaemia relatively well.
[A: 531; B: 23.100; C: 527; D: 85; E: 185; F: 447; G: 1988]

649 If there is evidence of progression of simple retinopathy, early use of photocoagulation is indicated. Leaking vessels in the perimacular area may be destroyed, thus reducing oedema in the area. In proliferative retinopathy the aim should be to destroy new vessels before vitreous haemorrhage, macular damage or retinal detachment occur. The blue-green argon laser appears to be more effective than the white xenon.
[B: 23.97; C: 525; E: 188; F: 446; G: 1977; H: 1750]

650 Pulmonary tuberculosis may occur, and pulmonary symptoms, weight loss or increased insulin requirements are indications for radiological examination of the chest. Urinary tract infections are common in diabetics and catheterization of the bladder should be avoided if at all possible. *Candida* infections of the genitalia producing balanitis in the male and vulvitis in the female are frequent presenting features of diabetes. They usually respond to control of the diabetic state.
[A: 522; B: 23.97; C: 525; D: 160; F: 444–5; G: 1977–80]

651 Loss of vibration and proprioceptive sense in the feet are characteristic. In addition deep pain sense may be lost and in severe cases there may be impairment of the sensory modalities, producing anaesthesia in the stocking area. Wasting and foot drop may occur.
[A: 521; B: 23.98; C: 735; D: 160; F: 446; G: 1979]

652 Patients with this problem characteristically complain of difficulty in reading. They may also have difficulty in reading the marks on an insulin syringe. The symptom usually improves over a few weeks and patients should be advised not to have refraction carried out during this period.
[B: 23.97; F: 445; G: 1976]

653 Precipitating factors include infection, myocardial infarction and treatment with drugs such as thiazide diuretics, steroids and diphenylhydantoin. The situation may be exacerbated by the drinking of large volumes of sugar-containing fluids.
[B: 23.95; C: 521; D: 164; F: 443; G: 1985; H: 1749]

654 Administration of bicarbonate to a patient with diabetic ketoacidosis accelerates the rate of fall of serum potassium during rehydration. Iatrogenic hypokalaemia is one of the principal causes of cardiac arrhythmias and sudden death during treatment of diabetic ketoacidosis. Excessive administration of

sodium bicarbonate may also cause hypernatraemia and cerebral oedema.
[A: 529; B: 23.92; C: 519; D: 162; E: 187; F: 443; G: 1983–4; H: 1748]

655 The finding of elevated serum iron, total iron binding capacity and ferritin with a positive iron excretion test support the diagnosis. Diagnosis is confirmed by liver biopsy which shows iron deposition in liver cells, with fibrosis and cirrhosis.
[A: 110; B: 20.32; C: 410; F: 1128; G: 1982; H: 489]

656 Pituitary gonadotrophin levels are characteristically low in anorexia nervosa with amenorrhoea, and this finding is associated with low oestrogen levels in the blood. Other pituitary hormone levels, including growth hormone and ACTH are normal.
[A: 571; B: 35.43; C: 767; E: 446; F: 1415; G: 1700–1; H: 417]

657 Adrenal causes of hirsutism include congenital adrenal hyperplasia, Cushing's syndrome and adrenal carcinoma. These conditions (and polycystic ovarian syndrome) may be accompanied by virilization (deepening of the voice and clitoral enlargement).
[A: 564; B: 29.5; E: 179; F: 537; G: 2271; H: 227]

658 Digitalis and spironolactone have some structural similarity to sex steroids and may cause gynaecomastia. A number of drugs may be associated with increased prolactin release from the anterior pituitary, and with gynaecomastia. These include the phenothiazines, tricyclic preparations, methyldopa and reserpine.
[A: 577; B: 30.24; F: 526; H: 1788]

659 The ovaries fail to produce oestrogens and progesterone after the menopause. As a result the pituitary gland becomes more active and circulating gonadotrophin (FSH and LH) levels are elevated.
[A: 568; B: 26.10; C: 499; D: 169; F: 536; G: 2190; H: 1850]

660 Survival following diagnosis and following recurrence is longer in receptor-positive patients. Patients with receptor-negative tumours are unlikely to respond to endocrine therapy in the form of oophorectomy or with drugs such as tamoxifen, whereas those with receptor-positive tumours may respond.
[G: 1919; H: 1792]

661 This is an autosomal recessive disorder, so that any family in which the trait has appeared in one child has a 1 in 4 chance of each additional child being affected. [B: 47.6; E: 621; F: 425; G: 2024; H: 462]

662 Sinus tachycardia and systemic hypertension are the usual features. Hypertension may be severe enough to cause left ventricular failure and papilloedema. [A: 539; B: 47.23; C: 736; D: 165; E: 422; F: 421; G: 2045; H: 497]

663 Grand mal seizures and cranial nerve palsies may occur. Psychiatric features include depression, hysteria and a transient paranoid psychosis, which may lead to admission to a mental hospital. [A: 540; B: 47.23; C: 736; D: 165; E: 422; F: 421; G: 2045–6; H: 497]

664 Elevated urinary delta-aminolaevulinic acid and urinary porphobilinogen are characteristically found in this condition. Porphobilinogen in the urine produces a red colour when Erlich's aldehyde reagent is added. In contrast to that produced by urobilinogen, this colour is not extracted when chloroform is added. [A: 540; B: 47.24; C: 427; F: 420–1; G: 2046; H: 497–8]

665 An acute attack of primary gout may be precipitated by dietary indiscretion and overindulgence in alcohol in particular. Other precipitants include injury, surgical operations, excessive exercise and intercurrent infections. [A: 418; B: 25.41; C: 635–6; D: 177; E: 40–1; F: 947; G: 2031–4; H: 479–80]

666 Ten per cent of all gout is associated with myeloproliferative disorders which cause increased purine turnover. These include leukaemia, myelofibrosis and polycythaemia rubra vera. Secondary gout may also occur in multiple myeloma and Hodgkin's disease. Treatment of these disorders with antimetabolites causes tissue destruction and a further rise of serum uric acid, and is especially likely to precipitate an acute attack of gout. Prophylactic treatment with allopurinol is usually advisable in this situation. [A: 419; C: 636; D: 177; E: 41; F: 947; G: 2032–3; H: 479]

667 Polymorphonuclear leucocytosis and raised ESR frequently accompany an acute attack of gout. The plasma urate is also raised, but may fall to normal when the attack subsides. [A: 419; C: 636; D: 177; E: 41; F: 947; G: 2034; H: 479]

668 The finding of negatively refractile crystals of monosodium urate, which are seen under polarized light is characteristic of gouty arthritis.
[A: 419; C: 637; D: 178; E: 41; F: 948; G: 2038; H: 482]

669 Hypertension and coronary artery disease are more common in individuals with gout than in the normal population.
[A: 418; C: 637; D: 178; F: 1073; G: 2037; H: 481]

670 Chronic gouty arthritis produces punched-out bony erosions near, but not usually involving, articular margins. Tophi may be seen on X-ray if they are calcified. In the later stages, osteoarthritic changes may appear in gouty joints.
[A: 419; C: 637; D: 178; E: 41; F: 948; G: 2036–7]

671 Calcification of joint capsules is frequently found in chondrocalcinosis. Joint cartilages, especially those of the knee, are frequently calcified. Joint damage may progress to osteoarthritis.
[A: 419; B: 25.44; C: 638; D: 179; E: 42; F: 949; G: 201; H: 1888]

672 In this situation eruptive xanthomas may occur on the buttocks. Lipaemia retinalis may be seen in the retina. Acute recurrent abdominal pain and acute pancreatitis are frequent complications. The plasma has a cloudy appearance—milky plasma syndrome.
[A: 537; C: 531; D: 168; E: 622–3; F: 429; G: 2006; H: 509]

673 Fasting hypoglycaemia is common and is frequently associated with ketonuria. It may result in convulsions and brain damage. Hyperglycaemia may occur immediately after meals. Other metabolic problems include hyperuricaemia, lactic acidosis and hyperlipidaemia. Platelets may be damaged by glycogen accumulation resulting in a haemorrhagic tendency.
[B: 47.13; C: 636; E: 624; F: 450; G: 1999; H: 500]

674 Screening tests include a bacterial inhibition test which may be performed on a sample of blood obtained by heel prick of newborn infants. In addition, the urine may be tested for reducing sugars and the galactose oxidase paper strip test may be used. Cord blood red cell enzyme test may be diagnostic.
[B: 47.10; E: 622; F: 449; G: 1997; H: 505]

675 In galactosaemia there is a renal tubular abnormality which causes glycosuria, galactosuria, proteinuria and

aminoaciduria. Up to 50 per cent of cases develop cataracts. These may disappear following treatment. [B: 47.10; F: 449; G: 1998; H: 505]

676 Osteoporosis is common and there may be kyphoscoliosis with thoracic cage deformities, flat feet, and genu valgum. Fingers and toes tend to be long. Joint mobility is reduced, and despite the presence of spinal curvature, the height tends to be increased. [B: 47.9; E: 621; G: 2028; H: 464]

677 Marfan's syndrome produces a somewhat similar picture to homocystinuria but the lens of the eye is displaced upwards and mental retardation does not occur.
[G: 2028; H: 533]

678 Gastric surgery including gastrectomy, gastrojejunostomy and pyloroplasty may cause reactive hypoglycaemia, usually $1\frac{1}{2}$–3 hours after a meal.

Early diabetes mellitus occasionally causes reactive hypoglycaemia 2–4 hours after a meal.

Idiopathic reactive hypoglycaemia may also occur, but tends to be markedly overdiagnosed.
[A: 533; D: 162; E: 188; F: 448; G: 1990; H: 1759]

679 Alcoholics who do not eat may develop fasting hypoglycaemia due to depletion of glycogen stores by starvation and inhibition of hepatic gluconeogenesis by alcohol.

Other causes of fasting hypoglycaemia include hypopituitarism, Addison's disease and severe liver disease. Self-administration of insulin or sulphonylureas may cause factitious hypoglycaemia. Finally hepatic carcinomas, mesotheliomas or retroperitoneal fibrosarcomas may cause hypoglycaemia due to secretion of a proinsulin-like peptide.
[A: 534; D: 162; E: 188; F: 448; G: 1992; H: 1759]

680 A low fasting blood glucose level with inappropriately high plasma insulin levels confirms the diagnosis (providing factitious hypoglycaemia has been outruled). Finding a high proinsulin level in the plasma will also confirm the diagnosis of insulinoma. [A: 534; E: 188; F: 448; G: 1993–5; H: 1762]

681 Failure of serum lactate to rise after ischaemic exercise; myoglobinuria after exercise.
[B: 47.13; E: 625; F: 450; G: 1999; H: 504]

682 24-Hour urinary 5-hydroxyindole acetic acid; bananas and walnuts.
[A: 541; B: 19.72; C: 359; D: 164; E: 89; F: 656; G: 2208–9; H: 476]

683 For every millimole of bicarbonate, one millimole of sodium has to be given, and fluid overload may ensue. Concurrent diuretic therapy is often necessary.
[B: 49.40; C: 141; D: 164; F: 403–5; G: 1964; H: 1755]

684 Ordinary clinical thermometers do not read below 35°C. Whenever hypothermia is a possibility, a low reading thermometer must be used.

Blood gases must be corrected for the patient's body temperature. The oxyhaemoglobin dissociation curve is shifted to the left by cold. This results in higher readings for Po_2, Pco_2 and oxygen saturation, and lower readings for pH and bicarbonate than would in fact be found if the blood were at 37°C.
[A: 750; C: 786; F: 292; G: 86; H: 58]

685 Bradycardia, atrial fibrillation, J waves (at the junction of the QRS complex with the ST segment) and other arrhythmias.
[A: 750; F: 293; G: 86; H: 58]

686 Kayser–Fleischer rings in Descemet's membrane of the cornea (best demonstrated with a slit-lamp); increased copper content in liver biopsy tissue.
[A: 543; B: 47.25; C: 719; E: 72; F: 411; G: 2049–50; H: 492–3]

687 Resting tremors, intention tremors, spasticity, rigidity, chorea, dysarthria and dysphagia.
[A: 543; B: 47.25; C: 410; E: 72; F: 573; G: 2050; H: 492]

688 Chylomicrons, formed in the cells of the intestinal epithelium, contain mainly dietary triglyceride but also some dietary cholesterol. Discharging triglyceride to adipose and muscle cells converts a chylomicron to a remnant particle which has an electrophoretic mobility between that of very low and low density lipoproteins. Very low density lipoproteins (VLDL) or prebetalipoproteins contain an excess of triglycerides. Low density lipoproteins (LDL) or betalipoproteins contain an excess of cholesterol. High density lipoproteins (HDL) are also known as alphalipoproteins.
[A: 536–9; D: 167; F: 426–7; G: 2002–3; H: 509–12]

689 In diabetes mellitus there is an increase in very low density lipoproteins (type 4 hyperlipoproteinaemia)

due to increased hepatic secretion and reduced peripheral catabolism.

The same change in lipoproteins occurs with alcohol consumption and oral contraceptive use. Where there is an underlying genetic predisposition to hyperlipoproteinaemia, both of these agents may cause massive elevation of plasma lipoproteins with the additional presence of chylomicrons (type 5 hyperlipoproteinaemia).
[A: 536–9; C: 532; D: 166–8; F: 430; G: 2004; H: 517]

690 Dietary alteration to reduce intake of cholesterol and saturated fats and increase intake of polyunsaturated fats. The second step is to give cholestyramine. Both of these measures may fail to give useful reduction in serum cholesterol levels. Plasmapheresis is a further resort.
[A: 536–9; B: 47.14–15; C: 532; D: 168; E: 622–3; F: 431; G: 2005–8; H: 510–18]

Bone & Calcium Metabolism

691 1,25-DHCC stimulates the synthesis of a specific calcium transport protein in the small intestinal epithelial cell. This protein facilitates calcium absorption.
[A: 431; C: 101; D: 173; E: 191; F: 464; G: 2232–3; H: 1847]

692 The most characteristic biochemical feature of vitamin D deficient rickets is an elevated serum alkaline phosphatase level. As the disease progresses serum calcium and phosphorus tend to fall, the latter more markedly.

In vitamin D resistant rickets due to renal phosphate loss, a low serum phosphate is the primary biochemical abnormality.

In the rare condition of rickets due to alkaline phosphatase deficiency, levels of this enzyme will be abnormally low and hypercalcaemia may be present.
[A: 439; B: 24.21; C: 102; D: 170; E: 197; F: 465; G: 2248; H: 1857]

693 Radiographs of the wrist show a broadened epiphyseal line with blurring of the joint. In addition the appearance of ossification centres is delayed. In older children characteristic cupping of the epiphyses occurs.
[A: 440; B: 24.22; C: 103; D: 170; E: 198; F: 465; G: 2247–8; H: 1856]

694 Serum alkaline phosphatase will usually not fall for several weeks after initiation of vitamin D therapy in

rickets, but is a good guide by which to adjust therapy. Vitamin D should be continued in therapeutic dosage (25–125 μg/day) until plasma alkaline phosphatase returns to normal for age. Therafter it may gradually be reduced to the prophylactic dose of 10 μg per day. [A: 440; B: 24.23; C: 103; F: 465; H: 1859]

695 Common causes of osteomalacia include malabsorption, which may follow partial gastrectomy, dietary deficiency, especially in elderly women, and chronic renal failure.

Obstructive jaundice may also cause osteomalacia due to impaired fat absorption. Epileptics on long-term anticonvulsants may develop osteomalacia due to induction of increased catabolism of cholecalciferol by liver microsomes.
[A: 440; B: 26.14; C: 105; D: 170; E: 198; F: 467; G: 2247; H: 1856]

696 Common sites for Looser's zones are areas of bones exposed to stress, for example, the ribs, axillary borders of scapulae, pubic rami and the medial cortex of the upper femur. They are often found in symmetrical positions.
[A: 440; B: 26.14; C: 105; D: 170–1; E: 198; F: 467; G: 2248; H: 1857]

697 Histological examination of an undecalcified stained bone biopsy specimen is the only way of confirming the diagnosis of osteomalacia. This will show an excess volume of osteoid tissue with a normal number of bony seams. The essential feature is reduction in the proportion of osteoid covered surfaces with stainable calcification fronts to below 60 per cent.
[A: 439; B: 26.13–14; C: 105; D: 171; F: 466; G: 2248; H: 1854]

698 Elderly people living alone, inmates of geriatric and mental homes, all of whom may have limited exposure to sunlight. In addition those who have had gastric surgery should be followed and epileptics on long-term anticonvulsants should receive prophylactic vitamin D supplements.
[C: 105; D: 171; F: 467; G: 2249; H: 1857]

699 Osteoporosis is associated with Cushing's syndrome, hypogonadism and thyrotoxicosis. It frequently follows prolonged treatment with corticosteroids.
[A: 442; B: 26.9; C: 106; D: 169; E: 196; F: 975; G: 2244; H: 1851]

700 Bone biopsy in osteoporosis shows a reduction in trabecular bone volume but the trabeculae are normally calcified.
[B: 26.10; C: 106; D: 169; F: 975; G: 2242–3; H: 1850]

701 Trauma usually produces anterior wedging of vertebrae rather than total collapse and usually only affects one or two vertebrae. There is usually a clear history of trauma. Secondary malignancy may produce symptoms similar to osteoporotic vertebral collapse. It most commonly originates from the breast. Myelomatosis may produce generalized vertebral rarefaction with compression fractures. It is associated with Bence Jones protein in the urine. Osteogenesis imperfecta may also cause vertebral fractures but is usually associated with a lifelong history of fractures, a familial tendency and bluish sclerae.
[A: 442; B: 26.11; C: 106; D: 169; E: 196; F: 976; G: 2243; H: 1851]

702 Radiological changes suggestive of osteoporosis include loss of bone density, reduction in number and density of trabeculae and thinning of the cortex. The upper and lower surfaces of thoracolumbar vertebrae may become biconcave. Later compression or collapse may occur.
[A: 442; B: 26.12; C: 106; D: 169; E: 196; F: 976; G: 2243; H: 1851]

703 Paget's disease is characteristically associated with very high serum alkaline phosphatase levels, reflecting increased osteoblastic activity. Urinary hydroxyproline is frequently elevated. Serum calcium and phosphorus are normal but may be elevated during periods of immobilization.
[A: 443; C: 644; D: 174; E: 197; F: 978; G: 2258–9; H: 1861]

704 Enlargement and deformity of bones is frequently found. The normal trabecular pattern of bone is replaced with areas of rarefaction and increased density.
[A: 444; B: 26.17; D: 174; F: 977–8; G: 2258; H: 1861]

705 Headache may be troublesome. Involvement of the skull base may cause compression of cranial nerves—particularly the second, eighth, seventh and fifth. Softening of the bone may allow protrusion of the cervical vertebrae into the skull base—platybasia. This may be followed by obstructive hydrocephalus.
[A: 444; C: 644; D: 173; E: 197; F: 977; G: 2258; H: 1861–2]

706 The shafts of long bones such as femur, tibia and humerus are typically the sites of pathological

fractures in Paget's disease. In addition spine and pelvis may be affected.
[A: 444; B: 26.17; D: 173; F: 977; G: 2258; H: 1862]

707 Rapidly worsening pain in a previously pain-free Pagetic bone is the usual presentation. A tender and pulsatile mass may form in the affected area. However, a pathological fracture may be the first sign of osteosarcoma, and delayed healing of a fracture should also suggest the diagnosis of osteosarcoma.
[A: 444; B: 26.17; C: 644; D: 173; E: 197; F: 978; G: 2258; H: 1862]

708 The vascularity of pagetic bone is markedly increased, thus raising the temperature of the overlying skin. This leads to increased cardiac output and may result in high output cardiac failure. This complication, however, is not common.
[A: 443; B: 26.17; C: 644; D: 173; E: 197; F: 977; G: 2258; H: 1862]

709 Corneal calcification is the only true physical sign of hypercalcaemia. This is a thin granular band best seen on the medial side of the cornea. It is separated from the sclera by a clear band of cornea, unlike arcus senilis.
[A: 435; D: 175; E: 192; F: 409; G: 2215; H: 1835]

710 Carcinoma of the breast is the commonest cause of hypercalcaemia due to bony metastases. Multiple myeloma may also cause hypercalcaemia and bony involvement.

Humoral hypercalcaemia of malignancy is most commonly due to squamous carcinoma of the bronchus or carcinoma of the kidney.
[A: 437; B: 23.52; C: 481; D: 176; E: 194; F: 369–70; G: 2233; H: 1837]

711 Subtle psychological disorders have been found in patients with mild hypercalcaemia and occasionally psychotic behaviour occurs. Difficulty in concentration may progress in some cases to disorientation, drowsiness and coma.
[A: 435; B: 23.51; E: 192; F: 408; G: 2238–9]

712 A mild hyperchloraemic acidosis is common in primary hyperparathyroidism whereas a mild hypokalaemic alkalosis is frequently found in humoral hypercalcaemia of malignancy.
[B: 23.52; D: 177; E: 193–4; F: 408–9; H: 1837]

713 Characteristic X-ray findings in hyperparathyroidism include a pepperpot appearance of the skull,

subperiosteal erosions of the phalanges and occasionally bone cysts in the long bones. In addition plain films of the abdomen may show nephrocalcinosis or renal calculi.
[A: 436; B: 26.15; C: 480; E: 193; F: 505; G: 2214–15; H: 1834]

714 Steroids seldom lower serum calcium in hyperparathyroidism but do produce a fall in serum calcium in most cases of hypercalcaemia due to malignancy, sarcoidosis, vitamin D intoxication, immobilization and milk–alkali syndrome.
[A: 436; D: 177; E: 194; F: 506; G: 2217; H: 1835]

715 No. Hypercalcaemia may persist for months after stopping vitamin D administration, due to high body stores. A low calcium diet should be prescribed and steroid administration may be necessary.
[A: 437; B: 24.23; C: 104; D: 176; E: 194; G: 2234; H: 1848]

716 If hypercalcaemia remains severe despite rehydration, intravenous phosphate may be necessary. However, it is contraindicated in the presence of renal impairment as it may cause general tissue calcification in this situation. Peritoneal or haemodialysis with low calcium exchange fluids may then be useful.

Intravenous mithramycin is very effective in lowering serum calcium rapidly but carries some risk of haemorrhage or renal damage.
[A: 437; B: 23.53; D: 177; E: 194–5; F: 507; G: 2239–40; H: 1839]

717 As albumin accounts for most of the protein-bound calcium in the blood, total serum protein and albumin levels should be checked whenever serum calcium is being estimated. Elevated serum albumin will produce a corresponding rise in total serum calcium, and a fall in albumin values will produce a corresponding fall in serum calcium. Serum calcium may be corrected to take into account variations of serum albumin above or below normal.
[A: 431; B: 26.7; D: 176; E: 190; F: 503; G: 2226; H: 1826]

718 Blood urea and creatinine are elevated due to the renal failure. Serum calcium is frequently low. The resulting osteomalacia is associated with raised serum alkaline phosphatase. Glomerular damage produces phosphate retention with an elevated serum phosphate.
[A: 441; B: 22.9–10; C: 438; D: 171–2; E: 198; F: 1010; G: 2254–5; H: 1303]

719 Clinical features of idiopathic hypoparathyroidism include tetany, psychosis, cataracts, papilloedema and moniliasis involving nails or tongue. Radiological changes include calcification of the basal ganglia seen on skull X-ray. The serum calcium is below normal, with elevated serum phosphate and unmeasurable serum parathormone levels.
[A: 433; B: 23.53–4; C: 481; D: 175; E: 195; F: 508; G: 2220–1; H: 1840]

720 Alkalosis is the commonest cause of tetany and thus tetany frequently results from hyperventilation in anxious or hysterical individuals. Tetany due to hypocalcaemia may result from post-thyroidectomy hypoparathyroidism, idiopathic hypoparathyroidism, and vitamin D deficiency due either to intestinal malabsorption or dietary deficiency.
[A: 432; B: 23.54; C: 481–2; D: 176; E: 195; F: 408; G: 2221–3; H: 2070]

Infectious Diseases & Immunization

721 A polymorphonuclear leucocytosis commonly occurs in bacterial infections such as a subphrenic abscess. Leucopenia is found in typhoid fever and SLE. Monocytosis is found in infectious mononucleosis. Atypical white cells may be found in leukaemia.
[A: 643; B: 12.2–4; C: 47; E: 30–1; F: 28–9; H: 643]

722 Blood culture is the most important diagnostic test in typhoid fever and blood should be repeatedly cultured if the diagnosis is strongly suspected. The finding of *Salmonella typhi* in cultures of stool and urine does not unequivocally confirm the diagnosis, as the patient may be a carrier suffering from an unrelated illness.
[A: 632; B: 12.47; C: 55–6; E: 26–7; F: 40–1; G: 446–8; H: 642]

723 The most common serious complications of typhoid fever are bleeding or perforation of the small intestine.
[A: 632; B: 12.46; C: 55–6; D: 298; E: 26–7; F: 40–1; G: 447; H: 643]

724 Both tetanus and peritonitis produce board-like rigidity of the abdominal wall, but in tetanus there is little or no tenderness.
[A: 649; B: 2.18; C: 61–2; E: 552; F: 83; G: 437–8; H: 685]

725 Unlike meningitis, in tetanus there is no fever, headache or pain on flexion of the neck. Lumbar

puncture will show an increased number of leucocytes in the CSF in meningitis but not in tetanus.
[A: 649; B: 2.19; C: 61; E: 552; F: 83; G: 438; H: 686]

726 The meningococcus is a Gram-negative intracellular diplococcus. The pneumococcus is a Gram-positive diplococcus and *Haemophilus influenzae* is a small Gram-negative bacillus.
[A: 357–8; B: 12.26; C: 63; F: 59–60; G: 411–16; H: 1961]

727 A widespread petechial or purpuric rash is a major feature of meningococcal meningitis but not of the others.

Haemophilus influenzae meningitis almost always occurs in children under the age of 6 years.

Pneumococcal meningitis is frequently associated with a preceding focus of infection such as sinusitis or otitis media. It may also occur following head injury or splenectomy.
[A: 634; C: 63; F: 59–61; G: 411–16; H: 1961]

728 *Salmonella* gastroenteritis is due to ingestion of living organisms which multiply within the bowel and enter the gut mucosal cells prior to causing symptoms. Staphylococcal food poisoning is due to ingestion of an enterotoxin which is produced by staphylococci multiplying in food usually contaminated by a person with a septic lesion. Cooking of the affected food may kill the staphylococci, but the enterotoxin is relatively heat-stable.
[A: 744; B: 12.58–60; C: 57–8; E: 25; F: 267; G: 64–6; H: 586]

729 Diarrhoea is the major feature of *Salmonella* gastroenteritis. Fever is frequent and vomiting usually less prominent than in staphylococcal food poisoning. Abdominal pain is common.
[A: 744; B: 12.58–60; C: 57–8; E: 25; F: 268; G: 64–6; H: 586]

730 He has been in one of the areas where plague occurs and a mass of lymph nodes, usually in the groin but in other regions also, is the first sign of the disease following the bite of an infected flea, but the presentation is wrong. The incubation period is usually 2–4 days and the onset is marked by high fever, chills and prostration. The bite, surrounded by haemorrhage and oedema, is painful.

Streptomycin, tetracycline and co-trimoxazole are all effective.
[A: 678; B: 12.71; F: 46; G: 464; H: 663]

731 The incubation period of amoebic dysentery varies from 2 weeks to many years, and is usually several months. Bloody diarrhoea is the main feature but it may only be moderately severe. Lower abdominal pain is frequent. Fever, malaise and vomiting, which may occur in bacillary dysentery are uncommon in amoebic dysentery.
[A: 745; B: 12.39; C: 59; D: 299; E: 25; F: 38; G: 458–9; H: 650]

732 Confirmation of a diagnosis of amoebic dysentery is by finding amoeboid trophozoites with ingested red cells in the stool, in mucosal biopsy material or in scrapings taken from an ulcer at sigmoidoscopy. Specimens should be examined immediately after they are collected as amoebae rapidly stop moving following cooling.
[A: 693; B: 12.41; C: 813; D: 299; E: 589; F: 201; G: 592; H: 864–5]

733 Fever, sweating and pain in the right hypochondrium are the usual symptoms. Pain may also be felt in the right shoulder due to diaphragmatic irritation. On examination, enlargement and tenderness of the liver with marked pyrexia are the main findings. Diarrhoea is unusual. Jaundice may occur occasionally, but only in a small percentage of cases.
[A: 693; B: 12.41–2; C: 813; D: 299; E: 589; F: 200; G: 591; H: 865]

734 Radioisotope scanning of the liver will show a filling defect, and ultrasound examination will distinguish between a cystic and solid lesion.

In areas where investigational facilities are minimal a therapeutic trail or metronidazole is quite justifiable, and will produce a rapid response if the abscess is amoebic.

Finally, in cases of genuine doubt, aspiration through a fine bore needle may be necessary. Amoebic abscesses usually contain a brownish 'anchovy sauce' type pus, and only rarely are amoebae found in this pus.
[A: 693; B: 12.42; C: 814; D: 299; E: 590; F: 201; G: 591–2; H: 865]

735 Koplik's spots may be seen on the buccal mucosa prior to the apperance of the rash. They resemble grains of salt surrounded by an erythematous zone. They are most common around the opening of the parotid duct, but they may be widespread throughout the buccal mucosa. They disappear with the onset of the rash.
[A: 639; B: 12.28; C: 68; E: 15; F: 138; G: 247; H: 794]

736 The differential diagnosis of measles includes rubella, scarlet fever, infectious mononucleosis and drug rashes. The rash of rubella usually occurs on day one of the illness. Conjunctival suffusion and tender suboccipital lymphadenopathy are characteristic of rubella.
[A: 641; B: 12.29; C: 68–9; E: 15–16; F: 137; G: 249; H: 795]

737 A membrane covering the pharynx, tonsils and neighbouring structures. At first whitish, soft and easily removed, later it becomes grey or black, tough and firmly adherent to the underlying mucosa. It can encroach on the airway and cause death. The toxin may affect the myocardium and peripheral nerves.
[A: 624; B: 12.21–3; C: 53; E: 24; F: 75; G: 430–1]

738 Infectious mononucleosis may be associated with fever, sore throat and morbilliform rash. An exudative tonsillitis may be seen, but lymphadenopathy is often generalized and may be associated with splenomegaly. A petechial rash on the palate is characteristic. There may be clinical or biochemical (elevated SGPT) evidence of hepatitis. Blood film shows an atypical lymphocytosis. The Paul–Bunnell test is positive in infectious mononucleosis, but not in scarlet fever.
[A: 629; B: 12.25; C: 50; E: 23; F: 65–8; G: 371; H: 615]

739 The cough spasms of whooping-cough are typically followed by vomiting, and they are worst at night.
[A: 627; B: 12.24; C: 52; E: 22; F: 49; G: 427; H: 655]

740 Pulmonary complications include pneumonia, segmental or lobar collapse and bronchiectasis. The most dangerous complication, however, is the occurrence of apnoeic attacks which may cause convulsions, neurological damage, and death in infants.
[A: 628; B: 12.24; C: 52–3; E: 22; F: 50–1; G: 427; H: 655]

741 Complications include orchitis (which occurs in 25 per cent of males who get the disease after puberty and may lead to sterility if bilateral), oophoritis and pancreatitis. Encephalomyelitis occasionally occurs.

An increased lymphocyte count in the CSF is an extremely common finding and mumps is one cause of acute lymphocytic meningitis.
[A: 641; B: 12.27; C: 69; E: 17; F: 160–1; G: 262; H: 815]

742 Sarcoidosis may cause painless parotid enlargement, frequently associated with uveitis. Unilateral parotid enlargement may be due to a tumour the most

common of which is a sialoma (mixed salivary tumour). This is usually painless, benign and slow-growing. Enlargement of the parotid gland due to calculous obstruction of the duct is rare. In this condition swelling and pain are exacerbated by mastication.

Parotid enlargement also occurs in hepatic cirrhosis and during treatment with some drugs, e.g. guanethidine.
[F: 161; G: 263; H: 817]

743 Complications include encephalomyelitis, with cerebellar ataxia, chickenpox pneumonia, myocarditis and secondary skin infection with staphylococci or streptococci. The disease may be fatal in patients on steroids or in those suffering from leukaemia.
[A: 638; B: 12.31; C: 70; E: 17; F: 133–4; G: 253; H: 802–3]

744 Smallpox is associated with a 2–4 day prodromal illness before the rash appears. The rash is maximal peripherally, i.e. on face and extremities, and axillae are almost always spared. The vesicles are deep-set, circular, multilocular and usually present at one stage of development (i.e. no cropping).
[A: 636; B: 12.34; E: 18–19; F: 130; G: 254; H: 803]

745 The complications of *P. falciparum* malaria are:
(a) cerebral malaria which is frequently preceded by confusion and may progress to coma, convulsions, focal neurological signs and death.
(b) severe haemolytic anaemia which may produce haemoglobinuria ('blackwater fever') with oliguria and acute renal failure.
(c) jaundice and hepatic failure may lead to misdiagnosis of viral hepatitis.
[A: 653–7; B: 12.68–9; C: 809; D: 298; E: 588; F: 182–3; G: 571–2; H: 870]

746 First, severe falciparum malaria will require parenteral therapy with antimalarials. Chloroquine is the drug of choice.

Secondly, *Plasmodium falciparum* is resistant to chloroquine in certain areas, including South America, South-east Asia and East Africa, and patients from these areas should be treated with quinine dihydrochloride.

Antimalarial chemoprophylaxis must be continued for 4 weeks after leaving an endemic area.
[A: 656; B: 12.70–1; C: 810; D: 298; E: 588–9; F: 185; G: 572–3; H: 871–2]

747 Fourteen days of primaquine treatment is effective in eradicating the liver form of the disease. However, primaquine may cause severe haemolysis in individuals with glucose-6-phosphate dehydrogenase deficiency, usually persons of African, Asian or Mediterranean origin. These individuals should have a glucose-6-phosphatase assay performed before primaquine therapy is suggested.
[A: 655; B: 12.69; C: 808; D: 297–8; F: 181; G: 568–72; H: 870–2]

748 Severe leucopenia, thrombocytopenia and normocytic anaemia are characteristic. IgG is markedly increased.

Diagnosis depends on demonstrating the parasite in stained smears of bone marrow or lymph node aspirate (or less safely in spleen or liver biopsy specimens). It may also be cultivated from these sources on special 'NNN' medium.
[A: 657; G: 12.81–2; C: 815–16; F: 188; G: 585; H: 874]

749 Massive splenomegaly is also caused by chronic myeloid leukaemia, myelofibrosis and the tropical splenomegaly syndrome which is associated with chronic malaria.
[A: 657; B: 12.81; C: 816; F: 189; G: 585–6; H: 874]

750 Sleeping sickness due to *T. gambiense* has a chronic course, leading to death after a few years. On the other hand, *T. rhodesiense* may cause death within a few months.

The disease is spread by the bite of an infected tsetse fly. Antelopes are a reservoir of *T. rhodesiense* infection.
[A: 661; B: 12.77; C: 818; E: 590; F: 193–4; G: 576; H: 876]

751 Neurological features develop within a few weeks or months in the Rhodesian form of the illness, and up to several years after infection in the Gambian form. The early features include headache, insomnia and personality changes. Frequently there is a period of improvement followed by tremor, ataxia, slurring of speech, mental deterioration and choreiform movements. Later there is an irresistible desire to sleep, followed by convulsions occasionally, but coma and death invariably, if treatment is not instituted.
[A: 661; B: 12.77; C: 819; E: 590; F: 194–5; G: 577; H: 877]

752 The most serious effect of chronic *T. cruzi* infection is cardiomyopathy which may cause cardiomegaly,

arrhythmias and sudden death of young adults during exercise.

Damage to Auerbach's plexus results in dilation of the oesophagus with dysphagia, and dilation of the colon with constipation and possibly obstruction.
[A: 662; B: 12.78; C: 821; E: 591; F: 198; G: 581; H: 879]

753 Diagnosis may be confirmed by finding *T. cruzi* in blood smears. In chronic cases organisms may be very scanty and animal inoculation, blood culture on 'NNN' medium or xenodiagnosis may be successful. Xenodiagnosis involves the use of clean laboratory bred reduviid bugs which are allowed to feed on blood from the suspected case. Two weeks later the intestinal contents of the bugs are examined for *T. cruzi*.
[B: 12.79; C: 821; F: 198–9; G: 582; H: 879]

754 Treatment is supportive. The disease is virtually always fatal.

Control of infected animal populations is by far the most important aspect of prevention. Pre-exposure prophylaxis is available. Following suspected exposure to rabies, local wound debridement, active immunization and passive immunization are the three main aspects of management. Initial results with the new human diploid cell vaccine appear to be excellent.
[A: 682; B: 12.94–7; C: 848; E: 21; F: 147–8; G: 834; H: 821]

755 Chronic cases may be afebrile and frequently the only clinical feature is generalized lymphadenopathy. An atypical lymphocytosis similar to that found in infectious mononucleosis may occur. However, in toxoplasmosis the Paul–Bunnell test is negative, and antibodies to *Toxoplasma gondii* may be found in the serum using the dye test or a fluorescent method.
[A: 650; B: 12.101; C: 822; D: 82; E: 30; F: 207; G: 596; H: 881]

756 In tuberculoid leprosy there is vigorous cell-mediated immunity to *M. leprae*. Organisms are scanty in the tissues and these patients are probably non-infectious.
[A: 677; B: 14.18–19; C: 825; E: 586; F: 93; G: 502–3; H: 712]

757 Peripheral nerve trunks such as radial and ulnar may be markedly thickened. Damage to these nerves results in severe sensory loss in the extremities. As a result of this, the digits and limbs suffer repeated traumatic damage and burns, and frequently require amputation.
[A: 677; B: 14.18; C: 826; F: 93; G: 502; H: 712]

758 Tuberculoid leprosy may also damage the trigeminal nerve and lead to anaesthesia of the cornea thereby further increasing the risk of traumatic damage. [C: 826; F: 93; H: 712]

759 In advanced lepromatous leprosy nodular lesions appear on the face and ears. Eyebrows may be lost. Occasionally, diffuse thickening of the facial skin produces a 'leonine facies'. Ulceration of mucosae of nose and mouth and necrosis of the nasal cartilage and bones may produce very severe tissue destruction and deformity in the later stages.
[A: 677; B: 14.19; C: 826; F: 93; G: 503; H: 712]

760 Tissue juice obtained from a small slit over a skin lesion or from the ear lobe may be stained by a modified Ziehl–Nielsen method. This will reveal *M. leprae* in cases of lepromatous leprosy, but not in tuberculoid leprosy. Alternatively the organism may be found in nasal mucus in lepromatous leprosy. This finding is a good index of infectivity.
[B: 14.21–2; C: 826–7; F: 93–4; G: 503; H: 713]

761 Cholera begins suddenly with massive diarrhoea (rice water stool), with vomiting but no abdominal pain. Hypotension rapidly develops due to dehydration. Severe muscular cramps occur but the patient remains fully alert. Death occurs within a few hours due to acute circulatory failure, unless effective treatment is given.
[A: 687; B: 12.49; C: 830; E: 27; F: 32–3; G: 461; H: 676]

762 Culture of stool or rectal swab is the most important diagnostic test but a quick method is to examine the stools for *Vibrio cholerae* by dark-ground microscopy or a fluorescent antibody technique.
[B: 12.49; C: 831; E: 27; F: 33–4; G: 461]

763 Rehydration and electrolyte replacement is the major factor in treatment. A large bore intravenous cannula is essential and a cut-down or femoral vein cannulation may be necessary. Ringer lactate is a satisfactory replacement solution. Very large amounts of intravenous fluid may be required for initial rehydration. As soon as possible oral tetracycline should be started. It will shorten the course of the illness.
[A: 688; B: 12.49–50; C: 831; E: 28; F: 34; G: 462; H: 676]

764 Septicaemia and meningitis are extremely serious complications. In addition, patients who inhale the

organism may develop a virulent haemorrhagic bronchopneumonia.

Penicillin is the drug of choice if the organism is sensitive.
[B: 12.97; C: 832; F: 80; G: 470–1; H: 668]

765 A blood film reveals an atypical lymphocytosis. The Paul–Bunnell test for heterophile antibodies is positive. The Monospot test is similar to this. Additional serological findings may include positive results for syphilis tests, positive rheumatoid factor and cold agglutinins.

The main complications are hepatitis (usually anicteric), autoimmune haemolytic anaemia, thrombocytopenic purpura, myocarditis and benign lymphocytic meningitis. The Guillain–Barré syndrome may occur.
[A: 643; B: 12.35; C: 570; D: 291; E: 20; F: 1174–6; G: 265–6; H: 855]

766 Painless terminal haematuria is the cardinal symptom of this disorder, especially following exercise.
[A: 674; B: 12.53; C: 860; D: 300; E: 591; F: 217; G: 615; H: 910]

767 The diagnosis is confirmed by finding the characteristic egg with a terminal spine, in the urine. The chances of finding the eggs are increased by collecting the urine following exercise.
[A: 675; B: 12.53; C: 860; F: 218; G: 615; H: 910]

768 Itching of the area of skin through which the infective cercariae entered the body may be followed by allergic manifestations. These include urticaria and eosinophilia, headache and sweating, abdominal pain and splenomegaly. Patches of pneumonic consolidation may be seen on X-ray and are associated with cough. These allergic phenomena are known as the Katayama syndrome.
[A: 675; B: 12.54; C: 860; D: 300; F: 218; G: 613–14; H: 908]

769 In heavy infections of *S. mansoni* the characteristic laterally spined eggs are found on stool microscopy. In light infections, repeated stool examination may be necessary. The eggs may also be found in specimens of rectal mucosa obtained at sigmoidoscopy.
[A: 675; B: 12.54; C: 860; F: 218–19; G: 613–15; H: 908]

770 Hepatic fibrosis with portal hypertension, splenomegaly, ascites and haematemesis due to rupture of oesophageal varices are serious

complications. Prominent collateral veins on the abdomen may be seen.

Neurological features include Jacksonian epilepsy, hemiparesis and blindness. These are due to deposition of eggs in the central nervous system.
[A: 676; B: 12.54; C: 861; E: 592; F: 219–20; G: 614; H: 910]

771 In Q fever, the test is negative. In Rocky Mountain spotted fever and typhus, positive titres develop to OX-19 and OX-2. In scrub typhus, OX-K antibodies develop.
[A: 280; B: 12.98; C: 856; E: 29–30; F: 118–19; G: 329–30; H: 757]

772 Pleurodynia or Bornholm disease; myocarditis and pericarditis; meningitis or encephalitis; orchitis.
[A: 645; B: 12.15–21; E: 20; F: 149–51; G: 269; H: 809]

773 Clinically the illness presents with high fever, headache, limb pains and bronchitis. On the fifth day a morbilliform rash appears, which may later become petechial. Splenomegaly may occur and the patient frequently becomes delirious.
[A: 681; B: 12.72–3; C: 853; F: 116; G: 318–19; H: 748]

774 Infection is due to drinking water containing a small crustacean known as *Cyclops* or the water flea, which is the intermediate host of the worm.
[B: 12.50; C: 879; E: 593; F: 230; G: 633; H: 893]

775 Eggs of the parasites are passed in the stool of an infected person. In warm, moist soil these develop into infective filariform larvae which can penetrate intact human skin, usually that of the feet of individuals walking barefoot on soil contaminated by faeces.
[A: 668; B: 12.51; C: 869–70; D: 300; E: 593; F: 231–2; G: 624; H: 903]

776 The characteristic egg is found in the stool. The egg yolk may contain 2–8 lobes.
[A: 669; B: 12.51; C: 869–70; E: 593; F: 232; G: 264; H: 903]

777 Fever, severe headache and bone pains are the main symptoms. A morbilliform rash is common and cervical lymphadenopathy may occur. The most serious complication is dengue haemorrhagic fever, in which disseminated intravascular coagulation, fever and shock develop with a high mortality, especially in children.
[A: 685; B: 12.85; C: 845; E: 585; F: 154; G: 277; H: 830]

778 An acute episode of haemolysis is a well recognized sequel to *Mycoplasma pneumoniae* infection. Haemoglobinuria with sudden development of anaemia may occur. The cause of this haemolysis is the development of cold agglutinins which may be detected in the serum. The direct Coombs' test becomes positive.
[A: 280; D: 233; F: 114; G: 344–6; H: 760]

779 The conjunctiva of the upper eyelid should be inspected for the characteristic follicles which may deform the upper tarsal plate and cause ptosis. However, even before this, slit lamp examination of the cornea may reveal increased vascularity and cellularity. Trichiasis, entropion and ectropion also contribute to corneal scarring, which is the cause of blindness in this disease.
[B: 33.8; C: 852; F: 122; G: 332–3; H: 763]

780 Adherent yellow oropharyngeal exudates with lethargy and lymphadenopathy are characteristic. Intercostal myalgia may be severe and bleeding may develop secondary to thrombocytopenia and hypoprothrombinaemia. Leucopenia and proteinuria are usually found.
[A: 684; C: 849; E: 21; F: 163; G: 299; H: 843]

781 Major features of yellow fever are fever, jaundice, leucopenia and proteinuria.
[A: 684; B: 12.83; C: 843; E: 585; F: 155; G: 295; H: 835]

782 The definitive host is the one in which the parasite reproduces.

Finding segments of the adult worm or ova in the stool makes the diagnosis.

T. saginata does not cause cysticercosis, which occurs only in *T. solium* infections.
[A: 663; B: 12.62–3; C: 865; E: 601; F: 220–1; G: 607–8; H: 914]

783 In most cases there is a single cyst in the right lobe of the liver and this produces pain and hepatomegaly. Leakage of hydatid fluid into the tissues may cause urticaria, asthma and anaphylaxis.

Significant eosinophilia is usual. X-ray may show calcification of the cyst, and ultrasound examination will confirm the cystic nature of the lesion. The Casoni skin test is frequently positive.
[A: 665; B: 12.99–100; C: 866; F: 222; G: 609–10; H: 917]

784 The main symptom is severe pruritis ani, which is worse at night.

If cellophane adhesive tape is applied to the perianal skin in the morning, the ova will adhere to it and may be identified by microscopic examination.
[A: 669; B: 12.43; C: 868; D: 300; E: 600; F: 233; G: 629; H: 899]

785 A solitary granuloma of the eye may develop and lead to strabismus and blindness. This granuloma is usually visible near the macula and must be distinguished from retinoblastoma.
[A: 667; C: 869; E: 600; F: 234; G: 628; H: 902]

786 *Strongyloides stercoralis* is unique among intestinal nematode infections in that diagnosis is made by finding motile rhabditiform larvae in the faeces. In the case of other intestinal worms, the diagnosis is confirmed by finding ova in the stool.

Inadvertent use of steroids in a case of *Strongyloides* infection may cause fatal systemic strongyloidosis.
[A: 696; B: 12.55; C: 871; E: 593; F: 231; G: 622; H: 905]

787 Initial symptoms are nausea and diarrhoea. These are followed by evidence of larval invasion, including fever, oedema of face and eyelids and myalgia. Muscles of limbs and jaw may be painful, stiff and tender. Cough, chest pain and dyspnoea may occur due to diaphragmatic invasion.
[A: 670; B: 12.62; C: 880; D: 118; E: 600; F: 235–6; G: 630; H: 894–5]

788 *Wuchereria bancrofti* is transmitted by night-biting *Culex fatigans* mosquitoes. The life cycle of the parasite is well adapted to the habits of the vector, in that the microfilariae which infect the mosquitoes appear in the blood of the human host only at night. This is nocturnal periodicity. The clinical importance of this is that it is essential to examine a thick blood smear taken as near as possible to midnight in order to confirm the presence of the microfilariae.
[A: 672; B: 12.87; C: 873; E: 593; F: 223; G: 633; H: 896]

789 The commonest late complication is hydrocele. Elephantiasis is less common and usually affects the legs.
[A: 672; B: 12.87; C: 874–5; F: 224–5; G: 634; H: 896]

790 The diagnosis may be confirmed by removing one of the characteristic skin nodules which occur in this condition and finding the adult worm within it.

In the absence of nodules, examination of a skin-snip, especially from thigh or shoulder, may reveal the characteristic microfilariae. Finally,

slit-lamp examination of the eye may reveal microfilariae in the cornea or anterior chamber.
[A: 673; B: 12.88–9; C: 877; E: 594; F: 227; G: 636; H: 898]

791 Pus containing 'sulphur granules' draining from the skin through indurated sinuses. The commonest site is below the jaw in the neck, but infection of the appendix can break through the abdominal wall in the right iliac fossa and pulmonary disease may cause thoracic sinuses. It is a chronic disease but systemic spread may be fatal.

Actinomyces israeli is sensitive to penicillin, which should be given for 6 weeks.
[A: 651; C: 243; F: 95; G: 474; H: 734]

792 Antivenom should not be given routinely in cases of snake bite. The majority of cases recover without specific treatment. Indications for antivenom administration are, first, evidence of systemic envenomation which includes the features noted above, with in addition vomiting or leucocytosis. Secondly, antivenom should be used when severe local swelling develops as this may precede local necrosis.

The major side-effect of antivenom is immediate anaphylaxis. This may be effectively treated by intramuscular adrenaline.
[C: 889–90; E: 213; F: 242–6; G: 121; H: 921]

793 Transmission is via the faecal–oral route and only cysts of *G. lamblia* are infective. The disease is usually water borne.

Diagnosis is confirmed by finding the characteristic cysts in iodine stained stool preparations.

Metronidazole is the drug of choice for eradication of the infection.
[A: 695; B: 12.44; C: 814; D: 299; E: 604; F: 204; G: 602; H: 887]

794 Protozoal diseases which are transmissible by blood transfusion include malaria, Chagas' disease, visceral leishmaniasis, and rarely sleeping sickness. Syphilis is also transmissible by this route but chilling of the blood will rapidly kill the spirochaetes.
[A: 104; C: 396; F: 1117; G: 1785; H: 1576]

795 The usual blood picture in acute brucellosis consists of a low white cell count with polymorphonuclear leucopenia and a lymphocytosis.
[A: 648; B: 12.61; C: 62; E: 28; F: 52; G: 476–8; H: 659]

796 Patchy consolidation on chest X-ray may be segmental or lobar, and may spread to more than one lobe. It

differs from that found in other bacterial pneumonias in that it may persist for months and may be followed by fibrosis.
[A: 278; C: 244; D: 232; G: 359; H: 683]

797 Early treatment with erythromycin is usually associated with a reasonably good recovery. Cases with respiratory failure require assisted ventilation.
[A: 278; D: 232; G: 360; H: 684]

798 Radiological changes take at least 10 days to develop and should not be relied upon to confirm the diagnosis. Delay in diagnosis and treatment will allow irreversible bone necrosis to occur. Isotope bone scanning may localize the lesion early, and supporting evidence for the diagnosis may be obtained by culturing the infecting organism from the blood or from pus obtained by aspiration or drainage of the affected bone.
[B: 26.22–3; C: 643; F: 985; G: 2260; H: 1890]

799 Leptospirosis is a bacterial disease and usually produces a polymorphonuclear leucocytosis, whereas viral hepatitis is associated with a normal or low white cell count. Penicillin therapy carries significant benefit for a patient with leptospirosis if started early in the disease, whereas viral hepatitis does not respond to antibiotic therapy.
[A: 646; B: 12.56; C: 67; E: 28; F: 112–13; G: 534; H: 729]

800 *Treponema carateum*. It is quite common in adult immigrants from the West Indies. There is cross-reaction in the serological tests for venereal syphilis.
[B: 12.14; C: 838; F: 111; G: 524; H: 728]

801 Babies born to mothers who develop hepatitis B during the last 3 months of pregnancy or early in the puerperium should receive monthly injections of anti-hepatitis B immunoglobulin, starting as soon after birth as possible. Workers in dialysis units in which hepatitis B is prevalent should also receive the immunoglobulin. Sexual contacts of cases of acute hepatitis B may be given short-term protection by this immunoglobulin.
[A: 106; C: 396; D: 197; E: 14; G: 1655; H: 559]

802 Antibody production in response to pertussis vaccine is poor under the age of 3 months. Vaccination of children over this age should, in addition to protecting them from the disease, diminish the prevalence of the

disease in the community, and hence lessen the risk of smaller infants contracting pertussis.
[C: 53; E: 14; F: 51; G: 428; H: 656]

803 There has been an increasing tendency to use live attenuated vaccines as they theoretically will produce better immunity than killed vaccines. Live vaccines in common use include polio, rubella, measles, yellow fever, and BCG. Smallpox vaccine (vaccinia) is also a live vaccine. It should be noted that routine immunizations with live vaccines should be avoided in pregnancy.
[H: 595]

804 Pertussis immunization should not be given to children with a history of convulsions or with evidence of disorders of the central nervous system or to those having first degree relatives with idiopathic epilepsy. In addition the vaccine is contraindicated in children with acute illness, especially respiratory infections, and in those who have had severe local or systemic reaction to a previous dose of the vaccine.
[C: 53; E: 14; F: 51; G: 428; H: 656]

805 In the UK, only to females. Those to whom it is normally offered include girls aged 11–13 years, seronegative women with an occupational risk of contracting rubella (e.g. nurses), and postpartum women who were found to be seronegative during pregnancy. It is essential that women take efficient precautions to avoid pregnancy for at least 2 months after immunization, due to the risk of fetal infection with the vaccine virus.
[A: 640; B: 12.30; C: 69; E: 14; F: 137; G: 252; H: 597]

Venereal Diseases

806 False positive serological tests for syphilis may occur in infectious mononucleosis, leptospirosis, malaria and viral pneumonia. In these cases the false positive test usually lasts less than 6 months. In chronic infections such as leprosy and TB and in SLE the false positive test may last for more than 6 months.
[A: 720–1; B: 13.8; C: 66; D: 112; E: 157; F: 108–9; G: 514; H: 722]

807 The superficial lesions of early syphilis, whether congenital or acquired are infectious. The superficial lesions of late syphilis are non-infectious.
[A: 719; C: 65; F: 102–3; G: 507–12; H: 718–19]

808 Some serum should be squeezed from the ulcer and examined with a microscope fitted with a dark-ground

condenser. In primary syphilis motile *Treponema pallidum* organisms will be seen.
[A: 720; B: 13.4–8; C: 66; F: 102–3; G: 513–15; H: 721]

809 Specific tests for syphilis include the Reiter protein complement fixation test (RPCFT), fluorescent treponemal antibody test (FTA), treponemal haemagglutination test (TPHA) and treponemal immobilization test (TPI). These tests appear to overcome the problems of false positive non-specific tests, but in fact they cannot differentiate the antibodies produced by the various treponemal diseases, a differentiation which must be done on clinical grounds.
[A: 720; B: 13.7–8; C: 66; D: 112; E: 157; F: 108; G: 513–15; H: 722]

810 The cardinal features of secondary syphilis include
(a) skin rash—macular and erythematous; scaly, but not itchy;
(b) condylomata—heaped up highly infectious lesions in areas such as the perineum;
(c) mucous patches—shallow whitish ulcers with a red margin found in the mouth. They are highly infectious;
(d) lymphadenopathy—may be generalized and is painless.
[A: 719; B: 13.2; C: 65; E; 153; F: 99; G: 508; H: 718]

811 Dysuria and a mucoid or mucopurulent urethral discharge are the main features of NSU in the male. Tetracycline is the most useful drug and should be used for 10–20 days. Symptoms may recur following treatment.
[A: 721; B: 13.15; C: 65; E: 152; F: 167; G: 408; H: 765]

812 Keratoderma blenorrhagica is the most distinctive feature of Reiter's disease, and consists of a rash resembling pustular psoriasis, which is usually limited to the soles of the feet and the toes. There may be severe arthritis of the feet resulting in permanent deformity. Plantar fasciitis is common.
[A: 411; B: 13.15–16; C: 620–1; D: 138; E: 39; F: 168–9; G: 197; H: 1883–4]

813 Complications in the female include acute salpingitis, and infants of infected mothers may develop ophthalmia neonatorum leading to corneal scarring and blindness.

Systemic complications include acute or chronic arthritis 2–3 weeks after the genitourinary symptoms start. Iritis, septicaemia and a vesicular rash may also occur.

Follow-up 3 months after treatment is essential so that serological tests for syphilis may be carried out.
[A: 717; B: 13.10–13; C: 64; E: 150–2; F: 62–3; G: 406–10; H: 624]

814 In chancroid there is a painful and soft ulcer on the genitalia with associated enlarged inguinal lymph nodes which may suppurate. (Note the name soft sore.)

In contrast, the genital lesion of primary syphilis is painless and indurated, and the regional lymph nodes, although enlarged, are painless, firm and rarely suppurate.
[A: 722; B: 13.13; C: 836; F: 54; G: 425; H: 658]

815 These women should be advised to have cervical smear examinations carried out at regular intervals.
[B: 13.17; G: 508; H: 850]

Haematology

816 Women in this age group suffer considerable loss of iron during menstruation, pregnancy and lactation. Dietary intake of iron, especially in the undernourished, may be inadequate to replace these losses and iron deficiency may result.
[A: 594; B: 21.20; C: 543–4; D: 284; E: 374; F: 1125; G: 1747–8; H: 1514]

817 The most likely site of blood loss in this situation is the gastrointestinal tract. Therefore the first test one should do is to check the stool for occult blood. If this is positive further investigations include sigmoidoscopy and barium enema to check for large bowel neoplasm or other lesion, and endoscopy or upper GI barium studies to check for peptic ulceration or gastric neoplasm.
[C: 544; E: 375; F: 1124–5; G: 1747–8; H: 1515]

818 The MCV separates anaemias into three categories—microcytic, normocytic and macrocytic, each of which has a separate group of causes. Having determined into which category a particular case falls, one can investigate further along standard lines.
[A: 593; B: 21.3; C: 908; D: 75; E: 373; F: 1111; G: 1717–18; H: 263]

819 Haemolytic anaemia, uraemia, widespread malignancy, rheumatoid arthritis, liver disease, leukaemia and pancytopenia.
[A: 595; B: 21.4; C: 539; D: 76; E: 373; F: 1111; G: 1718; H: 268]

820 An elevated white cell count with atypical cells suggests leukaemia. This may be associated with thrombocytopenia. Leucopenia and thrombocytopenia with normocytic anaemia imply pancytopenia which may be primary (aplastic anaemia) or secondary due to drugs, industrial chemicals, irradiation and replacement of marrow by malignant or fibrous tissue. Hypersplenism may produce a similar picture.
[D: 76; F: 1111; G: 1718; H: 270]

821 In macrocytic anaemia, macrocytes, i.e. abnormally large red blood corpuscles, are found in the peripheral blood. While these are found in B_{12} and folate deficiency also, there are a number of conditions associated with macrocytes in the peripheral blood, but not with megaloblastic change in the bone marrow. These include cirrhosis, hypothyroidism, haemolytic anaemia, leukaemia and pancytopenia.
[A: 599; B: 21.24; C: 547; D: 77; E: 377; F: 1129; G: 1719; H: 1518]

822 The marrow shows marked changes from a megaloblastic to a normoblastic state within 48 hours of the first hydroxycobalamin injection. Within 3 days the peripheral blood reticulocyte count rises, reaching its peak on the sixth day—with levels of up to 50 per cent being reached in severely anaemic patient
[A: 597; B: 21.24; C: 550; D: 77; E: 379; F: 1139; G: 1727; H: 1524]

823 Tropical sprue is always accompanied by folate deficiency which may also occur in coeliac disease in children and adults in non-tropical areas. Partial gastrectomy, Crohn's disease and small bowel resection may also cause folate malabsorption.
[A: 597; B: 21.26; C: 551; D: 285; E: 377; F: 1135; G: 1725; H: 1522]

824 Haemorrhage, tissue infarction (e.g. myocardial infarction), drugs (especially steroids), malignancy, diabetic ketoacidosis and uraemia.
[B: 21.3; C: 540; E: 391; F: 1172; H: 286]

825 Neutropenia is frequently due to drug-induced marrow depression. SLE and deficiency of vitamin B_{12} or folic acid may all cause neutropenia. Significant splenomegaly from any cause may produce neutropenia due to hypersplenism.
[A: 607; B: 21.3; C: 569; E: 391; F: 1172; G: 1808–10; H: 286]

826 Malignancy, especially Hodgkin's disease and polyarteritis nodosa.
[B: 21.5; C: 540; E: 391; F: 1173; G: 225; H: 290]

827 Investigation is indicated if the history of easy bruising is associated with a history of excessive bleeding following minor surgery, tooth extraction or menstruation. Slight bleeding of the gums following tooth brushing is usually not significant, whereas spontaneous gum bleeding is.
[E: 413; H: 278]

828 None. This disorder appears to be due to capillary damage, and in fact platelet count and coagulation studies are normal. The capillary resistance (Hess) test may be positive.
[A: 604; B: 21.46; D: 78; E: 411, 414; F: 1214; G: 1880; H: 1560]

829 The bleeding time will be prolonged in thrombocytopenia and the coagulation time will be normal provided there is no associated coagulation defect.
[A: 606; C: 592; D: 81; E: 411; F: 1206–7; G: 1872; H: 279]

830 Patients with defects of the coagulation system such as haemophilia develop deep haematomas which tend to spread, haemarthroses, haematuria and retroperitoneal haemorrhage. Following trauma, bleeding may not occur for several hours, and then may recur for several days.
[D: 79; E: 411; F: 1207–8; G: 1871–2; H: 278–9]

831 In haemophilia A partial thromboplastin time is prolonged and the diagnosis is confirmed by finding reduced levels of factor VIII coagulant in the plasma with normal or raised levels of factor VIII protein. Coagulation time may or may not be prolonged, and platelet count, prothrombin time and bleeding time are all normal.
[A: 604; B: 21.52; C: 596; D: 79–80; E: 418; F: 1208–9; G: 1884; H: 1561]

832 Parenteral administration of vitamin K is frequently effective in improving coagulation in obstructive jaundice and other forms of liver disease. However, this takes 6–12 hours to return the prothrombin time to normal. Fresh frozen plasma is effective in producing a rapid elevation of clotting factors in liver disease. However, this effect is short-lived.
[A: 605; C: 598; D: 81; E: 419; F: 1213–14; G: 1890; H: 1565]

833 In advanced DIC clotting time is prolonged, circulating fibrinogen levels low, fibrin degradation products elevated and platelet count low. In addition

the prothrombin time and partial thromboplastin time may be prolonged.
[B: 21.50; C: 601; D: 81; E: 420; F: 1212; G: 1891; H: 1566]

834 Major complications of splenectomy include postoperative haemorrhage, susceptibility to infection, especially pneumococcal infections, and a persistently raised platelet count (thrombocytosis) which is associated with an increased incidence of thromboses.
[F: 1176; G: 1871; H: 554]

835 Thalassaemia major gives rise to a severe hypochromic microcytic anaemia with large numbers of target cells and normoblasts in the peripheral blood. In contrast to iron deficiency anaemia, serum iron is raised in thalassaemia major. Haemoglobin electrophoresis reveals gross reduction in Hb A levels with markedly elevated levels of Hb F (up to 90 per cent of total) and frequently some elevation of Hb A_2.
[B: 21.33; C: 561; D: 288; E: 388; F: 1160; G: 1778; H: 1553]

836 Rapid rehydration is essential. Narcotic analgesics must be avoided despite severe pain, due to the real risk of addiction. Non-narcotic analgesics should be used instead. Oxygen and correction of acidosis may be required. Antibiotics are indicated if infection is present, as is often the case.
[A: 600; B: 21.34; C: 557; D: 288; E: 387; F: 1156; G: 1773–5; H: 1548]

837 Normocytic normochromic anaemia is profound and progressive. Thrombocytopenia is frequently found. The white cell count is usually elevated to $20–50 \times 10^3/\mu l$, 30–90 per cent of these white cells being immature lymphoblasts. In some cases the white cell count may be normal or low (subleukaemic leukaemia), but even in these cases immature cells will be found in the peripheral smear or buffy coat.
[A: 609; B: 21.61; C: 571–3; D: 289; E: 397–9; F: 1183–4; G: 1818; H: 1624]

838 In ITP, unlike in acute leukaemia, there is no splenomegaly, hepatomegaly or lymphadenopathy. The absence of splenomegaly is a particularly important feature of ITP. In addition, in ITP white cell count is normal and anaemia is absent unless there has been substantial bleeding. Bone marrow examination confirms the differentiation.
[C: 570; D: 291–2; E: 415; F: 1184; G: 1817; H: 1625]

839 The granulocytes of chronic myeloid leukaemia are deficient in alkaline phosphatase when compared to normal granulocytes.
[A: 610; C: 575; D: 291; E: 395; F: 1187; G: 1822; H: 1631]

840 Rejection of the donor marrow may occur. Attempts to prevent this by immunosuppression increase the risk of infection. Graft versus host disease may also occur. Features of this include fever, rash, liver damage, diarrhoea plus a further increase in susceptibility to infection.
[A: 607; B: 21.30; C: 552; E: 382; F: 1166; G: 1738; H: 1526–9]

841 Invasion of marrow by metastatic carcinoma, multiple myeloma, and myelosclerosis are the usual causes.
[B: 21.5; C: 568; E: 384; F: 1168; G: 1742; H: 1530]

842 Thrombotic complications include cerebral thrombosis, myocardial infarction and peripheral vascular disease.

Haemorrhagic complications include haematemesis or melaena, haematuria and menorrhagia. Peptic ulceration occurs in 10 per cent of cases.
[A: 611; B: 21.59; C: 567; E: 393; F: 1189; G: 1796–7; H: 1578]

843 Haemoglobin, haematocrit, red cell count, white cell count and platelet count are all usually elevated in polycythaemia rubra vera, whereas only the red cell values are elevated in secondary erythrocytosis.
[B: 21.60; C: 566–7; D: 76; E: 394; F: 1190; G: 1796; H: 1578]

844 It has been held that ^{32}P can increase the percentage of cases of polycythaemia rubra vera which convert to leukaemia, but this is questionable.
[A: 612; C: 567; E: 395; F: 1190–1; G: 1797; H: 1578]

845 The first aim is to induce a remission. This can be achieved in approximately half the cases. The second aim is to maintain remission. Remission maintenance consists partly of regular courses of treatment and partly of specific therapy aimed at sites where relapse is known to originate, for instance, the meninges and central nervous system.
[A: 608; B: 21.61; C: 571–3; D: 290; E: 397–9; F: 1183–4; G: 1819; H: 1624]

Immunology, Autoimmune Disease & Rheumatology

846 B cells are responsible for antibody formation. Under suitable stimulation they differentiate into plasma cells. On their cell membrane they carry membrane-bound immunoglobulins, receptors for the Fc portion of IgG and for some complement factors, particularly activated C3 (C3b).

T cells (thymus-dependent) are responsible for cell-mediated immunity and delayed hypersensitivity. Their surface receptors include immunoglobulins and specialized antigen-binding sites. In the immune response subsets of T cells may behave as helper cells, suppressor cells or killer cells.

[A: 385; C: 24; E: 116; F: 379; G: 128–9; H: 315–16]

847 Receptors for IgG and activated complement factor C3 (C3b). This enables macrophages to phagocytose immune complexes, which in turn enables the cells to present antigenic 'information' to the lymphocytes.

[A: 385; C: 25; E: 116; G: 129; H: 317]

848 Each immunoglobulin molecule consists of two heavy (H) chains and two light (L) chains. Schematically, the two heavy chains form the stem and arms of the letter Y and a light chain is linked by disulphide bridges to each arm of the Y. The arms form the antigen-binding sites.

The ends of the arms of the molecule vary in their amino acid sequence and the specificity of the antibody resides here. The stem of the molecule has a constant amino acid sequence and this determines the general properties of the antibody such as ability to bind to mast cells (IgE) or cross the placenta (IgG).

[A: 387–8; C: 27; E: 116; F: 380; G: 127; H: 317]

849 IgM also fixes complement. ABO blood group antibodies and cold agglutinins are examples of IgM molecules.

IgA is the predominant immunoglobulin in the membranes and secretions of the respiratory, gastrointestinal and genitourinary tracts, and also in colostrum.

IgE is present in very small quantities, most of it bound to mast cells. The arrival of antigen at the binding sites of two adjacent IgE molecules causes histamine release.

IgD is present in blood in small quantities. Its specific function is not known.
[A: 389; C: 27–8; F: 380; G: 127; H: 318]

850 Infections with viruses, mycobacteria, protozoa and fungi.

Transplant rejection and tumour cell destruction are other expressions of cell-mediated immunity.
[A: 387; C: 25–6; F: 383; G: 130; H: 319]

851 The substances are called lymphokines. They diffuse into the surrounding tissue space and attract macrophages, polymorphs, B cells and other T cells to the area. The substances include migration inhibitory factor (MIF) and interferon.
[C: 25; G: 129; H: 319]

852 In normal circumstances clones of cells capable of reacting with self-antigens appear to be rendered unresponsive by continuous exposure to the antigen. The B cells may lose their capacity to make autoantibody, or helper T cells may fail to help. In addition antibody production may be inhibited by suppressor T cells.

There are genetic factors predisposing to the breakdown of immune tolerance. Viral infections may provoke autoantibody formation. Overactivity of helper cells or failure of suppressor cells have also been demonstrated.
[A: 388; C: 25–6; G: 129; H: 321]

853 Complement activation is a central part of the normal immune response to infection. It is also involved in the damage inflicted by autoimmune disease.

Deficiency of complement factors or the inhibitors and cofactors which regulate the complement system can cause disease, often resembling SLE.

The complement fixation test has a central place in the laboratory detection of specific antibodies.
[C: 28; E: 126–7; F: 381; G: 135–7; H: 322–3]

854 Measurement of C3 and C4 is technically easy compared to measurement of the other factors.

The first steps of the classic pathway involve C1, C4 and C2 in that order. If both C4 and C3 levels are low, that suggests classic pathway activation. If C4 is normal but C3 low, alternate pathway activation is suggested. The finding of normal levels of C4 and C3 does not rule out complement activation.
[C: 29; E: 127; F: 381; G: 135–6; H: 323]

855 Assay of C1 esterase inhibitor reveals very low values. Danazol, a synthetic steroid with some androgenic properties, has proved effective in many cases. [F: 1233; G: 138; H: 324]

856 Many (but not all) cases of asthma, allergic rhinitis and conjunctivitis, urticaria, angio-oedema and contact dermatitis. Systemic anaphylaxis following insect bite or parenteral drug administration is a generalized type I reaction. [A: 393; C: 29; E: 125; F: 381; G: 131; H: 324]

857 Coombs' test. The test is positive if red cells are agglutinated by anti-IgG or anti-C3 antibodies. This is the direct Coombs' test.

The indirect Coombs' test is used in cross-matching blood for transfusion. Donor red cells are first incubated with recipient's serum before the direct test is performed. [A: 394; C: 31; F: 382; G: 132; H: 324]

858 SLE; infective endocarditis; malignancies, polyarteritis nodosa; rheumatoid disease; erythema multiforme. [A: 395; C: 32; E: 119; F: 382; G: 133–4; H: 324]

859 Hashimoto's thyroiditis; idiopathic adrenal failure; pernicious anaemia; graft versus host reactions in bone marrow transplants. [A: 397; C: 33; F: 383–4; G: 130; H: 325]

860 In myasthenia gravis, antibodies to the acetylcholine receptor sites on the muscle block the action of acetylcholine. [C: 34; F: 384; G: 133; H: 1754]

861 K or killer lymphocytes with receptors for the Fc portion of IgG bind to the IgG molecules, with ensuing lysis of the target cell. Complement is not involved. [C: 34; F: 384; H: 325]

862 Susceptibility to infection, autoimmune disease and lymphoreticular malignancy. [A: 390; C: 40; E: 116–17; F: 386; G: 150; H: 326]

863 Presence in the IgA-deficient recipient of anti-IgA antibodies. Blood can be safely transfused in such cases only from an IgA-deficient donor. [E: 117; F: 386; G: 143; H: 330]

864 Bone pain, especially arising from the vertebral column. Vertebral collapse with nerve root compression is a well recognized presentation.

Tiredness may result from anaemia. Pneumonia and other infections are common. Hypercalcaemia may be sufficient to cause lethargy, constipation, drowsiness and even coma. Headaches, dizziness and visual disturbance may result from hyperviscosity of the blood.
[A: 617; B: 21.78; C: 587; D: 292; E: 403; F: 1201; H: 333–4]

865 Plasma and urine protein electrophoresis must be done in every case of suspected myeloma. A paraprotein (monoclonal band of immunoglobulin) will be found in the serum of 80 per cent of myeloma patients. In the remaining 20 per cent it will be found only in the urine where it is known as the Bence Jones protein. Serum calcium is often elevated but alkaline phosphatase is usually normal. The ESR is usually high. A normocytic, normochromic anaemia is common. If renal impairment is present urea and creatinine will be elevated.

Bone marrow examination commonly shows increased numbers of plasma cells.
[A: 618; B: 21.79; C: 588; D: 292; E: 403; F: 1202; G: 1854–7; H: 334]

866 In several ways. The presence of large quantities of light chains in the glomerular filtrate (Bence Jones proteins) may block the tubules. This is more likely to occur if the patient becomes dehydrated. Hypercalcaemia and hypercalciuria can cause polyuria and nephrocalcinosis. Pyelonephritis results from impaired resistance to infection and vascular and tubular damage in the medulla.

Amyloidosis is a risk with chronic overproduction of immunoglobulins but it occurs in less than 5 per cent of cases of multiple myeloma.
[A: 618; B: 21.78–9; C: 587; E: 403; F: 1201–2; G: 1858–60; H: 334–5]

867 Chemotherapy commonly consists of melphalan and prednisone. Combination chemotherapy with several drugs is necessary when tumour cell mass is high.

Radiotherapy to painful bone lesions or fracture sites may be required. Plasmapheresis can remove excess circulating immunoglobulin in hyperviscosity states. Renal failure may need conventional dialysis until the disease responds to chemotherapy.
[A: 618–19; B: 21.80; C: 588–9; D: 292; E: 404; F: 1202; G: 1861; H: 335–6]

868 A florid picture of large retinal haemorrhages, exudates and patchy dilatation of retinal veins. The appearances are very striking.

Hyperviscosity is treated by plasmapheresis, anaemia by transfusion with washed red cells and the underlying malignant proliferation by chemotherapy. Chlorambucil is usually given first but multiple drug combinations are also being used.
[A: 619; B: 21.80; C: 589; E: 404; F: 1203; G: 1862–3; H: 336]

869 The abnormal alpha heavy chains may be missed on routine electrophoresis. Clinically there is severe malabsorption, the small intestinal mucosa showing a heavy infiltrate of plasma cells.
[B: 21.80; F: 1203; G: 1866; H: 337]

870 Amyloid is a protein consisting mainly of fibrils. These bear some resemblance in their amino acid sequence to immunoglobulin light chain in primary but not in secondary amyloidosis. There is also another molecular component similar in amino acid sequence to C reactive protein.

The exact cause of amyloid deposition is unknown but the presence of chronic antibody production appears to be a predisposing factor.
[A: 542; B: 25.17; C: 436; F: 415–18; G: 1863–4; H: 339]

871 Elevated ESR, anaemia and sometimes leucocytosis and eosinophilia. Serum complement levels of C3 and C4 may be low and the urine may contain protein and red cells.
[C: 33; E: 121; F: 1022–4; G: 134; H: 349–50]

872 Renal, mesenteric, coronary, vasa nervorum and the arteries supplying proximal muscles are commonly involved.

Renal impairment, gastrointestinal symptoms, myocardial infarction, mononeuritis multiplex and proximal myopathy can all occur. Other features of polyarteritis nodosa include gangrene of the digits and pericarditis.

A group of patients have pulmonary disease with asthma and eosinophilia but these may be classified separately, on the grounds of a different histology, as allergic granulomatosis.
[A: 414; B: 25.29; C: 215; D: 127; E: 121; F: 967; G: 181–2; H: 352]

873 Respiratory illness precedes disease in other parts of the body and comprises asthma, bronchitis and recurrent pneumonia. The asthma is usually steroid-dependent and a family history is lacking. Chest X-rays may show shadows consistent with patchy and recurrent consolidation. Fever is common.
[B: 18.105; D: 127; F: 967; G: 182; H: 352–3]

874 Headaches of a persistent, dull, throbbing nature with associated scalp tenderness; tender, thickened temporal arteries with reduced or absent pulsation; raised ESR and characteristic histology on temporal artery biopsy.
[A: 415; B: 25.30; C: 215; D: 130; F: 968–9; G: 217–18; H: 354]

875 Raised ESR. Like temporal arteritis, polymyalgia rheumatica responds well to corticosteroids. It may be possible to discontinue treatment after one year.
[A: 424; B: 25.31; C: 634; D: 129; E: 40; F: 969; G: 217; H: 355]

876 Lesions show a rough symmetry over the lower limbs, although other areas may be affected, including the palms.

Respiratory infections and drug ingestion are the two commonest aetiological factors. The condition also occurs in SLE and rheumatoid disease. Cryoglobulins (proteins which precipitate on cooling below 37°C) may also cause it.
[F: 1204; G: 166–7; H: 353]

877 There appears to be increased B cell activity and impaired T cell function. These may account for the increased incidence of drug reactions and lymphoproliferative malignancies in SLE.
[A: 412; B: 25.25; C: 628; D: 125–6; E: 119–20; F: 959; G: 175; H: 358]

878 Vasculitis.
[A: 412; B: 25.26; C: 628–9; E: 120; F: 960; G: 175–6; H: 356–9]

879 The arthritis of SLE resembles rheumatoid arthritis in its distribution but joint destruction and deformity are not usual.

The urinary sediment in SLE is typically 'telescoped', by which is meant that features of several stages of nephritis are present simultaneously. The sediment contains red cells, white cells, casts of all kinds, fat globules and tubular cells. This appearance, however, can occur in other collagen vascular diseases as well.
[A: 412–13; B: 25.27; C: 628–9; D: 125; E: 120; F: 960–1; G: 177; H: 357]

880 Renal involvement (in some cases steroids are given in conjunction with azathoprine and cyclophosphamide), central nervous system involvement, pleurisy,

thrombocytopenia, haemolytic anaemia and other life-threatening complications.
[A: 414; B: 25.28; C: 630; D: 126; E: 121; F: 962; G: 179–80; H: 359]

881 The HLA antigens appear to be markers for different immune responses. For some disease conditions there is a close association with particular antigens. The closest and best known association is between ankylosing spondylitis and HLA B27.
[C: 36–8; E: 127; F: 351–3; G: 39; H: 360–4]

882 Turbid fluid with a large fibrin clot, synovial fluid glucose less than half the blood level, white cell count greater than $50 \times 10^3/\mu l$ with more than 80 per cent polymorphs.

Normal synovial fluid contains less than 200 white cells per microlitre.
[A: 421; B: 25.7; C: 610; F: 944; G: 2356; H: 1871]

883 Yes. Rheumatoid is not the only diagnostic possibility, of course, but an asymmetrical pattern of joint involvement occurs in about a third of cases.
[A: 400; B: 25.12; C: 606; D: 131; E: 33; F: 934; G: 188; H: 1874]

884 Rheumatoid nodules, which most commonly occur over the elbows or other pressure areas, and vasculitis, which is due to deposition of immune complexes in vessel walls.
[A: 402; B: 25.16; C: 607; D: 132; E: 34; F: 934–5; G: 187; H: 1874–5]

885 Drugs, physiotherapy and orthopaedic surgery. Drugs include: salicylates and other non-steroidal anti-inflammatory drugs; gold or penicillamine, both of which may produce very good responses but require close monitoring of blood counts and renal function; immunosuppressive drugs such as azathioprine.
[A: 404; B: 25.19–24; C: 610–17; D: 133–5; E: 34–6; F: 937–9; G: 190–3; H: 1876–7]

886 Early changes comprise blurring of joint margins, erosions and patchy sclerosis of the articular surfaces. Later the joint space is lost and the characteristic 'bamboo spine' occurs.
[A: 408; B: 25.35; C: 618; D: 136; E; 37; F: 941; G: 194; H: 1881]

887 Uveitis is common and may be recurrent. Aortic regurgitation occurs in approximately 5 per cent of

patients. Heart conduction abnormalities are sometimes found. Amyloidosis also occurs.
[A: 409; B: 25.35; C: 618–19; D: 137; E: 38; F: 941; G: 194–5; H: 1881]

888 Labial gland biopsy (from the lip) is safer than salivary gland biopsy and histology shows lymphocytic infiltration.

Loss of tears leads to conjunctival irritation and corneal ulceration. Loss of saliva causes difficulty in swallowing and exposes the teeth to rapid decay.
[A: 403; B: 25.18; C: 607; D: 136; F: 964–5; G: 193; H: 1879]

889 Typically a (non-gonococcal) urethritis is followed by bilateral conjunctivitis and arthritis. The arthritis involves the joints of the legs and feet more commonly than those of the upper limbs.

Other features include keratoderma blenorrhagica (indistinguishable from pustular psoriasis), circinate balanitis and plantar fasciitis.
[A: 411; B: 13.15; C: 620; D: 138; E: 39; F: 168–9; G: 197; H: 1883]

890 Spondylitis, similar to ankylosing spondylitis; arthritis mutilans, a severe destructive polyarthritis.
[A: 410; C: 621; D: 136; E: 39; F: 942; G: 196; H: 1884]

891 Women are affected as often as men. A woman presenting with the symptoms and signs of ankylosing spondylitis may have inflammatory bowel disease.
[A: 411; C: 622; E: 39; F: 943; G: 198; H: 1885]

892 Arthritis, erythema nodosum, thrombophlebitis and central nervous system abnormalities. The underlying lesion is a vasculitis.
[A: 411; C: 623; F: 971; G: 199; H: 1886]

893 C—calcinosis; R—Raynaud's phenomenon; S—sclerodactyly; R—telangiectasia.
[A: 415–16; B: 25.32; C: 632; D: 128–9; E: 123; F: 963; G: 169; H: 1898]

894 The oesophagus (where the lower two-thirds become atonic with loss of peristalsis), the remainder of the gastrointestinal tract and the lungs. Pulmonary fibrosis may be compounded by aspiration pneumonia secondary to oesophageal reflux.
[A: 416; B: 25.32; C: 631–2; D: 129; E: 123; F: 963; G: 169; H: 1898]

895 Narrowing of the joint space, no evidence of local decalcification and a tendency to marginal bony outgrowths or lipping.

This is in contrast to the subarticular erosions and loss of bone density that occurs in rheumatoid arthritis.

[A: 422–4; B: 25.37; C: 639–42; D: 138; E: 43; F: 945; G: 203; H: 1894]

Muscle Disorders

896 The disease involves the shoulder girdle muscles and progresses to involve most muscles apart from the cranial muscles. By 7–12 years the patient is confined to a wheelchair. Later, contractures and scoliosis develop, and the patient dies in the late teens from respiratory infection or cardiac failure.

[A: 340; B: 34.29; C: 739; D: 120; E: 559; F: 1391; G: 916; H: 2060]

897 Creatine kinase (CK) levels may be elevated in cord blood and may reach extremely high levels as the disease progresses. Seventy per cent of female carriers of this disorder have raised CK levels, and this fact may be useful when giving genetic advice.

[A: 340; B: 34.29; E: 559; F: 1390; G: 915–16; H: 2060]

898 These include frontal baldness, cataract, gonadal atrophy, causing impotence and sterility in men and amenorrhoea in women. There is frequently a degree of intellectual deterioration and personality change.

[A: 341; B: 34.27; C: 740; D: 120; E: 560; F: 1393; G: 917; H: 2061]

899 The ESR is usually elevated, frequently exceeding 100 mm/hour. Polymyalgia may be associated with giant-cell arteritis, which may cause sudden blindness. Polymyalgia rheumatica responds dramatically to steroids.

[A: 424; B: 25.31; C: 634; F: 968; G: 217; H: 355]

900 About 10 per cent of the adults who develop polymyositis-dermatomyositis have underlying malignancy, usually of lung, breast, uterus, ovary or gastrointestinal tract.

[A: 417; B: 25.33; C: 633; D: 118; E: 561; F: 1395; G: 923; H: 2054]

901 Patients who do not have antistriated muscle antibody are very unlikely to have a thymoma, whereas 90 per cent of those with this antibody do have a thymoma.

About 15 per cent of cases of myasthenia gravis have a thymoma. These cases should have thymectomy as the tumour may be locally invasive. Myasthenic symptoms do not usually respond to this, but cases with thymoma usually respond better to immunosuppressive drug treatment than non-thymoma cases.
[A: 338; B: 34.31; C: 737; D: 119; E: 556–9; F: 1396; G: 925; H: 2066]

902 Involvement of limb muscles, bulbar muscles and respiratory muscles also occurs. Bulbar muscle involvement may cause dysphagia, dysarthria and difficulty chewing. Respiratory muscle disorders may cause dyspnoea and, in severe cases, respiratory failure.
[A: 338; B: 34.32; C: 737; D: 119; E: 556–9; F: 1396; G: 926; H: 2065]

903 Emotional stress, pregnancy and infection.
[C: 737; B: 34.31; D: 119; F: 1396; G: 926; H: 2065]

904 Malignant hyperthermia is a dominantly inherited disorder characterized by a rapid rise in body temperature, generalized muscle rigidity, tachypnoea, rapid heart rate and metabolic acidosis which are precipitated by general anaesthesia. It carries a high mortality. Halothane and suxamethonium are the usual precipitants. Susceptible cases may have elevated CK levels and subclinical myopathy.
[B: 34.30; C: 740; E: 562; F: 1398; G: 921; H: 2068]

905 Osteomalacia. A waddling gait is the usual presenting feature. Plasma alkaline phosphatase is elevated.
[B: 34.30; C: 740–1; D: 24; E: 562; F: 1398; G: 923; H: 2056–8]

Dermatology

906 (a) A vesicle is an elevated skin lesion containing fluid and may be up to 0.5 cm in diameter.
(b) A bulla is a large vesicle, i.e. one exceeding 0.5 cm in diameter.
(c) A pustule is a pus-filled vesicle.
[E: 128; G: 2272–3; H: 234–5]

907 Herpes zoster, varicella, smallpox and herpes simplex are all associated with a vesicular rash. The dominant lesion in impetigo may be bullae.
[F: 1279; G: 374; H: 240]

908 Pemphigus vulgaris is a disease of middle age. Diagnosis is confirmed by finding antibodies to the

intercellular substance of epidermal cells, using a fluorescent antibody technique.
[A: 715; B: 31.35; D: 282; E: 138; F: 1281; G: 2303; H: 240–1]

909 Sulphonamides and barbiturates may precipitate the Stevens–Johnson syndrome. Treatment with systemic corticosteroids may be life-saving in severe cases.
[A: 708; B: 31.33; D: 283; E: 144; F: 604; G: 2305–6; H: 190]

910 Barbiturates, phenothiazines, sulphonamides and sulphonylureas are the drugs most frequently implicated in iatrogenic light sensitivity.
[G: 2288–9; H: 255]

911 Scleroderma, dermatomyositis and SLE.
[G: 2273; H: 246]

912 Oral contraceptives, sulphonamides and dapsone may cause erythema nodosum. Bacterial infections of note which also cause it include streptococcal infections, tuberculosis, and leprosy.
[A: 708; B: 31.90; C: 254; D: 280; E: 144; F: 970; G: 2295; H: 244]

913 In dermatomyositis the erythema is usually situated over the dorsal metacarpophalangeal joints. In SLE the erythema is over the dorsal proximal phalanx with sparing of the knuckles.
[F: 1268; G: 173]

914 Pruritis is quite unusual in psoriasis. Psoriatic plaques may occur in the scalp. However, loss of hair from these areas is unusual.
[A: 704; B: 31.15; D: 275; F: 1227; G: 2280; H: 239]

915 Five to ten per cent of cases of psoriasis may develop joint involvement. Distal interphalangeal joint involvement is characteristic and large joints of the limbs are also affected.

The rheumatoid factor is not found in the serum in psoriatic arthropathy.
[A: 704; B: 31.17; C: 621; D: 275; E: 133; F: 942; G: 2280; H: 239]

916 Reiter's disease may be associated with palm and sole lesions, a condition known as keratoderma blenorrhagica.

Secondary syphilis may produce palm and sole lesions similar to those found in psoriasis.
[E: 133; F: 1227–8; H: 239]

917 The disease usually starts at about 3 months of age and the face is usually involved initially. Later the cubital and popliteal fossae and wrist flexures become the principal sites. The natural history is for the condition to improve as the child grows, but it rarely clears completely.
[A: 702; B: 31.10; C: 33; D: 276–7; E: 128–9; F: 1228; G: 2283–4; H: 241]

918 Lichen planus commonly affects the anterior aspect of the forearms, the legs, and the lower back. Buccal mucosae and genitalia are also frequently involved. Severe itching is common.
[A: 715; B: 31.20; D: 275; E: 134; F: 605; G: 2280; H: 190]

919 Many patients with dermatitis herpetiformis have changes in the villi of the duodenum and jejunum very similar to those of coeliac disease, and a malabsorption syndrome may be present in these cases.
[A: 716: B: 31.31; D: 282; E: 139; F: 1252; G: 2304; H: 1404]

920 Face, hands and buttocks are most frequently affected. The causative organism is *Staphylococcus aureus*, and it usually responds to gentamicin, neomycin or fusidate ointments.
[A: 709; B: 31.44; E: 142; F: 57; G: 374; H: 568]

921 By examination of scrapings of skin from the lesion. These should be stained with potassium hydroxide and examined microscopically for fungal hyphae. Culture will identify the particular species.
[B: 31.51; D: 278; E: 141; G: 2282; H: 746]

922 The severe itching, and the fact that other members of the family are similarly affected make scabies a likely possibility. Application of benzyl benzoate to the entire skin surface from the chin to the soles, following a bath, is the most effective treatment. All intimate contacts of the patient should be similarly treated.
[A: 711; B: 31.62; C: 886; E: 143; G: 110–11; H: 919]

923 Obstructive jaundice, leukaemia, Hodgkin's disease, uraemia and polycythaemia rubra vera. Diabetes mellitus produces pruritus which is usually localized to the genitalia and is caused by infection with *Candida*. [B: 31.39; F: 1239; G: 2296; H: 247]

924 Cytotoxic drugs may cause severe or complete alopecia. Heparin and thallium may also cause it. Irradiation to the scalp may be given during some

forms of cancer therapy, and it may cause complete alopecia.
[B: 31.37; E: 148–9; F: 1243–4; G: 2271]

925 The commonest pathological cause of pigmentation is jaundice. Haemochromatosis, porphyria, various internal malignancies and pellagra may also produce pigmentation.
[B: 31.40; D: 283; F: 1241; G: 2289–91; H: 250]

926 Addison's disease and pernicious anaemia.
[B: 31.42; C: 489; F: 1240; G: 2292; H: 251–2]

927 Deepening pigmentation, enlargement, itching, spontaneous bleeding and scaling in a previously asymptomatic mole. The occurrence of any of these features is an indication for immediate wide surgical excision and histological examination of the lesion.
[B: 31.86; E: 147; F: 1286; G: 2310; H: 1655]

928 Rodent ulcers usually appear on the face and neck of elderly individuals who have been heavily exposed to sunlight. This tumour is unique in that while it erodes tissue locally, it does not metastasize, and hence carries a good prognosis following excision or radiotherapy.
[B: 31.80; E: 147; F: 1231; G: 2308; H: 1653]

929 The juvenile form of this condition is benign. In adults, the development of acanthosis nigricans always indicates internal malignancy—most frequently stomach cancer.
[B: 31.41; D: 281; E: 146; F: 1284; G: 2285; H: 1650]

930 The commonest of these are carcinoma of the bronchus and breast. Malignant melanoma commonly produces black nodular skin secondaries. Hodgkin's disease and lymphocytic leukaemia may cause itchy, nodular lesions which may ulcerate.
[B: 31.89; F: 1284; H: 1647–8]

Iatrogenic Disease

931 There are a number of reasons for this. They include depletion of iron stores by preoperative haemorrhages, plus intermittent blood loss following the operation. Also the upper duodenum which is the main site of iron absorption may be bypassed. An additional factor may be achlorhydria which is associated with impaired iron absorption.
[A: 88; B: 21.21; C: 544; E: 61; F: 1134; G: 1520; H: 1381]

932 The usual cause of B_{12} deficiency in this situation is lack of intrinsic factor leading to deficient B_{12} absorption. Intrinsic factor is lacking because of atrophy of the remaining part of the stomach. Occasionally stagnant loop syndrome develops following a Polya (Billroth II) type operation, and this contributes to the B_{12} deficiency through bacterial overgrowth and bacterial consumption of vitamin B_{12}.
[A: 88; B: 19.41; C: 551; E: 61; F: 1134; G: 1520; H: 1381]

933 This is the radiological and biochemical picture of osteomalacia. A number of factors contribute. First, food intake is frequently diminished due to reduction in size of the stomach. Accordingly intake of calcium and vitamin D is reduced. A degree of malabsorption and steatorrhoea is frequent following partial gastrectomy, and this reduces vitamin D absorption. Finally, a rise in the pH of duodenal contents which follows this operation lessens calcium absorption.
[A: 88; B: 19.41; C: 336; E: 61; F: 627; G: 1520; H: 1381]

934 Chlorpromazine is the best known of these, and jaundice usually develops 3–6 weeks after commencement of the drug. Other drugs causing similar effects include other phenothiazines, sulphonylureas, phenylbutazone, and the antimicrobial preparations erythromycin estolate, sulphonamides, nitrofurantoin, PAS and rifampicin. The jaundice usually clears if the offending drug is discontinued.
[A: 112; B: 20.29–30; C: 391; D: 204–5; F: 568–9; G: 1659; H: 1457]

935 Diarrhoea following treatment with clindamycin and many other antibacterials may be due to development of pseudomembranous colitis. This is due to colonization of the bowel with the toxin-producing anaerobe, *Clostridium difficile.* Complications include toxic dilation and perforation of the colon. The disease usually responds to treatment with oral vancomycin.
[A: 745; C: 76; E: 611–12; F: 648; G: 1585; H: 1424]

936 Sulphonamides may cross the placenta and cause neonatal kernicterus by displacing bilirubin from serum proteins. Sulphonamides, trimethoprim and rifampicin have been associated with teratogenesis in animals, although not in man. None of these drugs should be used in pregnancy.
[G: 1649]

937 Important causes of drug-induced pancytopenia include chloramphenicol, phenylbutazone,

indomethacin, tolbutamide and rarely some sulphonamide preparations. Recovery is rare when pancytopenia is due to chloramphenicol or an analgesic.
[A: 727; B: 21.59; C: 569; D: 289; E: 382; F: 1164–5; G: 1808–9; H: 1526]

938 The anticonvulsant phenytoin causes hirsutism which may be quite marked. (Other drugs causing hirsutism include minoxidil, androgens, anabolic steroids, and some corticosteroids such as prednisone.)
[F: 1245; G: 859; H: 1176]

939 A frequently used chemotherapy regimen for tuberculosis consists of rifampicin, isoniazid and ethambutol which are used together during the initial 8 week phase of treatment. The most serious side-effect of ethambutol is optic neuritis, and patients should be warned to discontinue ethambutol immediately and report to their doctor should they notice any visual deterioration.
[A: 293; B: 14.13; C: 260; D: 240; E: 338; F: 20; G: 910; H: 709]

940 It is likely that she has developed vaginal candidiasis. Both broad spectrum antibiotics such as tetracycline and oral contraceptives may precipitate this. However, her urine should also be checked for glucose as pruritis vulvae due to candidiasis may be a presenting feature of diabetes mellitus.
[C: 317; E: 139–40; F: 600; G: 548; H: 741]

941 Lithium, which is used in the treatment of manic depressive psychoses, may cause enlargement of the thyroid gland. Other drugs which may cause thyroid enlargement include the antithyroid drugs carbimazole, thiomersal and potassium perchlorate; also phenylbutazone, para-aminosalicylic acid, sulphonamides and iodides which are present in some cough mixtures.
[B: 23.40; C: 759; E: 175; F: 1420; G: 2132; H: 1696]

942 The patient had been started on propranolol. Non-selective beta-adrenergic blocker drugs such as propranolol may blunt the adrenergic warning signals of hypoglycaemia. In addition they may interfere with the sympathetic stimulation of glucose release from muscle glycogen, thus reducing the body's ability to respond to hypoglycaemia. These drugs are thus better avoided if possible in patients on insulin.
[G: 1265; H: 1760]

943 Ototoxicity with aminoglycosides is more common in very young children, the elderly, those with renal impairment and those with pre-existing hearing loss. It is essential to monitor serum levels of aminoglycosides especially in cases with severe infections in whom renal function may deteriorate rapidly. Diuretics such as frusemide may exacerbate aminoglycoside ototoxicity and should be avoided if possible in patients on these antibiotics.
[A: 759; C: 77; E: 610; F: 15; G: 736; H: 580]

944 Vocal cord paralysis due to recurrent laryngeal nerve injury. Damage to the nerve is a recognized complication of thyroidectomy.
[B: 23.29; C: 472; E: 173; F: 496; G: 2125; H: 1707]

945 Sciatic nerve damage during surgery.

946 Oxygen toxicity. This is related to the fraction of inspired oxygen ($F_{\mathrm{i}}\mathrm{O}_2$) and the duration of oxygen administration. Since the limits of safety are not exactly defined, it is important to use the minimum adequate $F_{\mathrm{i}}\mathrm{O}_2$ for the shortest time necessary.
[B: 18.23; C: 235; E: 370; G: 1041; H: 1279]

947 The scar is likely to indicate thyroid surgery. Accidental parathyroidectomy or damage to the vascular supply of the parathyroid glands is a complication of thyroid surgery, and may cause hypoparathyroidism and tetany.
[A: 433; B: 23.54; C: 472; E: 173; F: 496; G: 2220; H: 1840]

948 Yes. Tissue removal inevitably results in scar formation and a scar can act as an epileptogenic focus.

949 Some patients with chronic lung disease require treatment with corticosteroids. Exacerbation of peptic ulceration and perforation are side-effects of steroid therapy.
[A: 752; C: 495; F: 551; H: 1384]

950 Hypertension secondary to her steroid therapy.
[A: 752; F: 551; H: 1735]

951 The risk of osteoporosis is less with an alternate day regimen. In addition, in a postmenopausal woman, hormone (oestrogen) replacement therapy should be considered.
[C: 495; E: 196; F: 551; H: 1735]

952 Creatine kinase and serum aldolase are both raised. Electromyography is also abnormal.
[D: 118; E: 562; F: 551; G: 924; H: 2057]

953 Damage to the innervation of the erectile tissue, the nervi erigentes.
[F: 545; H: 230]

954 General reluctance to discuss sex; low expectations of sexual satisfaction; inadequate time to discuss a possibly embarrassing subject in busy clinics.
[E: 293; F: 545; G: 2174; H: 230]

955 Cholelithiasis, for which cholesterol-lowering diets are a predisposing factor.
[C: 415; F: 582]

956 Protein–calorie malnutrition and zinc deficiency due to a failure to institute intravenous feeding and vitamin and trace element replacement.
[H: 408]

957 In experienced hands, the mortality is less than one in a thousand cases. Complications include ventricular fibrillation, myocardial infarction and coronary artery dissection.
[B: 16.29–30; E: 315; F: 683; H: 1021]

958 It is partly due to immobilization. Some patients suffer from diseases causing immobilization; others undergo surgery with postoperative restriction of movement. Apart from these situations many hospitals inadvertently encourage patients not to take exercise or move about.
[B: 18.99; C: 199; E: 305; F: 803; G: 1130; H: 1253]

959 Cardiac neurosis.
[F: 792; G: 1227; H: 33–4]

960 Ward rounds in which unexplained conferences take place in hushed tones at the foot of the bed.
[G: 2–3; H: 5]

961 Between 20 and 40 per cent of patients develop some features of hepatic encephalopathy. The incidence is related to the extent of the underlying liver disease.
[A: 107; B: 20.24; C: 409; E: 71; F: 575; G: 1641; H: 1481]

962 In view of her sex and age, it must be established that she is not pregnant. Similar caution should be exercised with all drugs.
[F: 372; G: 1930; H: 1617]

963 By siting intravenous drips on the back of the hand or in the antecubital fossa, but not on the forearms. This precaution should be observed in any patient with renal impairment.

964 The previous surgery may have led to adhesion. [F: 646; G: 1490; H: 1437]

965 Haemorrhage. Some bleeding is inevitable and occasionally it is heavy. Both procedures are potentially fatal. It is essential to exclude or treat any bleeding tendency and to have blood available for tranfusion before performing liver or renal biopsy. [B: 22.17; C: 430; F: 1002; G: 1648; H: 1453]

Poisoning and Overdoses

966 As little as 10 ml of the liquid concentrate may be fatal. Excessive quantities produce inflammation and ulceration of upper gastrointestinal tract with renal, hepatic and myocardial damage, convulsions and death. Smaller quantities produce less severe initial effects, but they are followed by a progressive pulmonary fibrosis with respiratory failure and death. [A: 739; B: 63.10; D: 295; E: 212; F: 266–7; H: 961]

967 (a) By measuring blood gases and by measuring respiratory minute volume with a Wright's spirometer. A minute volume of less than 4 litres indicates that artificial ventilation is urgently needed.
(b) Short-acting barbiturates are metabolized rather than excreted in the urine and therefore forced alkaline diuresis is ineffective. However, long-acting barbiturates such as phenobarbitone are excreted in the urine, and forced alkaline diuresis accelerates their excretion.
[A: 734; B: 63.5; C: 787; D: 295; E: 208; F: 259–60; G: 712–14; H: 982–3]

968 Initially there is confusion, photophobia and vomiting with severe abdominal pain. Kussmaul's breathing develops due to acidosis. Severe poisoning leads to coma, convulsions and respiratory arrest. Blood gas analyses reveal severe acidosis (pH as low as 6.8), with very low bicarbonate levels. Treatment includes gastric lavage and the administration of ethanol which delays metabolism of methanol into the toxic products.
[E: 209; F: 258; G: 75; H: 960]

969 The antidote consists of either oral methionine or intravenous *N*-acetylcysteine. Both prevent liver

damage provided they are administered within 10 hours of paracetamol ingestion.
[A: 740; B: 63.7; C: 788; D: 295; E: 207; F: 263; G: 1658; H: 953–4]

970 It is essential that gastric lavage is carried out on comatose patients only after the insertion of a cuffed endotracheal tube. Should this precaution be omitted, aspiration of stomach contents is likely to occur. Paraffin oil ingestion is a contraindication to gastric lavage, as even a small quantity of this substance entering the lungs causes severe pneumonia.
[A: 733; C: 784–5; D: 294; E: 204; F: 252; G: 74; H: 950]

971 Initially there is respiratory alkalosis due to stimulation of the respiratory centre by the drug. This produces a secondary hypokalaemia. Later, metabolic acidosis develops, partly due to the acidic nature of salicylates.
[A: 739; B: 63.7; C: 788–9; D: 295; E: 205; F: 262; G: 75–6; H: 963]

972 Naloxone given intravenously is an effective antidote to the depressant effect of narcotics and may restore spontaneous breathing. However, in severe cases artificial ventilation may also be necessary. Naloxone may precipitate acute withdrawal symptoms in narcotic addicts.
[A: 736; B: 63.6; C: 788; D: 295; F: 263–4; G: 75; H: 979–80]

973 Cobalt edetate 1.5 per cent should be given intravenously immediately.
[A: 741; C: 787; F: 255; G: 75; H: 957–8]

974 First, gastric lavage may be useful for up to 24 hours after ingestion. Secondly, cardiac monitoring is essential. Acidosis should be corrected and artificial ventilation may be necessary. Care is needed in the use of anti-arrhythmic drugs as they may worsen the situation if used in excessive quantities. Cardiac pacing may be necessary for conduction defects. Physostigmine salicylate may help restore consciousness.
[A: 737; B: 63.6; C: 789; D: 295; E: 208; F: 265; G: 712; H: 988]

975 Gastric lavage with a solution of desferrioxamine is the first aspect of management. At the end of the lavage some of the desferrioxamine solution should be left in the stomach. Intravenous or intramuscular desferrioxamine should be given also. Desferrioxamine is an effective chelating agent.

Supportive therapy for shock, acidosis, convulsions and haemorrhage is essential.
[A: 738; B: 63.11; C: 787; D: 295; E: 210; F: 270; G: 75; H: 959]

976 Clinical features of carbon monoxide poisoning include pink coloured skin despite coma, shock and dilated pupils. Tendon reflexes are increased and plantar reflexes are extensor due to cerebral oedema. There may be severe cardiac muscle failure. Diagnosis is confirmed by finding high levels of carboxyhaemoglobin in the blood on spectroscopic examination.
[A: 741; B: 63.8; E: 209; F: 253; G: 82–3; H: 956]

977 By inactivating body cholinesterases which allows a build-up of acetylcholine, resulting in all the cholinergic effects mentioned. As might be expected, atropine is an effective antidote.
[B: 63.10; C: 788; E: 212; F: 284; G: 75; H: 957]

978 Drunken behaviour in an individual who smells of solvent or who has solvent stains on his clothing suggests solvent abuse. Diagnosis may be confirmed by finding solvents in blood using gas-liquid chromatography.
[F: 282; G: 705; H: 962]

979 Ethylene glycol (antifreeze) causes severe metabolic acidosis and renal damage. Automatic dishwasher detergents may cause severe burning of mouth and throat. Descalers used for baths and kettles may contain formic acid which is extremely corrosive.
[B: 63.10; C: 787; F: 269; G: 75; H: 954–5]

980 Haematological features include a haemolytic anaemia and basophilic stippling of red cells. Radiological changes of lead poisoning include increased density of the metaphyses of bones.
[A: 743; E: 210; F: 271; G: 78; H: 967]

Genetics

981 An X-linked recessive condition is caused by a gene carried on the X chromosome and is manifest in females only in the homozygote. In males a mutant gene on the X chromosome is always manifest as there is no second (normal) gene to oppose its effect, males having only one X chromosome. X-linked recessive conditions therefore usually affect males and are transmitted by healthy female carriers, i.e. heterozygous females in whom the effect of the mutant

gene on one X chromosome is modified by the effect of a normal gene on the second X chromosome.
[A: 6; C: 15; E: 112; F: 344; G: 36; H: 300]

982 Autosomal recessive disorders affect both males and females. Unlike dominant traits, autosomal recessive traits are expressed only in individuals with a double dose of the mutant gene (i.e. homozygotes). Heterozygotes are usually healthy.

The parents of affected individuals are usually healthy themselves, but both are heterozygous for the mutant gene (i.e. carriers). Each child of heterozygous parents has a 1 in 4 chance of being affected (homozygous); a 1 in 2 chance of being a healthy carrier (heterozygous) and a 1 in 4 chance of being normal.
[A: 4; C: 13; E: 112; F: 343; G: 35; H: 299]

983 The main features of Turner's syndrome include short stature, primary amenorrhoea with 'streak' ovaries, lack of secondary sex characteristics, webbing of the neck, increased carrying angle of the forearm (cubitus valgus) and coarctation of the aorta. A mild degree of mental retardation is frequently present.
[A: 11; C: 11; D: 262; E: 108; F: 356; G: 52; H: 313–14]

984 Features of Klinefelter's syndrome include eunuchoid body proportions, azoospermia and sterility, hypogonadism, gynaecomastia and frequently a degree of mental retardation.
[A: 11; C: 11; E: 108; F: 357; G: 52; H: 313–14]

985 Autosomal dominant traits are usually transmitted from one generation to the next and affected individuals are usually found to have an affected parent.

Examples of such conditions are polycystic kidney disease and Huntington's chorea. However, autosomal dominant conditions which reduce the likelihood of reproduction by the affected individual, such as achondroplastic dwarfism, may appear suddenly in a family due to a spontaneous mutation.
[A: 2; C: 12; E: 111; F: 343; G: 34; H: 297]

986 Features of tuberous sclerosis include adenoma sebaceum (small papules over the nose and cheeks) with epilepsy and varying degrees of mental retardation. Altough this is an autosomal dominant condition some individuals with the gene may show minimal features of the disease, e.g. a few facial papules.
[A: 3; C: 13; E: 111; F: 343; G: 37; H: 298]

987 The Philadelphia chromosome is characterized by loss of some genetic material from the long arm of one of the two 22 chromosomes. This 'missing' material is usually translocated to chromosome 9. The Philadelphia chromosome may be seen in leukaemic precursor cells of granulocytes, erythrocytes, megakaryocytes and monocytes but not in other somatic cells.
[B: 21.15; C: 9; D: 291; E: 396; F: 357–8; G: 54; H: 1632]

988 Genes can exist in more than one form. The variants are called alleles. An example of an allele conferring a particular disease response is allele no. 27 at the B locus in the HLA system or gene complex, i.e. HLA B27 which is associated with ankylosing spondylitis.
[A: 9; C: 16–18; E: 113; F: 345; G: 44–5; H: 302]

989 Slow acetylation means that drugs such as isoniazid and hydralazine have a longer half-life, with increased incidence of side-effects.

Pseudocholinesterase deficiency causes an inability to metabolize the short-acting muscle relaxant succinylcholine. Prolonged apnoea following general anaesthesia results.
[A: 730; F: 350; G: 46; H: 303]

990 In the case of sickle-cell anaemia, the heterozygous state (sickle-cell trait) can be detected and the risk of having a child with sickle-cell disease can be established. Furthermore, sickle-cell anaemia is one of the conditions which can be detected antenatally by amniocentesis and fetal cell culture. Even in the homozygote, however, the likely severity of the disease cannot be predicted with certainty, and prognosis must be based on the medical histories of the family members with the condition.
[A: 14; C: 19–21; E: 114; F: 346–7; G: 56–9; H: 307]

Nutrition

991 Hypervitaminosis A may produce alopecia, generalized yellowish pigmentation and desquamation. Hepatomegaly and raised intracranial pressure may occur. This has been seen in individuals who ingest polar bear liver in large quantities.

Large doses of vitamin C may favour the formation of oxalate stones in the renal tract.
[B: 24.23–6; C: 97; F: 464; G: 1691; H: 432]

992 In kwashiorkor the child's weight is usually 60–80 per cent of the standard for age but the deficit may be masked by oedema due to hypoalbuminaemia. Serous effusions are usually minimal. Wasting of the muscles

of the upper arms is usual. The child is apathetic, and changes in hair are frequent. It becomes fine, straight and sparse and may turn a reddish colour. Pigmentation and desquamation of the skin are frequent. Hepatomegaly due to fatty infiltration may be present.

Mortality is around 20 per cent in severe cases even with proper management.
[A: 698; B: 24.8–9; C: 88; E: 102; F: 454; G: 1681; H: 408]

993 Features of chronic fluoride poisoning include mottling of the teeth (although they remain resistant to caries), and sclerosis of vertebrae, pelvis and limbs with calcification of ligaments.
[C: 97; G: 2262; H: 958]

994 Dryness of the conjunctiva (xerosis conjunctivae) is the earliest sign of conjunctival damage. Later dryness and dullness of the cornea develop and xerophthalmia is said to be present. Corneal involvement may progress to keratomalacia and blindness.
[A: 583; B: 24.24–6; C: 99–100; E: 104; F: 463; G: 1684–5; H: 431]

995 The pathognomonic sign is swollen spongy gums which are livid in colour and bleed on the slightest touch. Teeth may become loose and fall out. These changes are absent in edentulous individuals. Perifollicular haemorrhages on the legs are followed by purpura and ecchymoses which may become widespread. Haemorrhage under nails, conjunctivae and into joints and the gastrointestinal tract may occur. Wound healing is impaired.
[A: 587; B: 24.17–20; C: 108; D: 78; E: 103; F: 469; G: 1690; H: 429]

996 Korsakoff's psychosis is usually associated with Wernicke's encephalopathy and is caused by thiamine deficiency in alcoholics. Additional features of Wernicke's encephalopathy are nystagmus, loss of papillary reflexes and ophthalmoplegia. If untreated it may progress to coma and result in permanent neurological damage or death.
[A: 383; C: 111; F: 471; G: 774; H: 426]

997 Generalized oedema of legs, face, trunk and serous cavities is the essential feature of wet beriberi. This may be associated with cardiomegaly and cardiac failure. The failure is high output in type with warm extremities.
[A: 586; B: 24.26–8; C: 111; E: 104; F: 471; G: 1688; H: 426]

998 Beriberi is usually caused by a diet in which most of the calories are derived from polished rice. Early features of dry beriberi include weakness of the legs and paraesthesiae. Later there may be muscle wasting and tenderness and walking may become impossible. Hyporeflexia and anaesthesia over the tibiae is common.
[A: 586; B: 24.26–8; C: 111; E: 104; F: 471; G: 1688–9; H: 426]

999 Dermatitis, diarrhoea and dementia are the characteristic three D's of pellagra. The dermatitis occurs on sun exposed areas and resembles severe sunburn. Diarrhoea is frequent, and glossitis is often associated, giving the tongue a raw beef appearance. Anxiety and depression may progress to delirium and dementia in severe and chronic cases.
[A: 587; B: 24.28; C: 114; E: 104; F: 472; G: 1687; H: 424]

1000 Glossitis may be due to deficiency of folate, vitamin B_{12}, and iron. It also occurs in niacin deficiency (pellagra).
[B: 24.31; C: 116; D: 74; F: 475; H: 191]

1001 Fat-containing animal products are sources of dietary vitamin D. Butter and eggs contain moderate amounts, but the richest sources are liver oils derived from fatty fish such as cod and halibut. In Britain, margarine fortified with vitamin D is the most reliable source for adults.
[A: 586; B: 24.20; C: 101–2; F: 464; H: 1846]

1002 To maintain a steady weight, the average daily calories requirement is approximately 30 calories per kg body weight. This increases to 45 and 60 calories per kg body weight for septicaemia and pyrexia of 40°C respectively.
[B: 50.12; C: 316; G: 1706–8; H: 420]

1003 Hypertonic glucose, in 10 or 25 per cent solutions, is the most readily available form of sugar for intravenous feeding. It needs to be given into a central venous line to avoid thrombophlebitis. Insulin may also be needed. One gram of glucose provides 4 calories.

Intralipid is an emulsion of triglyceride and phospholipid. One gram provides 9 calories. It does not irritate peripheral veins and infusion can be abruptly discontinued without risk of reactive hypoglycaemia. Intralipid in serum can interfere with laboratory tests and measurements.
[G: 1707; H: 421]

1004 Delayed wound healing, increased susceptibility to skin infection with *Candida*, skin rash and loss of taste. Acrodermatitis enteropathica may occur. [H: 421]

1005 The gastrointestinal tract and the pancreas atrophy. Villi shorten and mucosal enzyme levels, including lactase, fall. Bacterial overgrowth in the small intestine may occur.

The onset of feeding may be marked by malabsorption, with fluid being drawn into the gut lumen by osmosis leading to copious diarrhoea. [B: 50.10; C: 316]

Multisystem Disorders

1006 Did he have any bleeding problems? The history and findings are in keeping with haemophilia. [A: 605; B: 21.52; C: 596; E: 417; F: 952; G: 1883; H: 1870]

1007 Anaemia. The lesson to be learned from this case is that the appearance of the complexion and mucous membranes can be a poor guide to the haemoglobin level. [A: 591; B: 21.20; C: 542; D: 284; F: 1110; G: 1748; H: 267]

1008 The failure to respond to treatment suggests malignancy. Five per cent of gastric malignancies are lymphomas. [B: 19.51; F: 631; G: 1603; H: 1387]

1009 Hyperlipidaemia or polyarteritis nodosa. [A: 198; B: 17.12; D: 58; E: 280; F: 431; G: 1220; H: 1162]

1010 Leukaemia, aplastic anaemia or idiopathic thrombocytopenic purpura. [H: 1939]

1011 Collagen vascular disorders; blood disorders, such as cryoglobulinaemia, macroglobulinaemia, hyperviscosity syndrome; Cushing's syndrome (or steroid therapy). [B: 31.92; F: 970; H: 1185]

1012 Yes. Myocardial infarction accounts for about a fifth of cases, by a mechanism known as reflex sympathetic dystrophy. [B: 25.67; C: 643; F: 801; G: 1237; H: 1135]

1013 Ehlers–Danlos syndrome. This syndrome manifests a number of different phenotypes but the main features are hyperelasticity of the skin and ligaments, recurrent dislocations of joints and easy bruising. A defect in collagen is present.
[B: 25.48; F: 1277; G: 2054; H: 530]

1014 (a) Marfan's syndrome. (b) Dissecting aortic aneurysm.
[A: 445; B: 25.47; C: 213; E: 627; F: 986–7; G: 2053; H: 532]

1015 Pseudoxanthoma elasticum. Yellowish papules and plaques occur in skin folds and angioid streaks are seen in the fundi.

A defect of elastin is present and the haematemesis is one manifestation of the vessel weakness which results.
[B: 25.48; E: 55; F: 1278; G: 2294; H: 535]

1016 Hereditary haemorrhagic telangiectasia. It is also known as the Osler–Rendu–Weber syndrome.
[B: 21.44; C: 594; D: 82; E: 412; F: 1211; G: 1880; H: 1560]

1017 Myxoedema; old age.
[A: 595; B: 24.31; C: 545; D: 74; E: 375; F: 1245; G: 1748; H: 1515]

Addendum

1018 Splenomegaly is the main physical finding and it may become massive. Haemorrhage, particularily from the gastrointestinal tract, gums and nose is a serious complication.
[A: 612; C: 568; E: 396; F: 1192; H: 1580]

1019 Because of the risk of 'coning'. Instead, diagnosis should be confirmed by CT or isotope scan. However, should marked neck stiffness accompany these physical signs, meningitis is likely and lumbar puncture should not be delayed.
[A: 360; B: 34.136; C: 701; E: 546; F: 1342; H: 1966]

1020 Bronchiectasis and cyanotic congenital heart disease.
[B: 34.135; E: 545; F: 1342; H: 1965]

1021 The non-Hodgkin's lymphomas usually originate from B lymphocytes.
[C: 580; E: 405; F: 1196; H: 1634]

1022 Hodgkin's disease is staged I, II, III, or IV, depending on the number and site of lymph node regions involved and the presence of extralymphatic organ involvement. The presence of systemic symptoms is denoted by the suffix B, their absence by the suffix A. [A: 613; C: 581; E: 407; F: 1197; H: 1635–7]

1023 The presence of symptoms usually indicates a greater volume of malignant tissue and this may be an adverse factor. The histological type also affects the response to treatment and the prognosis. [A: 615; C: 582; E: 408; F: 1198; H: 1639]

Index

Numbers in the index refer to question and answer numbers, not page numbers